Bone Tumours - A Comprehensive Review of Selected Topics

Edited by Hiran Amarasekera

Published in London, United Kingdom

Bone Tumours - A Comprehensive Review of Selected Topics
http://dx.doi.org/10.5772/intechopen.100923
Edited by Hiran Amarasekera

Contributors
Gonzalo Irizaga, Gonzalo Angulo, Jairo Garcia, Marcus Vetter, Ewelina Biskup, Diana Chiru, Ana Carolina Monteiro, Adriana Bonomo, Günther H.S. H Richter, Ingrid Plass, José M. García-Castellano, Borja Guerra, David García-Padrón, Nerea Martínez-Aragón, Margarita Ramírez-Sánchez, Vicente Vera-Gutiérrez, Gerardo Garcés-Martin, Leandro Fernández-Pérez, Dragana Gabrić, Roko Bjelica, Mato Sušić, Marko Vuletić, Nuno Bonito, Joana Monteiro

First published in London, United Kingdom, 2023 by IntechOpen
IntechOpen is the global imprint of INTECHOPEN LIMITED, registered in England and Wales, registration number: 11086078, 5 Princes Gate Court, London, SW7 2QJ, United Kingdom

British Library Cataloguing-in-Publication Data
A catalogue record for this book is available from the British Library

Additional hard and PDF copies can be obtained from orders@intechopen.com

Bone Tumours - A Comprehensive Review of Selected Topics
Edited by Hiran Amarasekera
p. cm.
Print ISBN 978-1-80356-929-1
Online ISBN 978-1-80356-930-7
eBook (PDF) ISBN 978-1-80356-931-4

For EU product safety concerns:
IN TECH d.o.o., Prolaz Marije Krucifikse Kozulić 3, 51000 Rijeka, Croatia,
info@intechopen.com or visit our website at intechopen.com.

Meet the editor

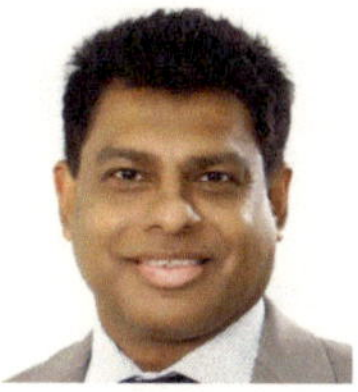

Hiran Amarasekera is a consultant orthopaedic surgeon currently practicing in Sri Lanka. He is a medical educator and an honorary senior lecturer at the University of Kelaniya and Kothalawela Defence University, Sri Lanka. He is also an examiner of medical students both in Sri Lanka and the UK, and a course provider for trauma courses run by the College of Surgeons. After obtaining his MBBS from Kasturba Medical College, Manipal, India, he completed an MS in surgical sciences from the University of Colombo. He was awarded an MPhil from the University of Warwick in 2015. Over a period of 20 years, his surgical training took him to many countries including India, Sri Lanka, Australia, United States, and the UK, and his many fellowships have included a travelling fellowship at the University of California Los Angeles, (UCLA), and a clinical fellowship to Melbourne Orthopaedic Group, Australia. In 2003, the same year that he became a trauma and orthopaedic consultant, he became a fellow of the Royal College of Surgeons of Edinburgh (FRCS Ed). He was awarded a fellowship from the Sri Lanka College of Surgeons in 2013 for his contribution to surgical education in the country. He is a member of the Swiss group AO (Association of Orthopaedics) and a faculty member of the teaching group AO Trauma. His special interests are in young adult hip and knee problems, sports injuries, lower limb arthroplasty, keyhole joint surgery, and revision arthroplasty. His present research is focused on non-surgical and minimally invasive alternative treatment for osteoarthritis, modern management of sports injuries and minimally invasive joint replacements. Dr Amarasekera is the editor of the *Journal of Sri Lanka Orthopaedic Association*, currently serves as a council member of the Association, and is its president-elect for 2024. He is a reviewer for the *Journal of Bone and Joint Surgery (Br)* and *Bone and Joint Journal (BJJ)* and a member of the editorial board of the *Sri Lanka Journal of Surgery (SLJS)*. He has over 50 international publications, presentations and several book chapters to his credit, and has reviewed over 100 papers for *BJJ* and *SLJS*. He has authored three book chapters and edited several open-access books with IntechOpen.

Contents

Preface

Bone Tumours - A Comprehensive Review of Selected Topics reviews key aspects of the management of bone tumours.

The contents are arranged in three sections. Section 1 discusses general topics and new research that help us to revisit the way we have been managing bone tumours. Chapter 1 discusses anaesthesia techniques to improve outcomes, while Chapter 2 explores new key concepts in the diagnosis of bone tumours. Chapter 3 is about the factors that influence the process of bone metastasis in solid tumours.

Section 2 is devoted to breast carcinoma, which remains one of the commonest malignancies globally. Chapter 4 presents new research on pre-metastasis in breast cancer and the interaction of bone tissue within a microenvironment. Chapter 5 comprehensively reviews modern management of bone health in breast cancer patients.

The subject of Section 3 is deep tumours, mainly sarcomas and blastomas that have been successfully managed with a good prognosis over the last decade thanks to a number of research successes. Chapter 6 discusses management of sarcomas in a challenging region of the body. Chapter 7 examines modern chemotherapy and gene therapy using drug targeting of chromosomal translocations, mainly in fusion-positive osteosarcoma. Chapter 8 discusses the general principles and the latest thinking behind the use of statins and other lipid-lowering drugs in the overall treatment of sarcomas. The final chapter looks at modern ameloblastoma management and describes future directions in management modalities.

All nine chapters are written by specialist researchers in key areas of bone tumour management, and discuss current research. New concepts and modern evidence-based research are presented against the background of existing principles.

I am sure this book will not only help researchers and scientists, but equally all clinicians including oncologists, radiotherapists, chemotherapists, orthopaedic surgeons and all involved in managing bone tumours. It will not only be useful as a quick read for individuals but also as a reference book that should have a place in all science and medical libraries. I thank all the authors for contributing their chapters, and Paula Gavran, Author Service Manager, and all the staff at IntechOpen for helping to make both electronic and printed versions of this book a success.

Hiran Amarasekera
Faculties of Medicine,
University of Kelaniya,
Kelaniya, Sri Lanka

General Sir John Kotelawala Defence University,
Dehiwala-Mount Lavinia, Sri Lanka

Neville Fernando Teaching Hospital,
Malabe, Sri Lanka

Section 1

General Concepts

Chapter 1

Anesthesia Management to Improve Outcomes

Gonzalo Irizaga and Gonzalo Angulo

Abstract

Neoplastic pathology is the second cause of death in developed countries. In our specialty, there is great concern about the implications of the anesthetic technique and the drugs used, present in the perioperative period of the cancer patient; as well as other perioperative factors. Among the latter, we highlight the management of psychological stress, adequate pain control, the type of surgery, avoiding hypothermia, and reducing transfusions of blood products. This concern is based on the fact that despite great advances in both surgical techniques for tumor resection and neoadjuvant and adjuvant polychemotherapy techniques; tumor recurrence rates have not decreased as desired. This suggests that the previously mentioned perioperative factors play an active role in tumor recurrence in cancer patients. Based on current evidence and our experience, we can affirm that the use of anesthetic/analgesic techniques based on the use of propofol, NSAIDs, and regional anesthesia with local anesthetics that achieve a decrease in the perioperative consumption of opiates, especially morphine, can be beneficial to protect the anti-metastatic immune response of the organism in a period of special protumoral susceptibility such as the perioperative period.

Keywords: Anesthesia, surgery, cancer recurrence, bone tumors, ostheosarcoma, regional anesthesia

1. Introduction

Neoplastic pathology is the second leading cause of mortality in adults in developed countries. The World Health Organization (WHO) as well as the Pan American Health Organization (PAHO) in their 2017 review, states that in 2015 cancer caused 8.8 million deaths worldwide. They stand out as the cancers with the highest number of deaths; lung cancer, hepatocarcinoma, colorectal cancer, gastric cancer, and breast cancer [1]. In Latin America, according to PAHO statistics, cancer is the second cause of death in the region, it is estimated that 2.8 million people are diagnosed each year and 1.3 million people die from this disease annually [1]. In about 50% of diagnosed cases, there is some degree of metastasis, this being responsible for more than 90% of cancer deaths. Surgical resection is the main treatment for malignant tumors, and in many cases; the only potentially curative treatment. Despite the constant development of new surgical techniques and both chemotherapy and radiotherapy treatments, the incidence of tumor recurrence has changed very little over time. This suggests that there could be other important factors, some of them apparently linked to the surgical procedure, which may play a fundamental role in the progression of neoplastic pathology and the appearance of metastases. There is a growing interest in understanding these factors and the potential effect that anesthesia and its different techniques may have on them [2, 3].

Anesthetic drugs can induce changes in cell pathophysiology such as cell proliferation, angiogenesis, and apoptosis, and may be determinant in the progression of oncological disease in patients. This is why we are interested in identifying the main perioperative factors that play a role in tumor recurrence in cancer patients who undergo surgery; as well as evaluating which drugs may or may not be beneficial in the perioperative period [3–5].

2. Bone tumors

Bone tumors are characterized by abnormal growth of tissue, which appears and develops into a defined tissue. In the musculoskeletal system, tumors can develop in both bone and soft tissue. Primary tumor lesions at the bone level are relatively infrequent, presenting an incidence of 0.2% of all malignant tumors in the body and preferentially affecting adolescents and young people [6]. Bone tumors can be benign or malignant and within these, primary or metastatic.

The most common bone tumors are bone metastases, multiple myeloma, and primary malignant bone tumors. The most common malignant bone tumor in adults is metastasis from lung, breast, and prostate carcinomas. These appear in advanced stages of the disease and mark a reduction in survival [6, 7]. There are three common primary bone sarcomas, Osteosarcoma, Ewing's Sarcoma, and Chondrosarcoma.

At the time of diagnosis, 15–20% of patients have metastases, of which 90% are pulmonary. This determines a significant drop in patient survival, which can reach 20 –25% at 5 years. Once diagnosed, treatment is classically based on neoadjuvant polychemotherapy, surgery, adjuvant polychemotherapy, and eventually radiotherapy. Survival has increased dramatically thanks to polychemotherapy based on different drugs. Tumor reduction induced by polychemotherapy makes limb preservation possible, using conservative surgery techniques; sometimes complex, which guarantee a satisfactory reception from the oncological point of view. When the surgical margins achieved are not satisfactory, radiotherapy could be considered [8, 9].

2.1 Osteosarcoma

Osteosarcoma is defined according to the WHO as a malignant tumor characterized by the formation of bone or osteoid substance by tumor cells. After myeloma, osteosarcoma is the most common primary bone tumor. It represents about 20% of malignant tumors and about twice as many cases as Ewin's sarcoma and chondrosarcoma [6]. Its clinical presentation is variable depending on the type, location, and age of the patient. It generally affects more men than women, between the ages of 10 and 25, with a higher peak in the second decade of life. It is very rare under 5 years of age. There is a second peak of incidence in people older than 35 years; almost always related to previous processes such as Paget's disease, fibrous dysplasia, or irradiation [7].

This malignant neoplasm is characterized by forming bone or osteoid substance directly and encompasses a wide variety of lesions that differ in their clinical and radiological presentation, microscopic appearance, and evolution. Depending on their location in the bone, 3 groups can be distinguished: superficial osteosarcomas, intracortical osteosarcomas, and intramedullary or central osteosarcomas; the latter being the most frequent. Among intramedullary tumors, various types of high-grade malignancy can be identified: the so-called classic or conventional form, telangiectatic osteosarcoma, and the small cell variant [8]. Although osteosarcoma can affect any bone; it is preferentially located in the metaphyses of long bones. It sits mainly on the knee; distal end of the femur (40%), proximal end of the tibia (15%), or upper end of the femur or humerus (14%), areas that correspond to the bone segments with the greatest growth of the skeleton [8]. (**Figures 1–4**) shows part of preparation of the bone piece in a knee osteosarcoma resection surgery in a young patient.

2.2 Ewing's sarcoma

Ewing's sarcoma is primarily a disease of adolescence, with a peak incidence of about three cases per million in the 15–19 year age group. Although rare, Ewing's sarcoma is the second most common bone sarcoma affecting children and adolescents. It is more frequent in men; mainly affects Caucasians; and frequently occurs in the spine, pelvis, arm, or leg [7, 8].

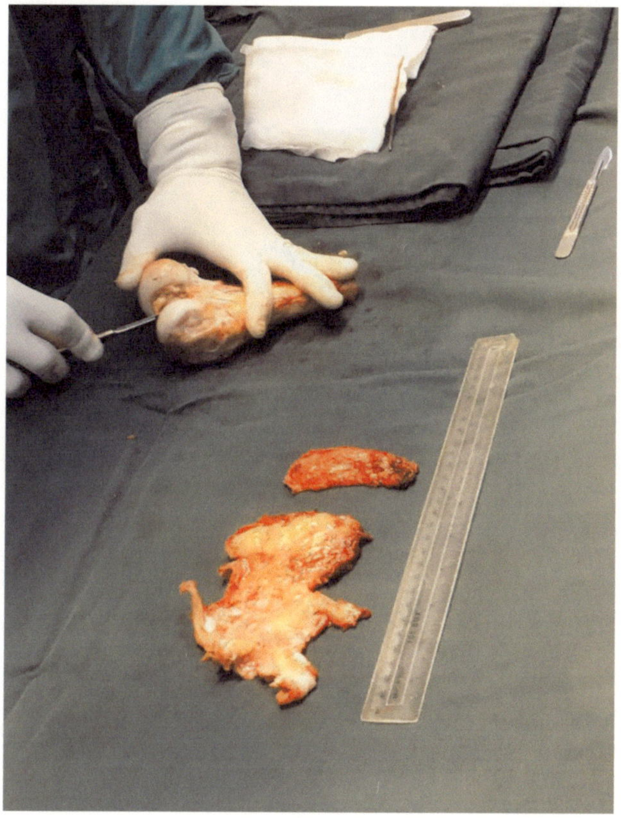

Figure 1.
Soft tissue removal.

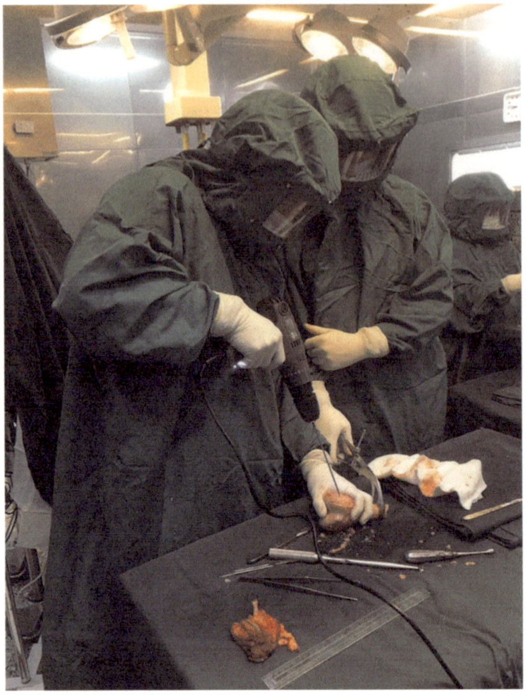

Figure 2.
Bone drilling.

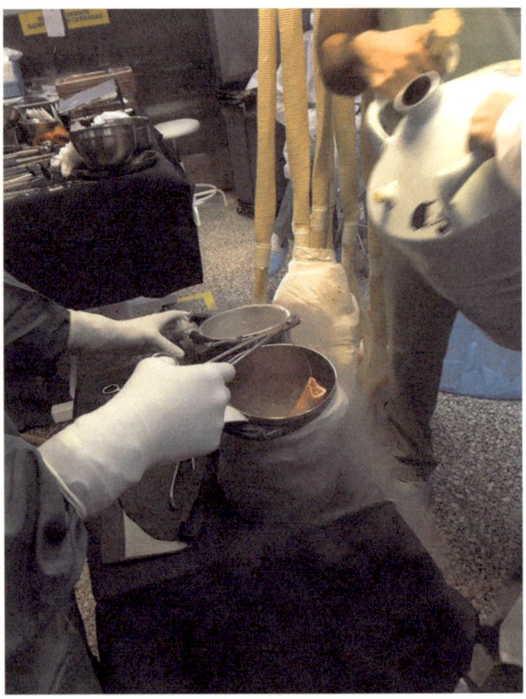

Figure 3.
Sterilization with liquid nitrogen.

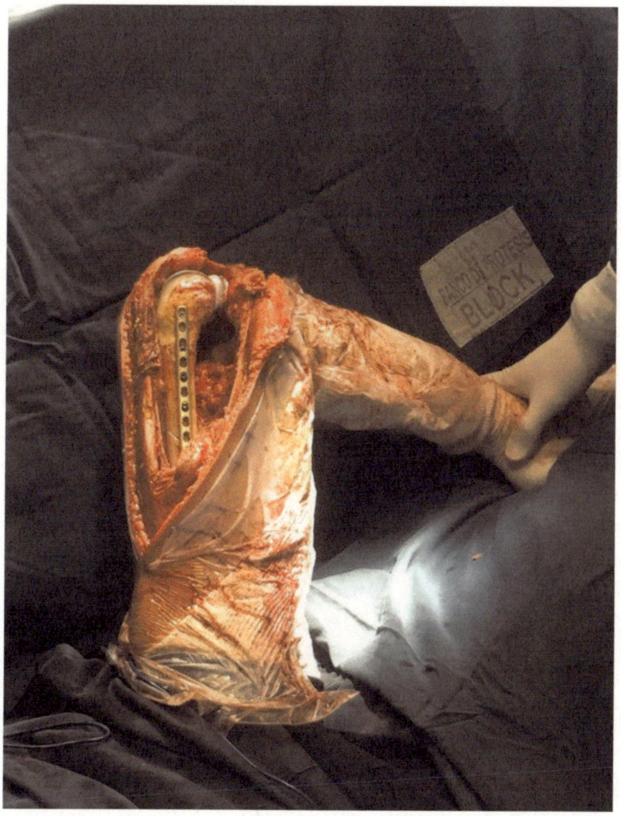

Figure 4.
Bone Reimplantation.

2.3 Chondrosarcoma

Chondrosarcoma is the most common bone sarcoma in adults. It mainly affects patients older than 50 years. The incidence is 8 per million inhabitants. Chondrosarcomas most commonly arise from the pelvis, upper femur, and shoulder girdle. The prognosis of chondrosarcoma varies depending on the primary location and the extent of spread [7, 8].

3. Antitumor immunity

The development of the primary tumor and its eventual ability to spread to a distance will depend on a balance between the potential for metastatic growth of the tumor and the immunity of antitumor host defense factors. The body's main anti-metastatic defense mechanism is the immune system, which is evident in the high frequency of malignant tumors that develop in immunosuppressed people or under immunosuppressive treatment [4, 10].

Helper T lymphocytes (Th) are the main intrinsic modulators of the immune system, regulating the two main pathways of specific defense: cellular and humoral, through the secretion of cytokines. The profile of cytokines secreted by Th lymphocytes polarizes the immune response towards a predominantly cytotoxic or cellular one (Th1) or towards the other end, fundamentally humoral (Th2). These responses are antagonistic. In surgical procedures, the balance is tilted towards increased Th2 production, which is detrimental to cellular immunity and, consequently, the ability of cytotoxic T lymphocytes (CD8+) to fight tumor cells that may have detached from the tumor or that were already present far from the tumor during the surgical procedure [11].

CD8+ T lymphocytes, mononuclear cells, dendritic cells, and especially natural killer (NK) cells are the components of immunity to which anti-metastatic action has been attributed. Cellular immunity at the expense of NK cells plays a fundamental role in tumor recurrence and survival [12]. NK cells are known to be the first line of defense against the development of primary tumors and cells with metastatic spread. They are cells with an immediate response, capable of spontaneously recognizing and destroying tumor cells, identifying the cells as their own or foreign, through the expression of the major histocompatibility complex type 1 (MHC-1). When a cell expresses MHC-1, it inhibits the action of NK cells; and when it is absent, as occurs in tumor cells, they release the content of their granules that destroy the tumor cell membrane [13]. The reduction of its activity can cause an increase in the development of tumors, both primary and facilitate distant dissemination [14]. Patients with low levels of NK cell activity preoperatively have a higher incidence of cancer-associated morbidity and mortality. In favor of the above, a better prognosis has been observed after tumor resection in patients with high levels of NK cell activity at the time of surgery [15]. After surgical damage, an inflammatory reaction occurs at the local level that produces the secretion of proinflammatory cytokines: tumor necrosis factor-alpha (TNF-α), interleukins IL-1b, IL-6, IL-12, IL-15, IL- 18, and interferon-gamma (IFN-γ). The primary objective of the inflammatory response that appears after any surgical intervention is to repair and heal damaged tissues. In response to the proinflammatory state, an anti-inflammatory state is then produced in order to restrict inflammation to the injured tissues. Anti-inflammatory mediators are interleukins IL-4, IL-6, IL-10, IL-11, IL-13, and transforming growth factor beta (TGF-β), as well as catecholamines, prostaglandin E2 (PGE2), glucocorticoids, alpha-melanocyte-stimulating hormone (α-MSH), interleukin-1 receptor antagonist (IL-1Ra), and soluble TNF receptors [3].

There is evidence that the inflammatory process is responsible for much of the immunosuppression that appears after surgery and that inflammation itself has a tumorigenic role [16].

Vasodilation that occurs during inflammation is primarily mediated by nitric oxide (NO) and prostaglandins (PGE2, prostacyclin), being a factor that facilitates the supply of soluble mediators and inflammatory cells to the damaged area. These lipid mediators are produced by arachidonic acid through the action of cyclooxygenase (COX) and are considered pro-angiogenic since they serve to heal damaged tissue through the neoformation of vessels, this effect favoring the development of micrometastases [3].

Tumors larger than 2 millimeters (mm) are dependent on the formation of new blood vessels to receive the oxygen supply necessary to continue growing; therefore, for a micrometastasis to develop, an angiogenic process is needed, which will invariably occur when tissue is damaged. It has been seen that overexpression of vascular endothelial growth factor (VEGF) in colorectal cancer is associated with increased invasiveness and metastatic potential of the tumor [17].

4. Perioperative factors that potentiate or inhibit immune responses

During surgical procedures, there are multiple factors related to surgery that determine secondary depression of immunity. Within these, we find psychological stress, tissue damage typical of the surgical act, pain, hypothermia, blood transfusion and factors related to the drugs used that generate alterations in immunity [3-5].

4.1 Non-pharmacological perioperative factors

4.1.1 Perioperative psychological stress

The psychological stress of the patient who is going to undergo surgery can contribute to producing immunological alterations. This happens through sustained activation of the sympathetic nervous system (SNS) and the hypothalamus-pituitary–adrenal axis (HPA). The perioperative activation of the HPA axis will determine the release of adrenocorticotropic hormone (ACTH) and cortisol, which will result in the release of glucocorticoids from the cortex of the adrenal glands with the consequent immunosuppressive effect; as well as an increase in the secretion of plasma catecholamines, adrenaline, and noradrenaline. The latter seem to be the key biomarkers in the relationship between stress and cancer progression [18]. The protumoral effect secondary to the elevation of plasma levels of catecholamines has been attributed to the fact that some tumors express β1 and β2 adrenergic receptors on tumor cells, which favor cell migration, angiogenesis and impair cellular immunity. This cellular immune depression begins preoperatively and can last for several days after surgery [19]. Bartal et al. found that the number of CD8+ T lymphocytes and CD4+ T lymphocytes was lower in patients in the hours prior to surgery compared to patients who were not going to undergo surgical procedures [16].

4.1.2 Surgical act

Surgery is the most effective treatment for cancer, but it is usually associated with systemic release of tumor cells. Tumor manipulation during resection may result in a "spill" of tumor cells into the bloodstream and lymphatic vessels. On the other hand, after surgery, the balance between pro- and antiangiogenic factors is shifted towards angiogenesis to facilitate tissue healing, which may favor tumor recurrence, metastasis formation, and activation of latent micrometastases [5]. The implantation of distant metastases focuses on the so-called "seed and soil" hypothesis; (seed and fertile land) described more than 100 years ago. It tries to explain the non-random location of the metastases of a primary tumor so that only certain tumor cells have the ability to colonize certain organs that have a suitable microenvironment for their growth [20]. It is known that the less aggressive the surgical trauma, the better preservation of the perioperative immune function, and therefore, the greater the trauma, the greater the probability of tumor recurrence; This is why it is proposed in some studies that the reduction of surgical trauma through the laparoscopic technique could reduce the probability of tumor recurrence in cancer patients [21, 22]. As previously mentioned, the surgical act encompasses multiple factors that favor tumor progression and dissemination. Among them, we highlight inadequate pain management, tissue injury related to surgery, hypothermia, and the need for transfusion of blood products.

4.1.3 Pain

Acute pain results in suppression of NK cell activity. It is a powerful stimulant of the HPA axis and its poor perioperative management could be of great importance in favoring tumor recurrence. Optimal pain control can attenuate postoperative immunosuppression and, therefore, tumor recurrence [3, 13, 14, 19, 23]. Postoperative pain in patients undergoing bone tumor resection surgery is significant. Chung et al. [24] examined pain patterns in the postanesthetic recovery unit and found that orthopedic patients had the highest incidence of pain in the outpatient setting. There are many approaches to postoperative pain management, each of which must be tailored to the patient's pre- and postoperative course. Cancer patients often have pain prior to their surgery and may also be receiving significant amounts of opioids to control it. We must have an accurate idea of our patient's tolerance and opioid requirements, and we must plan accordingly.

4.1.4 Hypothermia

Hypothermia can also influence the patient's immune system with the consequent impact on tumor recurrence. Impairs immune functions related to granulocyte chemotaxis and phagocytosis; as well as interfering with the production of antibodies [25]. An inhibition of the oxidative immune response on bacteria and a decrease in the phagocytic capacity of neutrophils and the generation of oxidative reaction intermediates have also been observed, in addition to exacerbating the immunosuppressive effects of surgery. Probably, the immunosuppressive effect of hypothermia is triggered by sympathetic discharge and consequent adrenal release of catecholamines, noradrenaline, and adrenaline, determining suppression of NK cells. Therefore, we believe that temperature monitoring, as well as the adoption of perioperative warming measures, will be extremely beneficial [26].

It has been shown that hypothermia increases the risk of requiring blood transfusions due to bleeding secondary to coagulopathies and platelet dysfunction; this is determinant of immunomodulation [17].

4.1.5 Perioperative transfusion of blood products

Perioperative anemia is present in 25–75% of cancer patients who are going to undergo surgery and is an independent risk factor for morbidity and mortality [27]. Tumors are relatively vascular structures and are therefore prone to bleeding throughout the intraoperative period. Metastases from kidney tumors and thyroid cancers cause significant neovascularization and can bleed dramatically during surgery, much more than other types of bone metastases. Optimizing preoperative hemoglobin values is of vital importance when it comes to reducing the need for transfusion of blood products [28].

Immunosuppression associated with blood transfusion is known in the literature as TRIM (transfusion-associated-immunomodulation) [29]. The effect of transfusion on immunity was suspected due to the better evolution of patients who underwent kidney transplantation and who had been transfused with more than 10 units of blood intraoperatively compared to patients who had not been transfused. In the transfused patients, the viability of the transplant was frankly higher [30]. Blood transfusions are associated with a reduction in Th cells and NK cells and a reduction in the production of cytokines, including IL-2 and IFN-γ [31]. Amato et al. [32] showed in a meta-analysis that perioperative blood transfusion was an independent risk factor for colorectal cancer recurrence.

4.2 Drugs

Anesthetic drugs can induce changes in cell pathophysiology, such as cell proliferation, angiogenesis, and apoptosis, which can be determinants of the progression of cancer in patients [4]. Anesthesia alters the functions of immune cells, including neutrophils, macrophages, dendritic cells, T lymphocytes, and NK cells [33]. Some of the drugs frequently used in general anesthesia have an inhibitory effect on natural-killer cell-mediated immunity, particularly morphine, ketamine, thiopental, and inhalational anesthetics [24], on the other hand, it would seem that propofol, non-steroidal anti-inflammatory drugs (NSAIDs) and local anesthetics have shown promising results (**Table 1**) [3-5].

Drugs	Family	Effects on immunity	Indications
Nitric oxide	Inhalation Anesthetic	• Inhibits the formation of hematopoietic cells that are important in cellular immunity. • Associated with an acceleration in the development of lung and liver metastases.	Anesthetic induccion
Sevoflurane/ Isoflurane	Volatile Anesthetics	Immunosuppression: • Decreases the number and function of NK cells, as well as induce lymphocyte apoptosis. • Determine an increase in HIF and angiogenesis.	Anesthetic induccion and maintenance
Etomidate	Imidazole	Reduces macrophage function	Anesthetic induccion
Propofol	Alkylphenol	• Promotes the cytotoxicity of NK cells. • Reduces the motility and invasiveness of tumor cells, inducing their apoptosis. • β adrenergic antagonism. Partial blockade of the HPA axis with the consequent immunoprotective response. • Inhibition of COX-2 (antiangiogenic).	Anesthetic induccion and maintenance
Thiopental	Barbiturate	Reduces both the number and activity of NK cells	Anesthetic induccion and maintenance
Ketamine	Phencyclidine	NK cell suppression	Anesthetic induccion and maintenance Analgesia

Drugs	Family	Effects on immunity	Indications
Midazolam/ Diazepam	Benzodiazepines	Inconclusive results	Anesthetic induccion and maintenance
Dexmedetomidine	α2 adrenergic agonist	• In tumors that express α receptors, it can enhance cell growth and proliferation.	Anesthetic induccion and maintenance
		• Inhibits the maturation and proliferation of dendritic cells.	Analgesia
Morphine	Opiates	**Morphine has been linked to immunosuppression through:**	Analgesia
		• Decrease in the number and activity of NK cells.	
		• Inhibition in the production of immunostimulatory cytokines such as IFN-γ and IL-2.	
		• Less T lymphocyte proliferation and activation.	
		Promotes angiogenesis by stimulating HIF secretion.	
Fentanyl/ Remifentanil		Inconclusive results	Analgesia
Tramadol		Stimulates the activity of NK cells	Analgesia
Ketoprofen/ Ketorolac	NSAIDs	COX-2 inhibition: • Increases the activity of NK cells.	Analgesia
		• Reduces angiogenesis.	
		• Increases cell apoptosis.	
COX 2 inhibitors			Analgesia
Lidocaine/ Bupivacaine	Local Anesthetics	Increase the activity of NK cells and cytotoxic T lymphocytes.	Analgesia
Cardioselective β blockers	β – adrenergic blockers	• Block β-receptors of tumor cells.	• Arterial Hypertension
		• Decrease catecholamine-associated immunosuppression.	• Ischemic heart disease
			• Heart failure
			• Arrhythmias
Atorvastatin	Statins	Anti-inflammatory, immunomodulatory and anti-angiogenic effect.	Lipid-lowering
Glucocorticoids	Dexamethasone	Inconclusive results	• Anti-iinflammatory
			• Analgesic
			• Antiemetic

NK- natural killer. HIF- Hipoxia inducible factor. HPA- Hypothalamus pituitary adrenal. NSAIDs- Non-Steroidal Anti-Inflammatory Drugs. COX-2- Cyclooxygenase 2.

Table 1.
Pharmacological implications in immunosurveillance.

4.2.1 Inhaled anesthetics

4.2.1.1 Nitrous oxide

Nitrous oxide interferes with DNA, purine, and thymidylate synthesis, depressing neutrophil chemotaxis. Thus, it inhibits the formation of hematopoietic cells which may be important in tumor surveillance. Additionally, neutrophil function is depressed, and mononuclear cell production reduced. In studies with mice, it has been seen that nitrous oxide is associated with an acceleration in the development of lung and liver metastases, being the most powerful stimulator of liver metastases of the anesthetics studied [34].

4.2.1.2 Volatile agents

In vitro and in vivo studies have shown that there is an association between inhalation anesthesia and increased tumor spread [35–37]. In a recent retrospective study, conducted in 2016 by Wigmore et al. [36] cancer patients were found to have a worse survival outcome if they received inhalation anesthesia. Inhalational anesthetics suppress the immune system by decreasing the function of NK cells, which play an important role in protecting against the proliferation of cancer cells. Inhalational anesthetics induce apoptosis in lymphocytes, reduce NK cell-mediated cytotoxicity, and alter the elevation of cytokines generated by NK cells in response to tumor cells.

4.2.2 Intravenous anesthetics

4.2.2.1 Etomidate

Etomidate has minimal effects on hemodynamics, therefore, it is considered for use, particularly in elderly, critically ill, and/or hemodynamically unstable patients. Due to its inhibition of the adrenal cortex, etomidate is not recommended for immunosuppressed or septic patients. Very few studies have investigated the effect of etomidate on cancer. In an in vivo study by Liu et al. [34] in 2016, it was found that etomidate significantly reduces the viability of macrophages in a dose-dependent manner.

4.2.2.2 Propofol

Propofol seems to have opposite effects to other general anesthetics as far as immunity is concerned. It seems that this drug does not suppress the immune system, but rather the opposite. It favors the cytotoxicity of NK cells, reduces the motility and invasiveness of tumor cells, inhibits COX and does not promote the synthesis of HIF (hypoxia-inducible factor), which is associated with a proven pro-angiogenic effect through the expression of vascular endothelial growth factor (VEGF) [28].

Different studies have observed beneficial anti-metastatic effects. It has been proposed that the inhibition of COX-2, and therefore of PGE2, could result in an improvement of the antitumor response of the immune system [38]. Other authors have proposed that propofol's weak β-adrenergic antagonist mechanism could be involved in its antitumor protection since many tumor cells have β-adrenergic receptors [39].

Zheng et al. [40] published 2018 a retrospective study of patients operated on for gastric cancer between 2007 and 2012, this study included 2856 individuals divided into 2 groups. Anesthetic maintenance was performed in one group based on total intravenous anesthesia (TIVA) with propofol plus remifentanil and the other with sevoflurane and remifentanil, showing greater survival in the group of patients that used TIVA.

Inada et al. [41] observed in patients undergoing craniotomy, how inhalational anesthesia with isoflurane compared with intravenous propofol produced a decrease in the ratio of Thr type 1 and 2 lymphocytes (Th1/Th2), which facilitates tumor progression, tilting the balance towards Th2 production; predominating therefore humoral immunity. On the other hand, Ren et al. [42] confirmed these findings with isoflurane versus propofol in lobectomy for lung cancer. They hypothesize that propofol promotes the activation and differentiation of peripheral Th cells to Th1, thereby favoring perioperative anti-metastatic cellular immunity.

In a study by Zhang Ye et al. [43] TIVA with propofol at therapeutic doses of 2–5 micrograms/milliliter (μg/ml) was found to inhibit tumor proliferation, induce apoptosis, and reduce invasion of osteosarcoma tumor cells (**Figure** 5).

4.2.2.3 Thiopental

Thiopental reduces both the number and activity of NK cells in animal models [24].

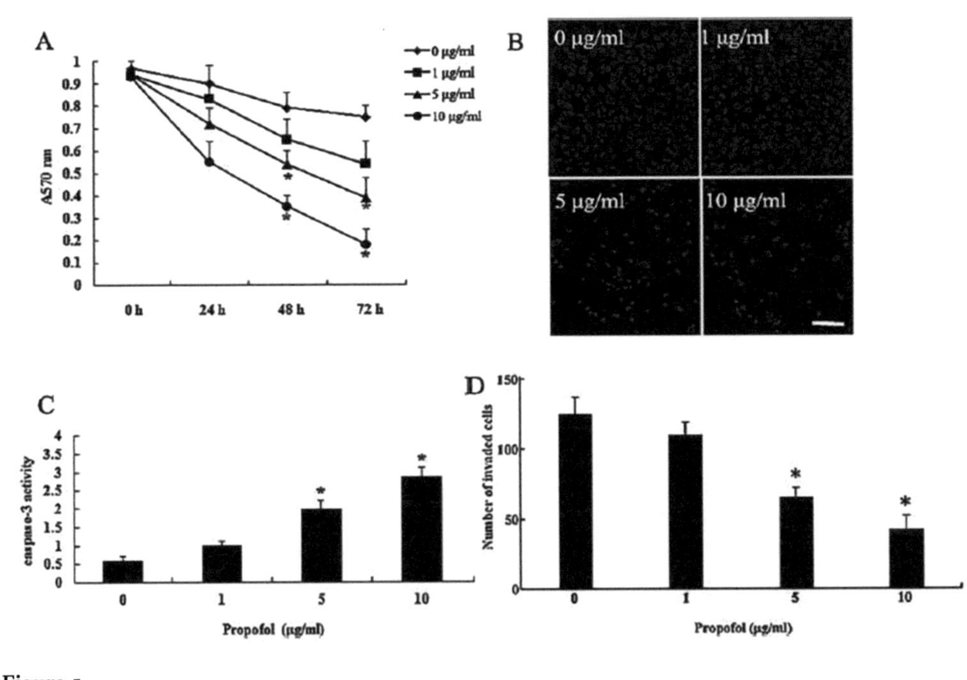

Figure 5.
*Propofol inhibits cell proliferation, promotes apoptosis, and reduces invasion. Propofol inhibits proliferation (A), promotes apoptosis (B-C), and reduces invasion (D) of MG63 osteosarcoma cell in a dose-dependent manner. *P < 0.01 compared with the control group without propofol treatment. Image taken from the article by Zhang Ye et al. [43]. With permission of the author.*

4.2.2.4 Ketamine

In a study in rats, Melamed et al. [44] determined that ketamine causes a significant decrease in the number and activity of NK cells, greater lung tumor progression as well as more numerous and aggressive lung metastases. Of the hypnotics analyzed in this study, ketamine showed the greatest immunosuppressive action, probably related to its potent adrenergic action. Recent studies support these conclusions and show not only decreased activity of neutrophils and NK cells, but also induces lymphocytic apoptosis in humans and inhibits the functional maturation of dendritic cells, interfering with other determinants of the immune reaction as in the production of cytokines that affect cellular immunity [44].

4.2.2.5 Benzodiazepines

Commonly used as anxiolytics, sedatives, anticonvulsants, and in the context of alcohol withdrawal. Among them, midazolam, lorazepam, clonazepam, and diazepam, are useful in anesthetic practice due to their properties, especially midazolam, for being a safe drug with a short half-life. The immune changes produced by the use of benzodiazepines have shown disparate results, and it has not been determined that they are drugs that produce significant variations in immunity and, therefore, in cancer recurrence. Negative results were obtained with supraphysiological concentrations, where the chemotaxis capacity was diminished; in another context, Marino et al. [45] found that single doses of diazepam and midazolam induced neutrophil migration and phagocytosis. In general, they are useful drugs in the practice of anesthesia in patients with neoplasia.

4.2.2.6 Opiates

One of the most frequent symptoms in cancer patients is pain, between 50 and 80% of patients experience some degree of pain. It is known that opiates are fundamental in the treatment of acute and chronic pain, as well as the perioperative period of oncological surgery. As the tumor progresses, it can cause severe pain related to the invasion of adjacent tissues, compromising nerves and bone structures [46].

The main concern regarding the effect that opiates may have; over the morphic in terms of oncological progression through the dissemination of tumor cells and the establishment of distant metastases, is mainly explained by 2 mechanisms; interactions with the immune system and stimulation of angiogenesis [47].

Impaired immune function is known to have a multifactorial etiology. On the one hand, the presence of uncontrolled pain generates activation of the SNS and the HPA axis with the consequent release of cortisol and catecholamines that determine immunosuppression [48]. On the other hand, there is both direct and indirect action of opioids on the immune system. Indirectly through the HPA axis and directly through specific receptors for opioids, such as μ3. These μ3 receptors and others such as OGFr (opioid growth factor receptor), are involved in cell signaling processes that mediate antibody production and NK cell-mediated cytotoxicity. The administration of opioids has been related to a decrease in the number and activity of NK cells, inhibition in the production of immunostimulatory cytokines such as IFN-γ and IL-2, less proliferation and activation of T lymphocytes, as well as less antibody production [49].

Opioids affect the integrity of the vascular endothelium, where they produce proliferation and migration of endothelial cells, a process known as angiogenesis [50]. Morphine administered in usual concentrations stimulates angiogenesis and proliferation of microvascular endothelial cells through a signaling pathway similar to that described for VEGF [51].

Binding to μ3 and OGF receptors by the synthetic opioids fentanyl and remifentanil occurs with much lower affinity [52].

Tramadol, in addition to its effect on the μ receptor, has adrenergic, serotonergic, and appears to preserve perioperative immune function compared to morphine. Studies have proposed that tramadol stimulates the activity of NK cells. Opioids with less structural similarity to morphine and less affinity for μ receptors are probably those that determine less immunosuppression [53].

Recent studies speak of a dual effect of morphine in the regulation of tumors, including its effects on proliferation, metastasis, angiogenesis, inflammation, and immunity.

In a review carried out in 2018; Tuerxun et al. [46] maintain that the main factors responsible for the dual role of morphine in terms of its activity on cancer lie in the dose and the type of tumor. In general terms; at high concentrations, morphine inhibits tumor cell growth, angiogenesis, invasion, and metastasis. However, low daily doses of morphine stimulate tumor cell proliferation, angiogenesis, and immunosuppression. Future studies will elucidate how true these claims are, but for now, they open a door to the analysis that will allow us to discuss how influential the use of morphine is in the perioperative period of cancer patients.

4.2.2.7 Non-steroidal anti-inflammatory drugs (NSAIDs)

NSAIDs inhibit COX-1 and COX-2, a fundamental enzyme of the arachidonic acid cascade that ends with the synthesis of the different eicosanoids (prostaglandins, thromboxanes, and leukotrienes). Overexpression of the enzyme cyclooxygenase 2 (COX-2) has been found in about 90% of lung tumors, 71% of intestinal adenocarcinomas, and 56% of breast cancer neoplasms, among other types of cancer. The hyperfunctioning of this enzyme results in increased synthesis of PGE2, which inhibits NK cell activity, increases angiogenesis, and decreases cell apoptosis, favoring tumor progression [54].

The influence of prostaglandins on cancer seems to be mediated by two mechanisms. The first is an indirect mechanism through its interaction with the antitumor immune system. PGE2, synthesized by macrophages, produces a decrease in the number of NK cells with a reduction in cytotoxic activity, also affecting the response mediated by CD8+ T lymphocytes, favoring the secretion of Th2-type cytokines compared to Th1, a phenomenon that occurs in the perioperative period. The second is a direct mechanism of interaction with tumor growth and spread [55]. HIFs are intracellular proteins that coordinate the cell's adaptive response to hypoxemia, regulating genes that act to promote angiogenesis, cell proliferation, and metabolism. These proteins are closely linked to mechanisms of cellular adaptation to hypoxia, also known as hypoxic preconditioning. PGE2 has proangiogenic effects on tumor cells [56]. Taking into account the pro-tumor effects of prostaglandins, it seems logical to think that NSAIDs could have an antitumor effect [57].

4.2.2.8 Local anesthetics and regional anesthesia

Both local anesthetics and regional anesthetic techniques seem to have a protective action against the progression of oncological disease. The justification for this statement is based on the attenuation of the endocrine-metabolic response to surgical stress and, consequently, on the reduction of the concentrations of glucocorticoids and endogenous catecholamines. On the other hand, local anesthetics favor the increased activity of CD8+ T lymphocytes and NK cells. In addition to regional anesthesia, less invasive surgical techniques reduce stress with the eventual decrease in SNS stimulation and decrease opioid requirements with the benefits that this entails. All of the above-mentioned favor the improvement of cellular immunity and could be associated with lower rates of cancer recurrence [58, 59].

Local anesthetics exert their effect by blocking voltage-gated sodium channels in the membrane of nerve cells, which are also found in the membrane of tumor cells and are thought to be involved in tumor cell invasion and metastasis [60].

In 2014 Scavonetto et al. [61] compared general anesthesia alone versus general anesthesia combined with epidural in a retrospective study in 1642 patients undergoing radical prostatectomy. This study demonstrated that supplementing general anesthesia with neuraxial analgesia for prostate cancer surgery was associated with decreased systemic cancer progression and improved overall survival compared with general anesthesia alone. This finding cannot be used to discriminate which element of anesthetic treatment (intrathecal opioids, local anesthetics) or mechanism (reduced stress response or systemic opioid reduction) may have contributed to the apparent benefit, but it is nevertheless a promising start for further research.

Recent studies have focused on the antitumor properties of local anesthetics; Wang HW et al. [60] in a study published in 2015, investigated the influence of local anesthetics on non-small cell lung cancer and found that lidocaine and ropivacaine can inhibit cell growth, invasion, and migration carcinogens, as well as induce their apoptosis. The antitumor properties of local anesthetics offer a potential opportunity for clinical application.

4.2.2.9 Glucocorticoids

Corticosteroids are commonly used in anesthesia for the prophylaxis of postoperative nausea and vomiting. When administered in a single dose, after the start of surgery, they attenuate the inflammatory response and the pain associated with the surgical procedure [62].

Although it is known that the prolonged use of these drugs worsens the prognosis of cancer patients, it is questionable whether their use limited to the perioperative period influences tumor proliferation and the appearance of metastases. There are conflicting results. Some studies show a reduction in tumor angiogenesis, levels of VEFG, and circulating interleukins with the use of single-dose corticosteroids [63]. Singh et al. [62] showed an increase in distant metastases in colon cancer when dexamethasone was used in a single dose, concluding that further studies are still needed to define the role of these drugs in tumor recurrence.

4.2.2.10 β-adrenergic blockers

β-adrenergic receptors have been associated with the progression of neoplasms; not only because of their presence in neoplastic cells and inducing changes in the dynamics of the immune system and tumor microenvironment, but also because they are active components of the endocrine-metabolic response and inflammation associated with surgical trauma. In an observational study carried out by Hiller et al. [64] in 2015, it was possible to demonstrate a reduction in the incidence of tumor recurrence and greater survival in patients who had indicated the use of β-adrenergic blockers. Another study carried out by Wang HM et al. [65] in 2012 concluded that β-adrenergic blockers are associated with an improvement in metastasis-free survival, disease-free survival, and overall survival in this cohort of patients with non-small cell lung cancer, who were undergoing radiotherapy. Most of the patients who had a beneficial outcome in the study were taking cardioselective β-adrenergic (β1) blockers, which is consistent with other findings indicating that β1 receptors are responsible for negative outcomes in lung adenocarcinoma.

However, there is currently little scientific evidence to support the perioperative use of these drugs to reduce the catecholaminergic response and improve cellular immunity; Therefore, these findings should be verified in future studies that guarantee their efficacy, always taking into account risk–benefit in each particular patient.

4.2.2.11 α 2 adrenergic agonists

Dexmedetomidine is a potent alpha 2 adrenergic agonist that exhibits sedative, hypnotic, analgesic, and sympatholytic effects. These characteristics make it possible to reduce the use of inhalation agents, opiates, and the sympathetic response in the perioperative period, with the consequent decrease in circulating catecholamine levels [66]. Based on the fact that both the sympathetic response and the pro-inflammatory state secondary to surgery, as well as the use of morphine, have been shown to accelerate tumor progression; It is believed that dexmedetomidine could reduce the progression of neoplastic disease secondary to the modulation of the inflammatory state typical of surgery, added to the reduction in the use of opiates and inhalational anesthetics [67].

It is known that surgery can determine immunosuppression, this is of vital importance in cancer patients.

Some studies have shown the role of dexmedetomidine in the immune response of cancer patients. Wang Y et al. [68] indicate that this drug maintains the Th1/Th2 ratio, which decreases the inflammatory response of patients who underwent gastric surgery with the consequent reduction in immunosurveillance alterations, which is of great importance in cancer patients. Due to the above, both in theory and in practice, dexmedetomidine is considered a very promising drug when it comes to the perioperative period of cancer patients. Unfortunately, recent studies show that this drug can promote tumor growth mainly secondary to direct stimulation of cancer cells. In an animal study, Lavon et al. [69] showed that dexmedetomidine at hypnotic doses may be related to the growth of metastases in the primary tumor of the breast, lung, and colon, although at sub hypnotic doses, that is, analgesic and sedative, the effect is not predictable; but not on all models. In addition, a study published by Gong et al. [70] showed that dexmedetomidine could negatively modulate human immunity by inhibiting the maturation and proliferation of dendritic cells, as well as by decreasing the activity and cytotoxicity of CD8+ T lymphocytes.

4.2.2.12 Statins

They have anti-inflammatory, immunomodulatory, and anti-angiogenic effect. They reduce the incidence of colon, prostate, and skin cancer. In a study by Rubin et al. [71] in 2005, a relative reduction of 47% in the risk of colorectal cancer was demonstrated.

5. Anesthetic management

Based on the latest evidence found in the literature, it is considered good anesthetic practice for resection of bone tumors to perform a TIVA based on remifentanil and

Preoperative	Psychological Stress			Its proper handling reduces the release of catecholamines and cortisol responsible for the consequent immunomodulation
	Blood Transfusions (Both pre- and intraoperative measures reduce the risk of transfusions and immunosuppression)	Hemotherapy		Application of blood saving techniques
		Hypothermia		Increases bleeding secondary to coagulopathies and platelet dysfunction
Intraoperative		Permissive hypotension		Reduces intraoperative bleeding
	Avoid Hypothermia			It decreases the chemotaxis and phagocytosis of granulocytes, as well as the production of antibodies
	Pharmacological management	Propofol		Favors the cytotoxicity of NK cells
				Reduces the motility and invasiveness of tumor cells, inducing their apoptosis
				Induces apoptosis of tumor cells
				β adrenergic antagonism. Partial blockade of the HPA axis with the consequent immunoprotective response
			Inhibits COX-2	Increases the activity of NK cells
				Reduces angiogenesis
		NSAIDs		Increases cell apoptosis
		Lidocaine		Included in a regional technique, allows us to maintain an adequate analgesic blockade; and reduce the doses of major intravenous opiates such as Morphine.
				Increases the activity of NK cells and cytotoxic T lymphocytes.
Postoperative	PAIN (Correct pain management attenuates sympathetic activation, decreasing the concentration of circulating catecholamines and cortisol)			**Multimodal analgesia:**
				• Regional analgesia based on peripheral nerve blocks with local anesthetics.
				• NSAIDs.
				• Dipyrone.
				• Paracetamol.

NK-natural killer. HPA- Hypothalamus pituitary adrenal. NSAIDs- Non-steroidal anti-inflammatory drugs. COX-2- Cyclooxygenase 2.

Table 2.
Perioperative strategies to reduce the risk of tumor recurrence.

propofol, in addition to adjuvant regional techniques according to the procedure to be performed (**Table 2**) [5]. We propose the example of a healthy young patient who undergoes resection surgery for osteosarcoma of the knee. After adequate standard ASA (American Society of Anesthesiologists) monitoring (**Figure 6**) [72], and monitoring of anesthetic depth through NINDEX monitor, (**Figure 7**) [73], the anesthetic technique that would provide the greatest benefits based on the previously mentioned; is combined general-epidural anesthesia. A propofol and remifentanil

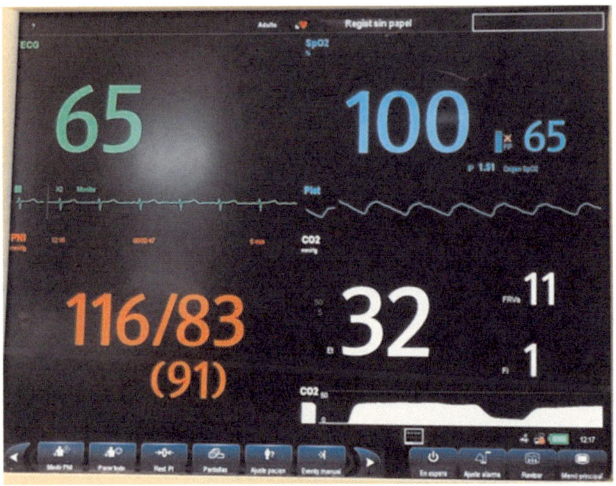

Figure 6.
Standard ASA monitoring (American Society of Anestesiologists).

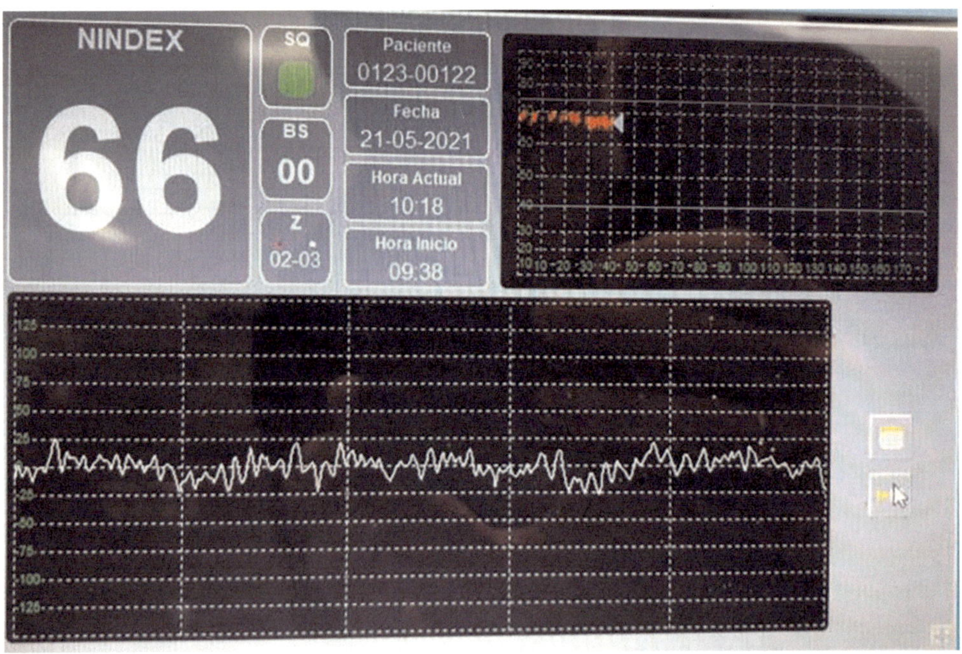

Figure 7.
Anesthetic depth monitoring NINDEX (Narcosis INDEX).

TIVA, target-controlled infusion in effect-site (TCIce), plus a continuous infusion of 1% lidocaine, 1 mg/kg/hour through the epidural catheter. It is also vitally important to help with NSAIDs such as Ketoprofen.

Through this anesthetic technique, multiple objectives are achieved:

Propofol:

- The use of propofol at the effect site at doses between 2 and 5 μg/ml determines the apoptosis of tumor cells that could detach from the tumor that is being resected and are found in the bloodstream. This was demonstrated in a work by Zhang Ye et al. [43] in 2014.

- It is believed that this drug does not suppress the immune system. Propofol favors the cytotoxicity of NK cells, reduces the motility and invasiveness of tumor cells, inhibits COX and does not promote HIF synthesis, thus having an antiangiogenic effect.

- It has been proposed that the inhibition of COX-2, and therefore of PGE2, could result in an improvement of the antitumor response of the immune system since prostaglandins are at the base of the formation of neovessels.

- The β-adrenergic antagonist of propofol could be involved in its antitumor protection, since many tumor cells have β-adrenergic receptors; this confers a partial blockade of the HPA axis with the consequent immunoprotective response.

Lidocaine:

Either in favor of opting for a regional technique that allows us to maintain an adequate analgesic blockade and allows, among other things, to reduce the dose of major intravenous opiates such as morphine, as well as for the benefits of local anesthetics per se; The use of lidocaine intraoperatively and postoperatively has great implications for tumor recurrence in cancer patients who undergo surgery. In the first place, it allows a marked reduction in plasma concentrations of cortisol and catecholamines secondary to the decrease in endocrine-metabolic responses triggered by tissue destruction related to surgery. Second, they act directly by increasing the activity of NK cells and CD8+ T lymphocytes; vital cells to maintain the integrity of cellular immunity.

NSAIDs:

The hyper-functioning of COX-2 secondary to its overproduction in some types of tumors; results in increased synthesis of PGE2, which inhibits NK cell activity, increases angiogenesis, and decreases cell apoptosis, favoring tumor progression. The use of COX-2 type NSAIDs reduces the synthesis of PGE2, favoring immunosurveillance with its positive effects on immunity.

6. Conclusions

Multiple clinical studies suggest that both anesthesia and surgery induce immunosuppression that can promote tumor recurrence through locoregional growth and distant spread; undesirable circumstance that reduces the survival of our patients and impoverishes their prognosis.

We believe that the anesthetic plan should include immunoprotective actions that fully cover the entire perioperative period. Among them we highlight minimizing the response to psychological and physiological stress, through medical stability and adequate pre, intra and postoperative analgesia.

An anesthetic-surgical technique that minimizes tissue injury, reduces bleeding and reduces the risk of blood transfusion will be beneficial in order to reduce tumor progression.

Although the evidence on the influence of anesthetic drugs on tumor progression is limited, it can be stated, based on recent experimental and clinical studies, that the use of anesthetic/analgesic techniques that reduce the perioperative consumption of opiates such as morphine, as well as other drugs with a proven negative profile, such as ketamine, are favorable to protect the anti-metastatic immune response in a period of special pro-tumor susceptibility such as the perioperative period.

We propose anesthetic techniques combined with the use of regional anesthesia and analgesia, preferring them to those based on the use of opioids and halogenated agents, since it has been shown that situations that determine greater activation of the SNS and the HPA axis, promoting a pro-inflammatory state, will generate a negative alteration of immunity with the consequent higher rate of tumor recurrence.

Therefore, based on current evidence and our experience, we recommend the use of supported analgesic/anesthetic techniques based on regional anesthetic blocks prior to surgical aggression, complemented by the administration of NSAIDs, dipyrone, paracetamol, and anesthetic maintenance with propofol. As well as an adequate management of psychological stress, the maintenance of normothermia and techniques that reduce the risk of blood transfusions in the perioperative period are related to the preservation of immunity and therefore with better results in cancer patients.

Acknowledgements

To Dr. Alejandro Corujo Núñez who carried out the revision of this chapter.

Conflict of interest

The authors declare no conflict of interest.

Author details

Gonzalo Irizaga and Gonzalo Angulo*
Departamento de Anestesiología del Hospital de Clínicas Dr. Manuel Quintela, Facultad de Medicina Universidad de la República, Montevideo, Uruguay

*Address all correspondence to: gonzaangulo91@gmail.com

References

[1] Organización Mundial de la Salud. Cáncer. Fecha de consulta: Enero de 2018. Disponible en: http://www.paho.org/

[2] Registro Nacional de Cáncer Comisión Honoraria de Lucha Contra el Cáncer. Situación Epidemiológica del Uruguay en Relación al Cáncer. Mayo 2020

[3] Orozco HD. Diseminación tumoral perioperatoria. Influencia de los factores Perioperatorios. In: Servicio de Anestesia y Reanimación. Madrid, España: Hospital General Universitario Gregorio Marañón; 2011

[4] Sánchez-Pedrosa G. Diseminación tumoral perioperatoria. 2. Efectos de la anestesia y analgesia. In: Servicio de Anestesia y Reanimación. Madrid, España: Hospital General Universitario Gregorio Marañón; 2011

[5] Irizaga G, Angulo G. Manejo anestésico del paciente sometido a cirugía de resección de osteosarcoma. In: Revista Chilena de Anestesia. Montevideo, Uruguay: Banco de Prótesis; 2021

[6] Davies AM, Petterson H. The WHO Manual of Diagnostic Imaging. 2002

[7] Fox MG, Trotta BM. Osteosarcoma: Review of the various types with emphasis on recent advancements in imaging. Seminars in Musculoskeletal Radiology. 2013;17(2):123-136. DOI: 10.1055/s-0033-1342969. Epub 2013 May 14. PMID: 23673544

[8] Guinebretière JM. Osteosarcoma clásico. Encyclopédie Médico – Chirurgicale – 14-165. Elseviere. 2001

[9] Badilla CR. Osteosarcoma. Revista Medica de Costa Rica Y Centroamerica LXXI (611). 2014. pp. 383-387

[10] Penn I. The effect of immunosuppresion on pre-existing cancers. Transplantation. 1993;**55**(4): 742-747. DOI: 10.1097/00007890-199304000-00011. PMID: 8475546

[11] Wada H, Seki S, Takahashi T, Kawarabayashi N, Higuchi H, Habu Y, et al. Combined spinal and general anesthesia attenuates liver metastasis by preserving TH1/TH2 cytokine balance. Anesthesiology. 2007;**106**(3):499-506. DOI: 10.1097/00000542-200703000-00014. PMID: 17325508

[12] Purtilo DT. Defective immune surveillance in viral carcinogenesis. Laboratory Investigation. 1984;**51**(4): 373-385. PMID: 6090808

[13] Herberman RB, Ortaldo JR. Natural killer cells: Their roles in defenses against disease. Science. 1981;**214**(4516):24-30. DOI: 10.1126/science.7025208. PMID: 7025208

[14] Brittenden J, Heys SD, Ross J, Eremin O. Natural killer cells and cancer. Cancer. 1996;**77**:1226-1243. DOI: 10.1002/(SICI)1097-0142(19960401)77:7<1226::AID-CNCR2>3.0.CO;2-G

[15] Levy SM, Herberman RB, Maluish AM, Schlien B, Lippman M. Prognostic risk assessment in primary breast cancer by behavioral and immunological parameters. Health Psychology. 1985;**4**(2):99-113. DOI: 10.1037//0278-6133.4.2.99. PMID: 4018006

[16] Bartal I, Melamed R, Greenfeld K, Atzil S, Glasner A. Immune perturbations in patients along the perioperative period: Alterations in cell surface markers and leukocyte subtypes before and after surgery. Brain, Behavior, and Immunity. 2010;**24**(3):376-386

[17] Kurz A, Sessler DI, Lenhardt R. Perioperative normothermia to reduce the incidence of surgical-wound infection and shorten hospitalization. Study of wound infection and temperature group. The New England Journal of Medicine. 1996;**334**(19): 1209-1215. DOI: 10.1056/NEJM199605093341901. PMID: 8606715

[18] Kurosawa S, Kato M. Anesthetics, immune cells, and immune responses. Journal of Anesthesia. 2008;**22**(3):263-277. DOI: 10.1007/s00540-008-0626-2. Epub 2008 Aug 7. PMID: 18685933

[19] Thaker PH, Sood AK. Neuroendocrine influences on cancer biology. Seminars in Cancer Biology. 2007;**18**(3):164-170. DOI: 10.1016/j.semcancer.2007.12.005. PMID: 18201896 PMCID: PMC2424028

[20] Fidler IJ. The pathogenesis of cancer metastasis: The "seed and soil" hypothesis revisited. Nature Reviews Cancer. 2003. Author manuscript; available in PMC 2012 Jun 1. Published in final edited form as: International Journal of Cancer. 2011;**128**(11):2527-2535. DOI: 10.1002/ijc.26

[21] Bouvy ND, Marquet RL, Jeekel J, Bonjer HJ. Laparoscopic surgery is associated with less tumour growth stimulation than conventional surgery: An experimental study. The British Journal of Surgery. 1997;**84**(3):358-361. PMID: 9117307

[22] Nakasaki T, Wada H, Shigemori C, Miki C, Gabazza EC, Nobori T, et al. Expression of tissue factor and vascular endotelial growth factor is associated with angiogenesis in colorectal cancer. American Journal of Hematology. 2002; **69**(4):247-254. DOI: 10.1002/ajh.10061. PMID: 11921018

[23] Palomero Rodríguez MA, Cacharro Moras LM, Mollinedo F. Inflamación, cáncer y, ¿anestesia? Revista Española de Anestesiología y Reanimación. 2008;**55** (3):135-136. ISSN: 0034-9356

[24] Chung F, Ritchie E, Su J. Postoperative pain in ambulatory surgery. Anesthesia and Analgesia. 1997; **85**(4):808-816. DOI: 10.1097/00000539-199710000-00017. [Erratum in: Anesth Analg 1997;**85**(5):986]. PMID: 9322460

[25] Van Oss CJ, Absolom DR, Moore LL, Park BH, Humbert JR. Effect of temperature on the chemotaxis, phagocytic engulfment, digestion and O_2 consumption of human polymorphonuclear leukocytes. Journal of the Reticuloendothelial Society. 1980; **27**(6):561-565. PMID: 7392012

[26] Shakhar G, Ben-Eliyahu S. *In vivo* beta-adrenergic stimulation suppresses natural killer activity and compromises resistance to tumor metastasis in rats. Journal of Immunology. 1998;**160**(7): 3251-3258. PMID: 9531281

[27] Shander A, Knight K, Thurer R, Adamson J, Spence R. Prevalence, outcomes of anemia in surgery: A systematic review of the literature. The American Journal of Medicine. 2004;**116** (Suppl 7A):58S-69S. DOI: 10.1016/j.amjmed.2003.12.013. PMID: 15050887

[28] Anderson MR, Jeng CL, Wittig JC, Rosenblatt MA. Anesthesia for patients undergoing orthopedic oncologic surgeries. Journal of Clinical Anesthesia. 2010;**22**(7):565-572. DOI: 10.1016/j.jclinane.2010.02.011. PMID: 21056818

[29] Blajchman MA. Transfusion-associated immunomodulation and universal white cell reduction: Are we putting the cart before the horse?. Transfusion. 1999;**39**(7):665-670. DOI: 10.1046/j.1537-2995.1999.39070665.x. PMID: 10413271

[30] Carpenter CB. Blood transfusion effects in kidney transplantation. The Yale Journal of Biology and Medicine. 1990;**63**(5): 435–443. PMCID: PMC2589367. PMID: 2149898

[31] Dixon E, Datta I, Sutherland FR, Vauthey JN. Blood loss insurgical oncology: Neglected quality indicator? Journal of Surgical Oncology. 2009;**99**(8):508-512. DOI: 10.1002/jso.21187. PMID: 19466741

[32] Amato A, Pescaroti M. Perioperative blood transfusions for the recurrence of colorectal cáncer. Cochrane Database of Systematic Reviews. 2006;**2006**(1): CD005033. DOI: 10.1002/14651858. CD005033.pub2. PMID: 16437512; PMCID: PMC6486137

[33] Bonilla Castillo L, Pérez Herrero MA, Torrent A. Efectos de la anestesia en la cirugía oncológica. Revista Electrónica de Anestesiar. 2017;**9**(10):2. DOI: 10.30445/rear.v9i10.337

[34] Liu M, Zhang Y, Xiong JY, Wang Y, Lv S. Etomidate mitigates lipopolysaccharide-induced CD14 and TREM-1 expression, NF-κB activation, and pro-inflammatory cytokine production in rat macrophages. Inflammation. 2016;**39**(1):327-335. DOI: 10.1007/s10753-015-0253-7. PMID: 26383906

[35] Iwasaki M, Zhao H, Jaffer T, Unwith S, Benzonana L, Lian Q, et al. Volatile anaesthetics enhance the metastasis related cellular signalling including CXCR2 of ovarian cancer cells. Oncotarget. 2016;7(18):26042-26056. DOI: 10.18632/oncotarget.8304

[36] Wigmore TJ, Mohammed K, Jhanji S. Long-term survival for patients undergoing volatile versus IV anesthesia for cancer surgery: A retrospective analysis. Anesthesiology. 2016;**124**(1): 69-79

[37] Kurosawa S, Kato M. Anesthetics, inmune cells, and immune respondes. Journal of Anesthesia. 2008;**22**(3):263-277. DOI: 10.1007/s00540-008-0626-2 Epub 2008 Aug 7

[38] Cuéllar-Garduño N. Impacto de la técnica anestésica en la recurrencia del cáncer. Revista Mexicana de Anestesiología. 2014;**37**(Supl. 1):S296-S298

[39] Zhou W, Fontenot HJ, Wang SN, Kennedy RH. Propofol induced alterations in myocardial beta-adrenoceptor binding and responsiveness. Anesthesia and Analgesia. 1999;**89**(3):604-608. DOI: 10.1097/00000539-199909000-00011. PMID: 10475288

[40] Zheng X, Wang Y, Dong L, Zhao S, Wang L, Chen H, et al. Effects of propofol-based total intravenous anesthesia on gastric cancer: A retrospective study. Onco Targets and Therapy. 2018;**11**:1141-1148. DOI: 10.2147/OTT.S156792. PMID: 29535538; PMCID: PMC5840299

[41] Inada T, Yamanouchi Y, Jomura S, Sakamoto S, Takahashi M, Kambara T, et al. Effect of propofol and isoflurane anaesthesia on the immune response to surgery. Anaesthesia. 2004;**59**(10):954-959. DOI: 10.1111/j.1365-2044.2004.03837.x

[42] Ren XF, Li WZ, Meng FY, Lin CF. Differential effects of propofol and isoflurane on the activation of T-helper cells in lung cancer patients. Anaesthesia. 2010;**65**(5):478-482

[43] Ye Z, Jingzhong L, et al. Propofol Inhibits Proliferation and Invasion of Osteosarcoma Cells by Regulation of

microRNA-143 Expression. Wuhan, Hubei, China: Hospital of PLA; 2014

[44] Melamed R, Bar-Yosef S, Shakhar G, Shakhar K, Ben-Eliyahu S. Suppression of natural killer cell activity and promotion of tumor metastasis by ketamine, thiopental, and halothane, but not by propofol: Mediating mechanisms and prophylactic measures. Anesthesia and Analgesia. 2003;**97**(5):1331-1339. DOI: 10.1213/01.ANE.0000082995.44040.07. PMID: 14570648

[45] Marino F, Catteneo S, Cosentino M. Diazepam stimulates migration and phagocytosis of human neutrophils: Possible contribution of peripheral-type benzodiazepine receptors and intracelular calcium. Pharmacology. 2001;**63**:42-49. DOI: 10.1159/000056111

[46] Tuerxun H, Cui J. The dual effect of morphine on tumor development. Clinical and Translational Oncology. 2019;**21**(6):695-701. DOI: 10.1007/s12094-018-1974-5. Epub 2018 Nov 23. PMID: 30470993

[47] Snyder GL, Greenberg S. Effect of anaesthetic technique and other perioperative factors on cancer recurrence. British Journal of Anaesthesia. 2010;**105**(2):106-115. DOI: 10.1093/bja/aeq164. PMID: 20627881

[48] Shen LD, Yang J, Li YX, et al. Correlation between senile cancer pain and depression and its effect on immune function. Journal of Kunming Medical College. 2011;**2018**(08):1263-1265. ISSN: 1672-4992/CN:61-1415/R

[49] Börner C, Warnick B, Smida M, Hartig R, Lindquist JA, Schraven B, et al. Mechanisms of opioid-mediated inhibition of human T cell receptor signaling. Journal of Immunology. 2009; **183**(2):882-889. DOI: 10.4049/jimmunol.0802763. Epub 2009 Jun 26. PMID: 19561113

[50] Moss J. Opiates may influence cancer outcome. The Official Journal of the Anesthesia Patient Safety Foundation. 2009;**24**(3):33-44

[51] Gupta K, Kshirsagar S, Chang L, Schwartz R, Law PY, Yee D, et al. Morphine stimulates angiogenesis by activating proangiogenic and survival-promoting signaling and promotes breast tumor growth. Cancer Research. 2002; **62**(15):4491-4498. PMID: 12154060

[52] Martin-Kleiner I, Balog T, Gabrilovac J. Signal transduction induced by opioids in immune cells: A review. Neuroimmunomodulation. 2006;**13**(1):1-7. DOI: 10.1159/000092107 Epub 2006 Apr 3

[53] Shirzad H, Shahrani M, Rafieian-Kopaei M. Comparison of morphine and tramadol effects on phagocytic activity of mice peritoneal phagocytes *in vivo*. International Immunopharmacology. 2009;**9**(7-8):968-970. DOI: 10.1016/j.intimp.2009.04.002 Epub 2009 Apr 8

[54] Soslow RA, Dannenberg AJ, Rush D, Woerner BM, Khan KN, Masferrer J, et al. COX-2 is expressed in human pulmonary, colonic, and mammary tumors. Cancer. 2000; **89**(12):2637-2645. DOI: 10.1002/1097-0142(20001215)89:123.0.co;2-b. PMID: 11135226

[55] Fujino H, Toyomura K, Chen XB, Regan JW, Murayama T. Prostaglandin E2 regulates cellular migration via induction of vascular endothelial growth factor receptor-1 in HCA-7 human colon cancer cells. Biochemical Pharmacology. 2011;**81**(3):379-387. DOI: 10.1016/j.bcp.2010.11.001 Epub 2010 Nov 9

[56] Singh B, Lucci A. Role of cyclooxygenase-2 in breast cancer. The

Journal of Surgical Research. 2002;**108** (1):173-179. DOI: 10.1006/jsre.2002.6532

[57] Koltai T. Voltage-gated sodium channel as a target for metastatic risk reduction with re-purposed drugs. F1000Res. 2015;**4**:297. DOI: 10.12688/f1000research.6789.1 eCollection 2015

[58] Esteve N, Ferrer A, Mora C, Gómez G, Ribera H, Garrido P. Influye la anestesia en los resultados de la cirugía oncológica?. Revista de la Sociedad Española del Dolor. [Internet] [citado 2022 Oct 03]; 2014;**21**(3):162-174. DOI: 10.4321/S1134-80462014000300007. Available from: http://scielo.isciii.es/scielo.php?script=sci_arttext&pid=S1134-80462014000300007&lng=es

[59] Shapiro J, Jersky J, Katzav S, Feldman M, Segal S. Anesthetic drugs accelerate the progression of postoperative metastases of mouse tumors. The Journal of Clinical Investigation. 1981;**68**(3):678-685. DOI: 10.1172/jci110303. PMID: 7276167; PMCID: PMC370849

[60] Wang HW, Wang LY, Jiang L, Tian SM, Zhong TD, Fang XM. Amide-linked local anesthetics induce apoptosis in human non-small cell lung cancer. Journal of Thoracic Disease. 2016;**8**(10): 2748-2757

[61] Scavonetto F, Yeoh TY, et al. Association between neuraxial analgesia, cancer progression, and mortality after radical prostatectomy: A large, retrospective matched cohort study. British Journal of Anaesthesia. 2014;**113** (Suppl 1):i95-i102. DOI: 10.1093/bja/aet467 Epub 2013 Dec 16

[62] Singh PP, Lemanu DP, Taylor MHG, Hill AG. Association between preoperative glucocorticoids and long-term survival and cancer recurrence after colectomy: Follow-up analysis of a previous randomized controlled trial. British Journal of Anaesthesia. 2014;**113** (Supplement 1):i68-i73

[63] Marshall L, Hameed A, Donal K. Can anaesthetic and analgesic techniques for cancer surgery affect cancer recurrence and metastasis? Current Anesthesiology Reports. 2015;**5**:190-202

[64] Hiller JG, Parat M-O, Ben-Eliyahu S. The role of perioperative pharmacological adjuncts in cancer outcomes: Beta-adrenergic receptor antagonists, NSAIDs and Anti-fibrinolytics. Current Anesthesiology Reports. 2015;**5**:291-304. DOI: 10.1007/s40140-015-0113-x

[65] Wang HM, Liao ZX, Komaki R, Welsh JW, O'Reilly MS, Chang JY, et al. Improved survival outcomes with the incidental use of beta-blockers among patients with non-small-cell lung cancer treated with definitive radiation therapy. Annals of Oncology. 2013;24(5):1312-1319. DOI: 10.1093/annonc/mds616. Epub 2013 Jan 8. PMID: 23300016; PMCID: PMC3629895

[66] Kewatramani A, Partani S, Sharma NP, Sharma V. Comparision of labetalol versus dexmedetomidina to assess the hemodynamic responses to laryngoscopy and intubation during induction of general anesthesia a prospective, randomized, controlled study. Indian Journal of Clinical Anesthesia. 2016;**3**(4): 512-517

[67] Herrera García AM, Domínguez Luis MJ, Arce Franco M, Armas González E, Álvarez de La Rosa D, Machado JD, et al. Prevention of neutrophil extravasation by α2 adrenoreceptor-mediated endothelial stabilization. Journal of Immunology. 2014;**193**(6):3023-3035. DOI: 10.4049/jimmunol.1400255. Epub 2014 Aug 11. PMID: 25114107

[68] Wang Y, Xu X, Liu H, Ji F. Effects of dexmedetomidine on patients undergoing radical gastrectomy. Journal of Surgical Research. 2015;**194**(1):147-153. DOI: 10.1016/j.jss.2014.10.008. Epub 2014 Oct 8. PMID: 25456116

[69] Cata JP, Singh V, Lee BM, Villarreal J, Mehran JR, Yu J, et al. Intraoperative use of dexmedetomidine is associated with decreased overall survival after lung cancer surgery. Journal of Anaesthesiology Clinical Pharmacology. 2017;**33**(3):317-323. DOI: 10.4103/joacp.JOACP_299_16

[70] Chen G, Le Y, Zhou L, Gong L, Li X, Li Y, et al. Dexmedetomidine inhibits maturation and function of human cord blood-derived dendritic cells by interfering with synthesis and secretion of IL-12 and IL-23. PLoS ONE. 2016;**11**(4):e0153288. DOI: 10.1371/journal.pone.0153288

[71] Rubin DT, Blumentals WA, Sheer RL, Steinbuch M, Law L. Statins and risk of colorectal cancer. American Journal of Gastroenterology. 2005;**100**:S394

[72] Monitorización estándar de la American Society of Anesthesiologists. Available from: https://www.asahq.org/standards-and-guidelines/standardsfor-basic-anesthetic-monitoring

[73] “NINDEX” (de: Narcosis INDEX. CONTROLES S.A, Dr. D. Cibils)

Chapter 2

Perspective Chapter: Bone Tumors – How to Make a Diagnosis?

Jairo Garcia

Abstract

The diagnosis of bone tumors begins with suspicion due to some clinical symptoms or due to image findings. From this point onwards, it should be understood the need for new imaging exams, usually based on whether the lesion is most likely benign or malignant. Some benign lesions have diagnosis defined by simple radiography; others need more detailed investigation. Malignant lesions always need a detailed location and systemic assessment. Malignant primary tumors occur generally in patients under 20 years, while secondary malignant lesions are usually related to patients over 40 years. Biopsy of a bone injury, when indicated, is always the last exam to be performed, generating a histological diagnosis and defining treatment.

Keywords: bone, cancer, biopsy, tumor, metastasis, diagnostic

1. Introduction

Bone tumor represents a variable entity of neoplasms, mostly benign, about 35–40% [1], or malignant, in this case, can be primary, that osteosarcoma is the only malignant primary tumor producing bone [2], or secondary due to bone metastases, and about 5% of all cancers have bone metastases to the initial diagnosis [3], most commonly from breast and prostate cancers [4]. Bone corresponds to the third most common site of metastases, after lung and liver [5–7], and the spine is the most common site of bone metastasis in the skeleton [8].

Due to the rarity of these lesions and the wide variety of possible diagnoses, the existence of a multi-professional team with orthopedists, radiologists, radiotherapists, oncologists, and pathologist is necessary for both the correct diagnosis and the proper treatment of the patient [9].

2. Clinical evaluation

History and physical examination are the initial approaches for any patient suspected of having a bone neoplasm (**Table 1**). Data, such as age (isolated corresponds to the most important data [10]), time of complaint, presence of pain, location of the lesion, and personal and family history of cancer, may provide important information for

What i need to consider for initial evaluation?	
• Patient age	
• Personal or familiar history of cancer	
• Symptomatic or only a imaging finding	
• About the lesion	• Which bone?
	• Where along the bone?
	• What is the density of the lesion?
	• What does the lesion do to the bone?
	• How the bone reacts?
	• Does the lesion invade adjacent tissues?
	• Single or multiple lesions?

Table 1.
Systematic evaluation.

clinical reasoning and diagnostic management [10–13]; although the physical examination is generally nonspecific [14]. Often the suspicion of a bone neoplasm occurs only due to an accidental finding of some imaging test [1].

About only malignant primary bone neoplasms, these are more common between 0 and 20 years of age (for patients under 5 years old, the diagnosis of metastases of neuroblastoma is more common). Osteosarcoma and Ewing's sarcoma are more common between 5 and 20 years of age. In patients over 40 years of age, secondary malignancies (metastases) and multiple myeloma are the most common diagnosis [15].

3. Imaging

3.1 Radiography

Every patient with suspected bone neoplasia should be initially evaluated by orthogonal radiography examination and, although the radiologist's report is of great value, the orthopedist must have the basic knowledge to recognize the information that the bone lesion can provide on radiography [10]. The correct diagnostic approach to a bone neoplasm cannot be adequately achieved without radiographic evaluation [14, 16, 17].

The radiographic findings provide important information about the nature of the bone lesion. We can observe if it is bone-forming (osteoblastic), if it promotes bone destruction (osteolytic) or if the lesion has areas of bone formation as well as areas of bone destruction (mixed). Second, the radiography will provide the lesion location (epiphysis, diaphysis, metaphysis, or surface), presence of periosteal reaction (spiculate, sunlight, onion skin, and Codman's triangle), presence of halo of sclerosis, presence of pathological fracture, extension to soft tissues (extra compartmental lesion), among other characteristics specific to each type of bone neoplasm that can even define the diagnosis (**Table 2**) [10, 11, 14, 18].

3.2 CT scan

Computed tomography can better delineate the information obtained on radiography, especially in lesions of bone sites with more complex anatomy, such as the pelvis

DOI: http://dx.doi.org/10.5772/intechopen.106673

Epiphyseal	Diaphyseal	Metaphyseal	Spine
• Chondroblastoma	• Ewing sarcoma	• Chondrosarcoma	• Metastasis
• Giant cell tumor	• Lymphoma	• Osteosssarcoma	• Multiple myeloma
• Clear cell chondrossarcoma	• Fibrous displasia	• Metastasis	• Chordoma (sacrum)
• Dysplasia epishysealis hemimelica	• Histiocytosis	• Infecction	• Histiocytosis
	• Adamantinoma	• Enchondroma	• Hemangioma
	• Osteofibrous dysplasia	• Osteochondroma	• Osteoma osteoide
		• Simple bone cyst	• Osteoblastoma
		• Aneurysmal bone cyst	• Aneurysmal bone cyst
		• Non-ossifying fibroma	

Table 2.
Differential diagnosis by lesion location.

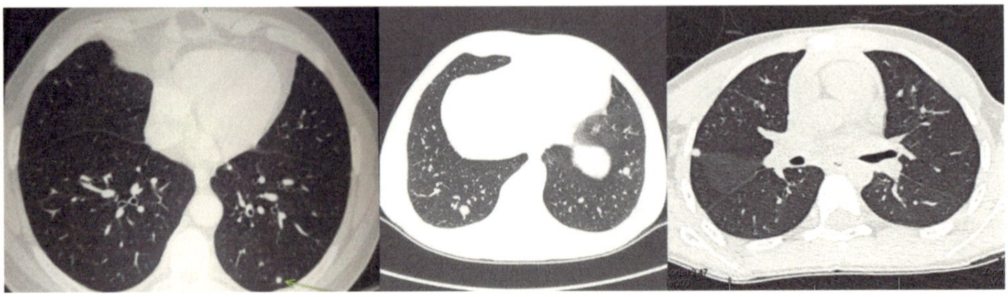

Figure 1.
Examples of CT-scan of pulmonary metastases in patients with osteosarcoma, in general the lesions are found in the periphery of the lung.

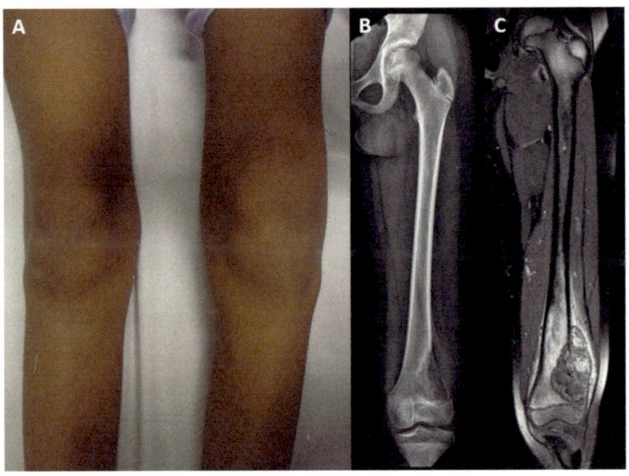

Figure 2.
(A) clinical aspect of the right knee, observing an increase in volume in the distal region of the femur, (B) radiographic appearance of aggressive bone lesion in the distal metaphysis of the femur, and (C) MRI demonstrating the full extent of the affected bone.

and spine. CT scan can observe the presence or absence of intralesional calcifications; it can be useful in the assessment of the risk of fragility fracture and used to guide biopsies. For lesions suspected of malignancy, CT scan is mandatory for the investigation of pulmonary metastases [11, 19]. In relation to osteoid osteoma, it is the exam of choice to locate the lesion niche (**Figure 1**) [2, 20].

3.3 MRI

Magnetic resonance imaging does not have a great diagnostic value in bone neoplasms, but it is the best test for local staging and surgical planning [17]. Evaluating structures adjacent to the lesion, such as the extension to soft tissues (most important sign of bone malignancy [16]) and the involvement of neurovascular structures, as well as the extent of spinal cord involvement and the presence of "skip" metastases (present in 25% of osteosarcomas) [14]. The examination should always include the two joints adjacent to the host bone (**Figure 2**) [10].

MRI is useful in assessing the response to chemotherapy, radiotherapy, and postoperative follow-up to detect mainly local recurrence [20, 21].

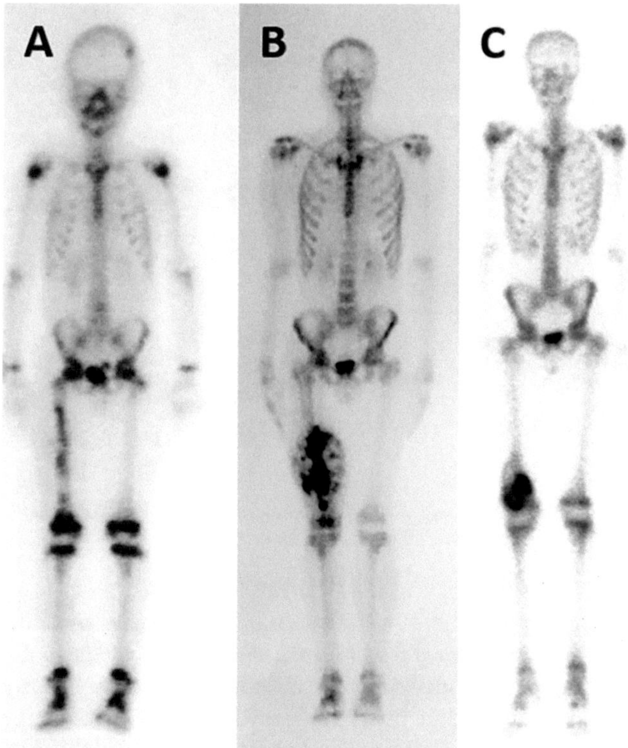

Figure 3.
(A) scintigraphy of a patient with Ewing's sarcoma affecting the entire femur, (B) patient with large-volume diaphyseal osteosarcoma, and (C) conventional osteosarcoma of the distal end of the femur.

3.4 Scintigraphy

Bone scintigraphy is routinely requested in the evaluation of malignant bone neoplasms, the exam measures changes in bone metabolism (increased turnover and osteoblastic activity), it is quite sensitive, but nonspecific (**Figure 3**) [16, 22].

Evaluation of bone metastases by scintigraphy is very useful since it can evaluate the skeleton in a complete way. The drug is well tolerated (technetium-99 m methylene diphosphonate [17]) and its analysis is not interfered with by metallic implants.

Osteoblastic lesions are easier to identify, while osteolytic lesions need a certain size to be detected [22]; examples of this are multiple myeloma and renal cell carcinoma metastases, which are usually negative in scintigraphy [23]. Non-neoplastic changes may appear in regions, for example, of degenerative disease in vertebrae and joints [22].

3.5 PET-CT

Corresponding to a procedure that combines the images of a positron emission tomography (PET) and a computed tomography (CT), there is no contraindication to the test, except in pregnant or breastfeeding patients. PET and CT scans are performed at the same time with the same machine using 18F-fluorodeoxyglucose (18F-FDG, surrogate analog in glucose metabolism) as a marker. The SUV (standard uptake value), calculated at the end of the exam, provides semi-quantitative

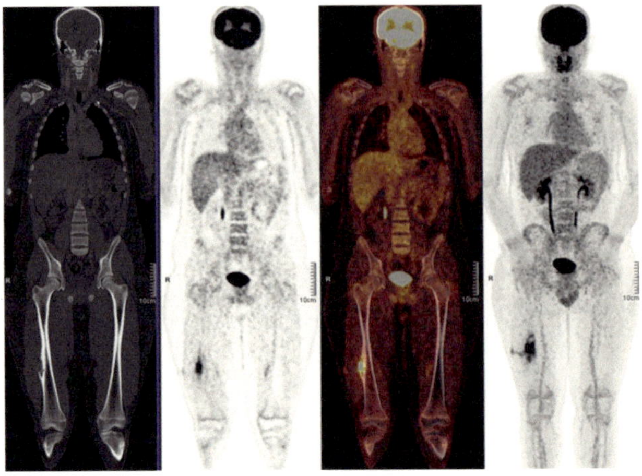

Figure 4.
Patient with Ewing's sarcoma in the diaphysis of the right femur, there is only uptake of the radiopharmaceutical in the region of the bone lesion, with no other changes in the exam.

information on glucose metabolism in the evaluated tissues, with a cut-off between 2.0 and 2.5 for defining benign and malignant lesions. PET-CT is evaluated for staging and monitoring the response to treatment of tumors, including detection of metastases and recurrence. Studies indicate that PET-CT shows sensitivity, specificity, and accuracy superior to scintigraphy to find metastases [24]. However, if it works according to the histological diagnosis, different results are observed. To screen for bone metastases in Ewing's sarcoma, PET-CT has better sensitivity than scintigraphy, whereas in osteosarcoma they are similar [25], although it has better accuracy than scintigraphy for the detection of approaching the growth plate in osteosarcoma [26]. PET-CT as a predictor of oncological response presents better results in Ewing's sarcoma than those presented in osteosarcoma [25] (**Figure 4**). In benign cartilaginous neoplasms, such as enchondromas or osteochondromas, the SUVmax value is generally less than 2, while in chondrosarcomas, most have values above 2, which represents a good tool for diagnostic differentiation [27, 28]. Patients with primary bone lymphoma and multiple myeloma have good applications for PET-CT for staging, follow-up, and prognostic evaluation [29].

3.6 Other modalities

PET-MRI is an examination modality where the metabolic phase of the study is performed using 18F-FDG/PET and the anatomical acquisition is performed by MRI. It has a good indication in tumors, such as lymphomas and sarcomas, but imaging protocols still need to be defined separately for each type of malignancy, both bone and soft tissue [30]. As advantages reduces radiation exposure, can optimize diagnostic accuracy, and is a good predictor of histological response. In addition, better delimitation of the primary tumor (invasion of soft tissues). As a disadvantage, there is still no diagnostic advantage in performing the staging of the patient by PET/MRI in relation to conventional exams [30, 31], it presents several results similar to PET-CT [32] and still has limitations for the evaluation of nodules. Lungs smaller than 5 mm in size, and chest CT is still superior in this regard [32, 33]. PET-MRI can even be used for radiotherapy planning and detection of tissue damage by chemotherapy.

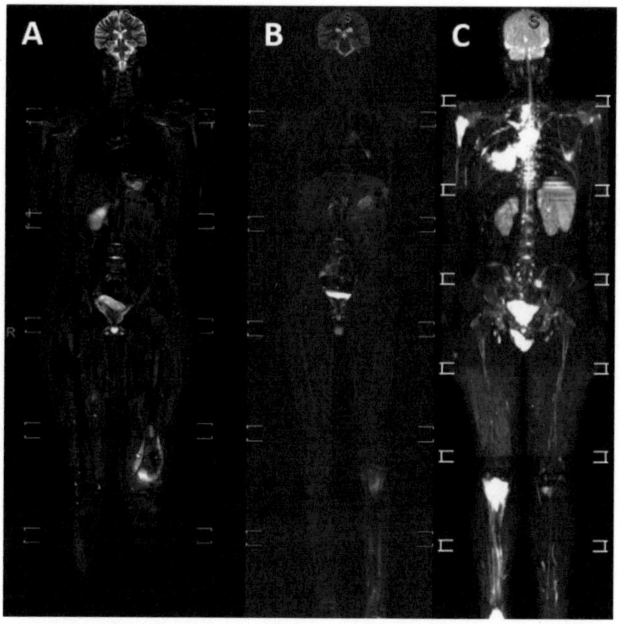

Figure 5.
Total body MRI. (A) patient with conventional osteosarcoma at the distal end of the femur, (B) patient with Ewing's sarcoma of the first metatarsal, observing metastasis in the proximal end of the tibia, and (C) patient with lung cancer and multiple bone metastases.

Regarding specific diagnoses, for example, in osteosarcoma, PET/MRI can better define the anatomical location of the lesion, but the lesion detection rate is similar to PET/CT. In Ewing's sarcoma, it is superior to PET-CT in the evaluation of an organ with high metabolic activity, such as the brain, probably the PET/MRI will become the exam of choice in these patients [29]. In the investigation of metastases for prostate and breast carcinoma, PET/MRI is presented as a great tool in the evaluation of these patients, but still not statistically superior to conventional methods [34]. However, although PET/MRI proves to be valuable, it cannot replace conventional exams if it is not accessible to most cancer patients [35].

Whole body MRI is an imaging method that uses a core protocol with essential imaging contrasts and it can be completed with sequences to evaluate other specific regions as needed, is a modality under evaluation for its applications and usefulness in bone sarcomas, however, it is observed that is better than scintigraphy to the screening for metastases [36] and is a good screening for cancer in patients with genetic syndromes, such as Li-Fraumeni, especially after the second test (lower false positive value, [37]) (**Figure 5**). In patients with prostate cancer, multiple myeloma and melanoma, whole body MRI is already introduced in international protocols, while its usefulness in neoplasms, such as breast cancer, ovarian cancer, and lymphoma is on the rise [38, 39]. WB-MRI is an excellent test for detecting bone metastases, especially in the spine region [40].

4. Metastases from unknown site

Patients over 40 years old who present with a painful new bone lesion should be investigated to mainly rule out bone metastasis or multiple myeloma [41].

Bone metastases occur in about 70% of advanced breast, lung, kidney, thyroid, and prostate carcinomas, while in gastrointestinal tumors, only 20% of patients have bone metastases, and among these patients, about half will present complications related to metastases, such as pathological fracture, spinal cord compression, pain requiring radiotherapy or surgery, and hypercalcemia, in about 10% of cases [42].

Breast and prostate cancers are the most common to generate bone metastases, however, when the patient has no diagnosis, the most common lesions to generate bone metastases are lung and kidney cancer [41]. Common sites of bone metastases are the proximal femur, pelvis, spine, ribs, and skull. Acral metastases are rare and they are usually related to lung cancer [42].

When evaluating patients with unknown site metastases, the focus is on finding the primary site of the neoplasm, and in about 85% of cases, a well-executed diagnostic evaluation can be successful to define de primary tumor. In the meantime, the evaluation begins with a comprehensive history and physical examination. Laboratory evaluation should include a complete blood count, erythrocyte sedimentation rate, alkaline phosphatase, liver function, renal function, thyroid function, electrolytes, PSA for men, and protein electrophoresis. Imaging evaluation begins with radiography of the lesion and the entire skeleton, as well as bone scintigraphy and CT scan of the chest, abdomen, and pelvis [41].

5. Staging

Tumors are proliferations of atypical, autonomous, irreversible cell clones with a tendency to lose cell differentiation. Tumors classified as benign are those that do not present cellular atypia, grow pushing the adjacent tissues, demonstrate the histological aspect of low aggressiveness, low tendency to local recurrence, and low tendency to spread (production of metastases). On the other hand, neoplasms considered malignant have a variable degree of cellular atypia, grow infiltrating adjacent tissues, demonstrate a more aggressive histological aspect, a high tendency to local recurrence, and a high tendency to spread.

The Enneking classification [43] (**Table 3**), for bone tumors has a first structure for the evaluation of benign tumors, a second structure defined for the evaluation of malignant tumors, and both in order to present an evolutionary degree of the lesions according to the increase in the stage in the classification.

The classification of the American Joint Committee on Cancer [44] (**Table 4**), defines only primary malignant bone neoplasms (except for primary bone lymphoma and multiple myeloma). This classification evaluates factors, such as histological grade, presence of regional metastases (lymph nodes), or distance (pulmonary and non-pulmonary), in addition to the size of the lesion. Related to the tumor size, it is observed that Ewing's sarcomas ≤8 cm have a better prognosis than those >8 cm, as well as in osteosarcoma that lesions ≤8 cm have a better prognosis in relation to osteosarcomas >8 cm greater in size.

Another staging related to primary bone sarcomas is in relation to the histological response to neoadjuvant chemotherapy. The surgical specimen is evaluated to analyze the degree of tumor necrosis and in patients with osteosarcoma and Ewing's sarcoma who present a degree of necrosis ≥90% are classified as good responders and who generally have good survival. This type of analysis was developed by Huvos [45, 46] (**Table 5**), initially for patients with osteosarcoma, however, it demonstrates to be applicable to Ewing's sarcoma [47].

Benign			
Stage	**Definition**	**Behavior**	
1	Latent or inactive	Static or heals spontaneously	
2	Active	Progressive growth but limited by natural barriers	
3	Aggressive	Progressive growth but not limited by natural barriers	
Malignant			
Stage	**Grade**	**Site**	**Metastases**
IA	low	Intracompartimental	None
IB	low	Extracompartimental	None
IIA	high	Intracompartimental	None
IIB	high	Extracompartimental	None
III	any	Any	Regional or distant

Table 3.
Enneking staging system for bone neoplams.

Stage	Grade	Size	Metastases
IA	Low	≤8cm	None
IB	Low	>8cm	None
IIA	High	≤8cm	None
IIB	High	>8cm	None
III	Any	Any	Skip
IVA	Any	Any	Pulmonary
IVB	Any	Any	Nonpulmonary

Table 4.
AJCC staging system – 8th edition.

Grade	Tumor response
1	None or minimal
2	Extensive necrosis with more than 10% of viable tumor
3	Extensive necrosis with less than 10% of viable tumor
4	Complete necrosis

Table 5.
Huvos's histologic grading of chemotherapy effect.

6. Biopsy

Biopsy of a bone neoplasm is a fundamental and final part of the diagnostic evaluation, with the objective of obtaining sufficient material for the histological diagnosis with minimal morbidity, limiting potential tumor spread, and not harming the surgical treatment [48, 49]. A surgeon experienced in the treatment of bone neoplasms or in Ref. centers must perform the biopsy in order to minimize the known complications of the method. A study showed that biopsies performed by other surgeons present up to 18% of diagnostic errors; 10% present as poorly planned biopsies or with insufficient material; 9% have some skin, bone, or soft tissue complication; 10% influenced the course of the disease and 3% resulted in unnecessary amputations [50]. Pathological fractures (**Figure 6**), are not common after biopsy procedures but may occur in about 10–25% of procedures performed in patients with osteosarcoma, 5% in chondrosarcomas, and 8–9% in Ewing's sarcomas (**Figure** 7) [51].

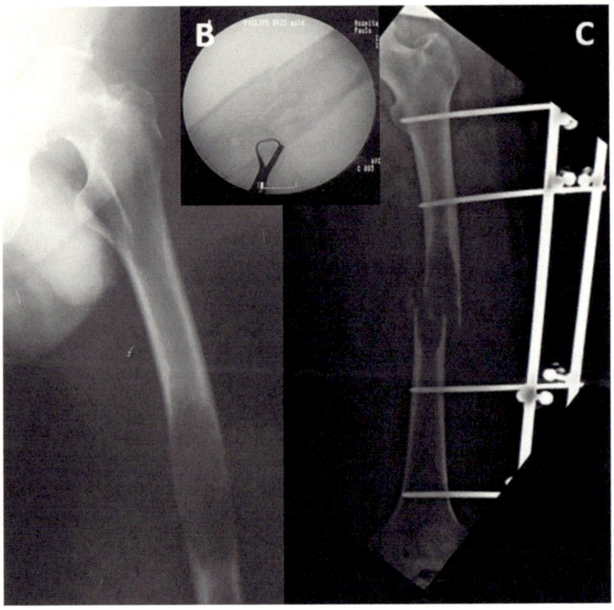

Figure 6.
(A) patient with an osteolytic lesion on the left femoral shaft, (B) fluoroscopy image of femur fracture during biopsy procedure, and (C) stabilization with external fixator was performed (patient with liver cancer).

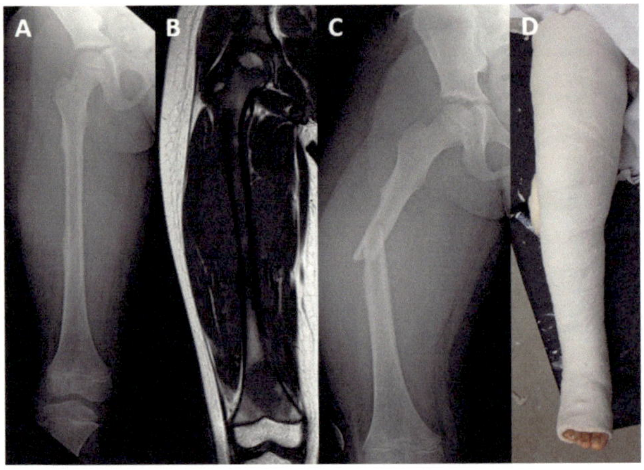

Figure 7.
(A) patient with a lytic lesion in the diaphysis of the right femur and an onion skin periosteal reaction, (B) extension femoral lesion with the presence of skip metastasis, (C) evolution to pathological fracture after biopsy procedure, and (D) stabilization with plaster cast.

There are two types of biopsy: open and percutaneous. Although for a long time the incisional (open) biopsy was considered the gold standard, the minimally invasive techniques (percutaneous – fine needle aspiration and core needle biopsy) have presented similar results [48, 49].

6.1 Fine needle biopsy/FNAC

High incidence of false negatives. Even when the result is positive, there is a great limitation in the diagnostic tissue evaluation due to the scarce specimen obtained by the procedure. The advantages of the method are that it is a procedure with minimal morbidity and is relatively inexpensive [48].

6.2 Core needle biopsy

Lower incidence of false-negative results when compared to fine-needle biopsy. The architectural structure of the tissue is preserved, so the tissue sample is suitable for histological evaluation and tumor grade, as well as for immunohistochemistry and molecular analysis. The procedure with minimal morbidity and low cost [48] (**Figure 8**).

6.3 Open biopsy

Indicated when a large volume of tissue is needed for proper diagnosis or when a percutaneous biopsy cannot be safely performed. Incisional biopsy is performed along the planned path in case of resection of the neoplasm and with the smallest incision compatible with the procedure. Transverse incisions should be avoided because their resection with a contaminated path during the treatment of the neoplasm, in addition to requiring a greater volume of excised tissue, can compromise the preservation of the limb. The formation of bruises and the use of drains that can contaminate the soft tissues should be avoided. The disadvantages of incisional biopsy are the possibility of contamination of soft tissues, complications with the operative wound, and is a more expensive procedure compared to percutaneous procedures [48].

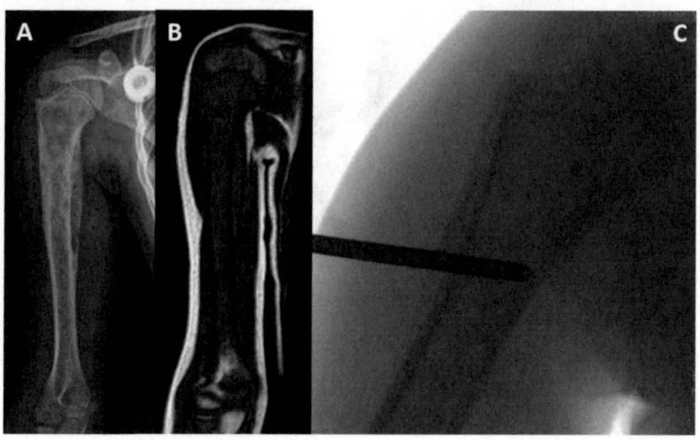

Figure 8.
Correct sequence for performing a biopsy procedure. (A) x-ray of the affected limb, (B) local staging (biopsy should be perform after complete systemic staging), and (C) core needle biopsy using fluoroscopy.

7. Biopsy imaging techniques

7.1 Fluoroscopy

Widely available, relatively inexpensive, and easy-to-use method. The lesion is evaluated in orthogonal positions with the needle being introduced perpendicular to the lesion, in the course of surgical planning and in order to contaminate the least amount of tissue possible (**Figure 8**) [52].

7.2 Ultrasound

Operator-dependent method requires some expertise to use, however, it exempts the patient from exposure to radiation, has a good evaluation of superficial lesions, is low cost, and presents a high image resolution [53–55]. The appropriate probe is chosen for the evaluation of the lesion and adjacent structures, once the probe achieves the right position at the region of choice for material acquisition; the needle is introduced parallel to the probe so that the entire path and tip of the needle can be observed.

7.3 CT

Relatively expensive method, greater exposure to ionizing radiation and in many places requires differentiated logistics, as the device is generally not limited only to biopsy procedures. Very useful in performing biopsies of complex structures, such as the pelvis or regions that require greater precision, from the surgeon, such as the spine. The accuracy of the CT-guided core-needle biopsy procedure is high, around 96%, and with a low complication rate, between 0 and 7.4% [56–59] (**Figure 9**).

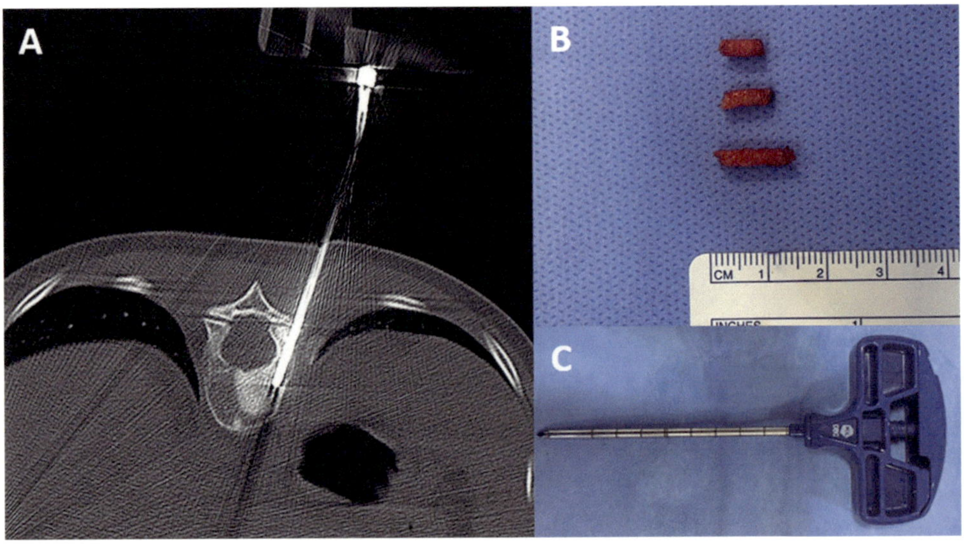

Figure 9.
(A) biopsy of osteoblastic lesion in vertebral body guided by CT scan, (B) bone fragments removed with a core needle, and (C) core needle.

8. Conclusions

The diagnostic evaluation of bone tumors, therefore, must be carried out systematically, starting with the history and physical examination, which will guide the diagnostic hypotheses and necessary complementary tests. A patient referred for specialized evaluation should not be delayed to obtain staging images for investigation, being standard radiography is sufficient for this purpose. A biopsy is the last procedure to be performed. It depends on the initial staging to be planned and should be performed at the service where the patient will start his treatment and preferably by the doctor responsible for the surgical treatment.

Conflict of interest

The authors declare no conflict of interest.

Appendices and nomenclature

CT	computed tomography
PET	positron emission tomography
MRI	magnet resonance imaging

Author details

Jairo Garcia[1,2,3]

1 Federal University of São Paulo, São Paulo, Brazil

2 GRAACC—Support Group for Adolescents and Children with Cancer, São Paulo, Brazil

3 Municipal Hospital Dr. Gilson Carvalho/Hospital Albert Einstein, São Paulo, Brazil

*Address all correspondence to: jairogreco@hotmail.com

References

[1] Schaser KD, Bail HJ, Haas NP, Melcher I. Behandlungskonzepte bei benignen Knochentumoren und tumorsimulierenden Knochenläsionen. Der Chirurg. 2002;**73**(12):1181-1190

[2] Greenspan A. Skeletal Radiology Benign bone-forming lesions: Osteoma, osteoid osteoma, and osteoblastoma Clinical, imaging, pathologic, and differential considerations. Skeletal Radiology. 1993;**22**:485-500

[3] Hsieh TC, Liao CW, Lai YC, Law KM, Chan PK, Kao CH. Detection of bone metastases on bone scans through image classification with contrastive learning. Journal of Personalized Medicine. 2021;**11**(12):1-13

[4] Moffi HL, HHM Y, Tsai YY, Hoffe SE. Overview of diagnosis and management of metastatic disease to bone. 2012;**19**. Available from: www.henrydomke.com

[5] Guillevin R, Vallee JN, Lafitte F, Menuel C, Duverneuil NM, Chiras J. Spine metastasis imaging: Review of the literature. Journal of Neuroradiology. 2007;**34**:311-321

[6] Ghanem N, Uhl M, Brink I, Schäfer O, Kelly T, Moser E, et al. Diagnostic value of MRI in comparison to scintigraphy, PET, MS-CT and PET/CT for the detection of metastases of bone. European Journal of Radiology. 2005;**55**(1):41-55

[7] Heindel W, Gübitz R, Vieth V, Weckesser M, Schober O, Schäfers M. The diagnostic imaging of bone metastases. Deutsches Ärzteblatt International. 2014;**111**:741-747

[8] Liu T, Wang S, Liu H, Meng B, Zhou F, He F, et al. Detection of vertebral metastases: A meta-analysis comparing MRI, CT, PET, BS and BS with SPECT. Journal of Cancer Research and Clinical Oncology. Springer Verlag. 2017;**143**:457-465

[9] Flanagan AM, Lindsay D. A diagnostic approach to bone tumours. Pathology. 2017;**49**(7):675-687

[10] Salom M, Chiari C, Maria Gómez Alessandri J, Willegger M, Windhager R, Sanpera I. Diagnosis and staging of malignant bone tumours in children: What is due and what is new?

[11] Caracciolo JT, Letson GD. Radiologic approach to bone and soft tissue sarcomas. Surgical Clinics of North America. W.B. Saunders. 2016;**96**(5):963-976

[12] Fritzsche H, Schaser KD, Hofbauer C. Benigne tumoren und tumorähnliche läsionen des knochens: Allgemeine behandlungsprinzipien. Orthopade. 2017;**46**:484-497

[13] Yaw KM. Pediatric bone tumors. Seminars in Surgical Oncology. 1999;**16**:173-183

[14] O'donnell P. Evaluation of focal bone lesions: Basic principles and clinical scenarios Evaluation of focal bone lesions part I: Basic principles

[15] Vanel D, Rimondi E, Vanel M, Gambarotti M, Alberghini M. Solitary bone lesions: Which ones to worry about? Cancer Imaging. 2012;**2**:409-413

[16] Thierfelder KM, Niendorf S, Gerhardt JS, Weber MA. dré. Bone tumors and metastases: Tips for initial diagnosis and follow-up: Update 2019. Der Radiologe. 2020;**60**(2):169-178

[17] Errani C, Tsukamoto S, Mavrogenis AF. Imaging analyses of bone tumors. JBJS Reviews. 2020;**8**(3):1-11

[18] Cerase A, Priolo F. Skeletal benign bone-forming lesions. European Journal of Radiology. 1998;**27**:S91-S97

[19] Sun W, Li M, Gu Y, Sun Z, Qiu Z, Zhou Y. Diagnostic value of whole-body DWI with background body suppression plus calculation of apparent diffusion coefficient at 3 T versus 18F-FDG PET/CT for detection of bone metastases. American Journal of Roentgenology. 2020;**214**(2):446-454

[20] Rana KA, Meyer J, Ibrahim S, Ralls M, Kent PM. The role of imaging of malignant bone tumors in children and young adults. Current Problems in Cancer. 2013;**37**(4):181-191

[21] Rajiah P, Ilaslan H, Sundaram M. Imaging of sarcomas of pelvic bones. Semin Ultrasound, CT MRI. 2011;**32**(5):433-441

[22] Sderlund V. Radiological diagnosis of skeletal metastases. European Radiology Springer-Verlag. 1996;**6**:587-595

[23] Ilaslan H, Schils J, Nageotte W, Lietman SA, Sundaram M. Clinical presentation and imaging of bone and soft-tissue sarcomas. Cleveland Clinic Journal of Medicine. 2010;**77**(SUPPL. 1)

[24] Kaste SC. Imaging pediatric bone sarcomas. Radiologic Clinics of North America. 2011;**49**:749-765

[25] Harrison DJ, Parisi MT, Shulkin BL. The role of 18 F-FDG-PET/CT in pediatric sarcoma. Seminars in Nuclear Medicine. 2017;**47**(3):229-241. Available from: https://linkinghub.elsevier.com/retrieve/pii/S0001299816301192

[26] Hurley C, McCarville MB, Shulkin BL, Mao S, Wu J, Navid F, et al. Comparison of 18 F-FDG-PET-CT and bone scintigraphy for evaluation of osseous metastases in newly diagnosed and recurrent osteosarcoma. Pediatric Blood & Cancer. 2016;**63**(8):1381-1386. DOI: 10.1002/pbc.26014

[27] Subhawong TK, Winn A, Shemesh SS, Pretell-Mazzini J. F-18 FDG PET differentiation of benign from malignant chondroid neoplasms: A systematic review of the literature. Skeletal Radiology. 2017;**46**(9):1233-1239. DOI: 10.1007/s00256-017-2685-7

[28] Jesus-Garcia R, Osawa A, Filippi RZ, Viola DCM, Korukian M, de Carvalho Campos Neto G, et al. Is PET–CT an accurate method for the differential diagnosis between chondroma and chondrosarcoma? Springerplus. 2016;**5**(1):236. Available from: http://www.springerplus.com/content/5/1/236

[29] Behzadi AH, Raza SI, Carrino JA, Kosmas C, Gholamrezanezhad A, Basques K, et al. Applications of PET/CT and PET/MR imaging in primary bone malignancies. PET Clinics. 2018;**13**(4):623-634. Available from: https://linkinghub.elsevier.com/retrieve/pii/S1556859818300749

[30] Kooraki S, Assadi M, Gholamrezanezhad A. Hot topics of research in musculoskeletal imaging. PET Clinics. 2019;**14**(1):175-182. Available from: https://linkinghub.elsevier.com/retrieve/pii/S1556859818301032

[31] Platzek I, Beuthien-Baumann B, Schramm G, Maus J, Laniado M, Kotzerke J, et al. FDG PET/MR in initial staging of sarcoma: Initial experience and comparison with conventional imaging. Clinical Imaging. 2017;**42**:126-132. Available from: https://linkinghub.elsevier.com/retrieve/pii/S0899707116301899

[32] Qi J, Thakrar PD, Browning MB, Vo N, Kumbhar SS. Clinical utilization of whole-body PET/MRI in childhood sarcoma. Pediatric Radiology. 2021;**51**(3):471-479. DOI: 10.1007/s00247-020-04834-7

[33] Baratto L, Hawk KE, States L, Qi J, Gatidis S, Kiru L, et al. PET/MRI improves management of children with cancer. The Journal of Nuclear Medicine. 2021;**62**(10):1334-1340. DOI: 10.2967/jnumed.120.259747

[34] Hancin EC, Borja AJ, Nikpanah M, Raynor WY, Haldar D, Werner TJ, et al. PET/MR imaging in musculoskeletal precision imaging - Third wave after X-Ray and MR. PET Clinics. 2020;**15**(4):521-534. Available from: https://linkinghub.elsevier.com/retrieve/pii/S1556859820300390

[35] Daldrup-Link HE. How PET/MR can add value for children with cancer. Current Radiology Reports. 2017;**5**(3):1-14

[36] Sun G, Zhang YX, Liu F, Tu N. Whole-body magnetic resonance imaging is superior to skeletal scintigraphy for the detection of bone metastatic tumors: A meta-analysis. European Review for Medical and Pharmacological Sciences. 2020;**24**(13):7240-7252. Available from: http://www.ncbi.nlm.nih.gov/pubmed/32706062

[37] Paixão D, Guimarães MD, de Andrade KC, Nóbrega AF, Chojniak R, Achatz MI. Whole-body magnetic resonance imaging of Li-Fraumeni syndrome patients: Observations from a two rounds screening of Brazilian patients. Cancer Imaging. 2018;**18**(1):27. DOI: 10.1186/s40644-018-0162-8

[38] Summers P, Saia G, Colombo A, Pricolo P, Zugni F, Alessi S, et al. Whole-body magnetic resonance imaging: Technique, guidelines and key applications. Ecancermedicalscience. 2021;7:15. Available from: https://ecancer.org/en/journal/article/1164-whole-body-magnetic-resonance-imaging-technique-guidelines-and-key-applications

[39] Petralia G, Padhani AR. Whole-body magnetic resonance imaging in oncology. Magnetic Resonance Imaging Clinics of North America. 2018;**26**(4):495-507. Available from: https://linkinghub.elsevier.com/retrieve/pii/S1064968918300436

[40] Nakanishi K, Kobayashi M, Takahashi S, Nakata S, Kyakuno M, Nakaguchi K, et al. Whole body MRI for detecting metastatic bone tumor: Comparison with bone scintigrams. Magnetic Resonance in Medical Sciences. 2005;**4**(1):11-17. Available from: http://www.jstage.jst.go.jp/article/mrms/4/1/4_1_11/_article

[41] Rougraff BT, Kneisl JS, Simon MA. Skeletal metastases of unknown origin. A prospective study of a diagnostic strategy. The Journal of Bone and Joint Surgery. 1993;**75**(9):1276-1281. Available from: http://journals.lww.com/00004623-199309000-00003

[42] Jehn CF, Diel IJ, Overkamp F, Kurth A, Schaefer R, Miller K, et al. Management of metastatic bone disease algorithms for diagnostics and treatment. Anticancer Research. 2016;**36**(6):2631-2637. Available from: http://www.ncbi.nlm.nih.gov/pubmed/27272771

[43] Enneking WF, Spanier SS, Goodman MA. A system for the surgical staging of musculoskeletal sarcoma. 1980. Clinical Orthopaedics and Related Research. 2003;**415**:4-18

[44] Amin MB, Edge SB, Greene FL, Byrd DR, Brookland RK, Washington MK, et al., editors. AJCC

Cancer Staging Manual. Cham: Springer International Publishing; 2017. DOI: 10.1007/978-3-319-40618-3. ISBN: 978-3-319-40617-6

[45] Rosen G, Caparros B, Huvos AG, Kosloff C, Nirenberg A, Cacavio A, et al. Preoperative chemotherapy for osteogenic sarcoma: Selection of postoperative adjuvant chemotherapy based on the response of the primary tumor to preoperative chemotherapy. Cancer. 1982;**49**(6):1221-1230. DOI: 10.1002/1097-0142

[46] Huvos AG, Rosen G, Marcove RC. Primary osteogenic sarcoma: Pathologic aspects in 20 patients after treatment with chemotherapy en bloc resection, and prosthetic bone replacement. Archives of Pathology & Laboratory Medicine. 1977;**101**(1):14-18. Available from: http://www.ncbi.nlm.nih.gov/pubmed/299812

[47] Js W, Paulian G, Ag H, Heller G, Pa M, Jh H. The histological response to chemotherapy as a predictor of the oncological outcome of operative treatment of ewing sarcoma*. Journal of Bone and Joint Surgery. 1998;**80**(7):1020-1033. Available from: http://journals.lww.com/00004623-199807000-00011

[48] Errani C, Traina F, Perna F, Calamelli C, Faldini C. Current concepts in the biopsy of musculoskeletal tumors. The Scientific World Journal. 2013;**2013**:1-7

[49] Traina F, Errani C, Toscano A, Pungetti C, Fabbri D, Mazzotti A, et al. Current concepts in the biopsy of musculoskeletal tumors: AAOS exhibit selection. Journal of Bone and Joint Surgery-American Volume. 2015;**97**(2):e7(1)

[50] Mitsuyoshi G, Naito N, Kawai A, Kunisada T, Yoshida A, Yanai H, et al. Accurate diagnosis of musculoskeletal lesions by core needle biopsy. Journal of Surgical Oncology. 2006;**94**(1):21-27

[51] Winkler D, Fritzsche H, Schaser KD, Hofbauer C. Biopsy of musculoskeletal tumors: Complications and avoidable errors. Orthopade. 2020;**49**:88-97

[52] Masood S, Mallinson PI, Sheikh A, Ouellette H, Munk PL. Percutaneous bone biopsy. Techniques in Vascular & Interventional Radiology. 2022;**25**(1):100800. Available from: https://linkinghub.elsevier.com/retrieve/pii/S1089251622000051

[53] Chira RI, Chira A, Manzat-Saplacan RM, Nagy G, Bintintan A, Mircea PA, et al. Ultrasound-guided bone lesions biopsies - A systematic review. Medical Ultrasonography. 2017;**19**(3):302-309. Available from: http://www.ncbi.nlm.nih.gov/pubmed/28845497

[54] Yeow KM, Tan CF, Chen JS, Hsueh C. Diagnostic sensitivity of ultrasound-guided needle biopsy in soft tissue masses about superficial bone lesions. Journal of Ultrasound in Medicine. 2000;**19**(12):849-855. DOI: 10.7863/jum.2000.19.12.849

[55] Torriani M, Etchebehere M, Amstalden EMI. Sonographically guided core needle biopsy of bone and soft tissue tumors. Journal of Ultrasound in Medicine. 2002;**21**(3):275-281. DOI: 10.7863/jum.2002.21.3.275

[56] Refaat Y, Gunnoe J, Hornicek FJ, Mankin HJ. Comparison of quality of life after amputation or limb salvage. Clinical Orthopaedics and Related Research. 2002;**397**(397):298-305

[57] Lack W, Donigan JA, Morcuende J, Buckwalter J, El-Khoury GY. Clinical utility of CT-guided biopsies in

orthopaedic oncology. Iowa Orthopedic Journal. 2010;**30**:76-79. Available from: http://www.ncbi.nlm.nih.gov/pubmed/21045975

[58] Hau MA, Il KJ, Kattapuram S, Hornicek FJ, Rosenberg AE, Gebhardt MC, et al. Accuracy of CT-guided biopsies in 359 patients with musculoskeletal lesions. Skeletal Radiology. 2002;**31**(6):349-353

[59] Puri A, Shingade VU, Agarwal MG, Anchan C, Juvekar S, Desai S, et al. CT-guided percutaneous core needle biopsy in deep seated musculoskeletal lesions: A prospective study of 128 cases. Skeletal Radiology. 2006;**35**(3):138-143

Chapter 3

Perspective Chapter: Bone Metastases of Solid Tumors

Joana Monteiro and Nuno Bonito

Abstract

Bone metastases are more common than primary bone cancers, especially in adults. Bone is the third most common organ affected by metastases, from many types of solid cancers but especially those arising in the breast and prostate. Besides the impact on survival, bone metastases may have a big impact on morbidity and represents a significant healthcare burden. Skeletal-related events (SREs) include pain, pathologic fracture, spinal cord compression, and hypercalcemia and can cause a deterioration of the quality of life. Detection of bone metastases is essential for accurate staging and optimal treatment; however, there is no consensus or standard approach for diagnosis, so the choice of imaging should be guided by clinical presentation. Treatment goals may consist of controlling pain and other symptoms, preserving and restoring function, minimizing the risk of SREs, stabilizing the skeleton, and enhancing local tumor control. Therapeutic options include pain management/ analgesia, osteoclast inhibitors, systemic anticancer therapy, radiation therapy, bone-targeting radiopharmaceutical therapy, surgery, and/or image-guided thermal ablation. The choice of treatment is influenced by factors like symptoms, impact on quality of life, performance status, estimated life expectancy, goals of treatment, and preferences of care.

Keywords: bone metastases, cancer pain, osteoclast inhibitors, bisphosphonates, denosumab

1. Introduction

Bone metastases are more common than primary bone cancers, especially in adults [1]. Bone is the third most common organ affected by metastases, from many types of solid cancers but especially those arising in the breast and prostate [1–3]. The most common locations for metastatic disease are the vertebral column, sacrum, pelvis, and proximal femurs [4].

The overall incidence of bone metastases is not known [1, 2]. It is estimated to have an incidence in about 70% of patients with breast and prostate cancer, which are the two most common cancers worldwide, but bone metastases can occur in a wide range of malignancies, described in **Table 1** [2, 3, 5].

In terms of prognosis, survival varies according to the tumor type, with the median survival of patients with breast and prostate cancer reaching years and of patients with lung cancer being measured in months, and it is also influenced

Primary tumor	Incidence of bone metastases (%)
Breast cancer	65–75
Prostate cancer	65–75
Thyroid cancer	40–60
Bladder cancer	40
Lung cancer	30–40
Renal cell carcinoma	20–35
Melanoma	15–45
Gastrointestinal cancer	5

Table 1.
Incidence of bone metastases in different cancers.

by coexisting non-osseous metastatic disease, which ends up being important in determining the prognosis [3]. However, bone metastases may have a big impact on morbidity and represents a significant healthcare burden [3, 6].

2. Mechanism of bone metastases

During metastatic dissemination, cancer cells from the primary tumor must first undergo epithelial-to-mesenchymal transition (EMT) to invade the surrounding tissue and enter the microvasculature (intravasation) of the blood and/or lymphatic systems. Once in the bloodstream, cancer cells may disseminate to distant organs, exit from blood vessels (extravasation), and settle in the foreign microenvironment, where they enter a dormant state or proliferate to subsequently form macroscopic secondary tumors (metastases) [7].

In the skeleton, the process of metastasis development begins with colonization, when circulating tumor cells enter the bone marrow and engage in specialized microenvironments or niches. Then, the colonizing tumor cells adapt to their new microenvironment, evade the immune system, and may reside in a dormant state for a long period of time until they reactivate and develop, escaping from the dormant state to actively proliferate and form micrometastases. With uncontrollable growth, the cancer cells become independent of the microenvironment and end up modifying the bone as metastases develop.

3. Type of bone metastases

In metastatic bone disease, the normal bone homeostasis that involves constant remodeling by the coordinated actions of osteoclasts and osteoblasts is disturbed [5, 7]. According to the primary mechanism of interference with normal bone remodeling, bone metastases can be classified as osteolytic, osteoblastic, or mixed [8].

Osteolytic lesions are characterized by the destruction of normal bone and are associated with high osteoclast activity and reduced osteoblast activity. Several factors secreted by tumor cells enhance osteoclast-mediated bone resorption, either directly (like interleukin-8) or indirectly [like the parathyroid hormone-related peptide (PTHrP), interleukin-6] via stimulation of the receptor activator of the nuclear factor kappa-B (RANK) ligand (RANKL) secretion and inhibition of osteoprotegerin (OPG) production by osteoblasts. In turn, the binding of RANKL to RANK on osteoclast precursors leads to the formation of new osteoclasts, increasing their activity [7]. This type of metastasis is characteristic of prostate cancer, small cell lung cancer, carcinoid tumors, and medulloblastoma.

Osteoblastic metastases are characterized by the deposition of new bone (osteosclerosis). Several factors secreted by tumor cells directly enhance osteoblast differentiation, like endothelin-1 (ET-1) and bone morphogenetic proteins (BMPs). The stimulation of osteoblast differentiation is associated with increased OPG production, whereas RANKL secretion is decreased, and tumor-derived ET-1 directly acts on mature osteoclasts to inhibit osteoclast activity. Therefore, there is a strong imbalance between bone formation and bone resorption, leading to aberrant bone formation [7]. This pattern is usually seen in renal cell cancer, non-small-cell lung cancer, melanoma, and thyroid cancer.

If a lesion has both osteolytic and osteoblastic components, it's classified as **mixed** and is usually seen in breast cancer, gastrointestinal cancers, and squamous cancers.

4. Clinical presentation

Bone metastases may cause few or no symptoms, being diagnosed incidentally during the initial staging of the primary cancer. However, they can represent a prominent source of morbidity because of skeletal-related events (SREs), which include pain, pathologic fracture, spinal cord compression, and hypercalcemia [3, 5].

Pain is the most common symptom of bone metastases and can have a significant impact on the quality of life [3, 9]. It could be of either biologic or mechanical origin. Biologic pain is related to the local release of cytokines and chemical mediators by the tumor cells, periosteal irritation, and stimulation of intraosseous nerves. Mechanical pain is related to the pressure or mass effect of the tumor tissue within the bone, with loss of bone strength, thus turning into activity-related pain. It's usually localized, but not rarely patients can complaint of pain in more than one site, and it might become severe and refractory to analgesia [7]. Sudden severe pain may be caused by a pathologic fracture, and prompt evaluation is necessary.

Pathologic fractures occur in 10–30% of all cancer patients, with proximal parts of the long bones being the most frequent fracture site and the femur accounting for over half of all cases [10]. Pain at the fracture site is the most common symptom, but other clinical features may be present depending on the fracture location, such as the inability to bear weight, point tenderness, pain that radiates, ecchymosis or skin discoloration, soft tissue mass or swelling at the site of pain, edema or joint effusion, loss of bony or limb contour, extremity shortening, open wound and bone exposure, decreased range of motion, significantly diminished mobility, and/or sensory disturbance of the distal extremity. The presence of neurologic symptoms should be a red flag for spinal cord compression.

Spinal cord compression can be caused by pathologic spine fracture, with the bone compressing the spinal cord or by tumor extension into the epidural space. Symptoms range from pain, which is usually the first symptom, to neurologic deficits, including motor weakness and paralysis, sensory deficits, bowel and bladder dysfunction, and ataxia [3, 11]. In terms of motor symptoms, these will depend on the site of compression – if it's at or above the conus medullaris, it generally produces fairly symmetric lower extremity weakness (if compression is above the thoracic spine, upper extremities may be affected too); if it's below the level of the conus medullaris, it may present with signs and symptoms of cauda equina syndrome, with asymmetrical and less severe weakness. Sensory findings are common and are usually present prior to the onset of weakness, with patients describing ascending numbness and paresthesia in a radicular distribution [11]. If the site of compression is above the conus medullaris, sacral dermatomes are usually spared, while in the cauda equina syndrome, a saddle sensory loss is common. Proprioceptive loss can also occur, although this is less common and usually occurs later.

Hypercalcemia is the most common metabolic complication of malignant disease, and it's usually caused by direct induction of local osteolysis by the tumor cells and generalized osteolysis by humoral factors secreted by the tumor [3, 7, 12]. Patients with mild hypercalcemia may be asymptomatic or have nonspecific symptoms, such as constipation, fatigue, and depression, while patients with higher serum calcium elevations may present polyuria, polydipsia, dehydration, anorexia, nausea, muscle weakness, and neuropsychiatric disturbances and may even lead to cardiac arrhythmias and acute renal failure [2, 7].

5. Diagnosis

Detection of bone metastases is essential for accurate staging and optimal treatment. There is no standard approach for the detection of bone metastases in patients with cancer, so the choice of imaging should be guided by the clinical presentation.

Radiographs are fast, cheap, and widely available and are recommended for the initial evaluation of symptomatic areas, particularly of the extremities [10]. The typical radiographic appearance of a lytic metastasis is a permeative lesion of the diaphysis or metadiaphysis of a proximal long bone or bone of the axial skeleton, while osteoblastic lesions are usually sclerotic in appearance, sometimes admixed with lytic elements. Although it can be specific, for a destructive lesion in trabecular bone to be recognized, it must be >1 cm in diameter with loss of approximately 50% of the bone mineral content, so the sensitivity is low [10, 13]. Therefore, if the clinical suspicion is high, then computed tomography (CT) or magnetic resonance imaging (MRI) should be done.

CT produces images with excellent tissue and contrast resolution [13]. Compared to MRI, it is superior in terms of the evaluation of structural integrity of the bone, and it can be used to diagnose bone metastases in situations in which MRI is contraindicated or not available. However, differentiation between metabolically active from inactive bone lesions cannot be made, limiting its use for the evaluation of treatment effect [13].

In general, **MRI** is more sensitive than CT to detect bone metastases, allows better delineation of the extent of tumor, and is particularly useful for patients with spine metastases to evaluate the extent of medullary and extraspinal disease [10, 14, 15]. Metastatic lesions display decreased signal on T1-weighted sequences, reflecting the replacement of normal fatty marrow with water-containing tumor, while on T2-weighted images, they usually have a higher signal than the surrounding normal bone marrow [14–16].

Whole-body skeletal evaluation with Tc-99 m **skeletal scintigraphy**, generally referred to as **bone scan**, is the most widely used method to detect bone metastases because it provides visualization of the entire skeleton [5, 15]. However, it lacks specificity, it has low sensitivity for tumors with little to no osteoblastic activity, and it is inferior to MRI on the evaluation of vertebral metastases [1, 10, 14, 15, 17].

Positron emission tomography (PET) scan is based on the preferential uptake of 18-fluorodeoxyglucose (18FDG) by tumor cells because of their increased glucose metabolism, so it detects the presence of tumor directly by quantifying the metabolic activity [5, 10, 16]. Therefore, it has high sensitivity and specificity for the diagnosis of distant metastases, including the bone, and it's use in initial staging and further evaluation for metastatic disease is increasing.

Definitive diagnosis requires histologic examination of **biopsy**. However, in patients with known cancer, a skeletal lesion with a typical appearance on imaging studies may be presumed to be metastatic, and there is no need for tissue diagnosis. For patients with bone-only disease, especially when there are few lesions or imaging tests are equivocal, histological confirmation of metastatic disease is strongly recommended [13]. The same holds true for patients with an unknown primary cancer who present with bone metastases and the initial evaluation fails to identify the primary site, where a biopsy is generally indicated to both confirm the malignant nature of the bone lesion and provide histologic information about likely primary sites. CT-guided fine needle aspiration biopsy (FNA) is easy to perform and accurate to document the presence of metastatic disease; however, it may not indicate the most likely site of the primary malignancy. Therefore, in this setting, a core biopsy may be needed, as it has higher diagnostic accuracy for determining the type, grade, and specific diagnosis of musculoskeletal tumors [18]. An open biopsy is required in a residual number of cases and may be done opportunistically in the operating room prior to possible internal fixation.

6. Treatment

Treatment goals may consist of controlling pain and other symptoms, preserving and restoring function, minimizing the risk of SREs, stabilizing the skeleton, and enhancing local tumor control. Therapeutic options include pain management/analgesia, osteoclast inhibitors, systemic anticancer therapy, radiation therapy, bone-targeting radiopharmaceutical therapy, surgery, and/or image-guided thermal ablation. The choice of treatment is influenced by factors like symptoms, impact on quality of life, performance status, estimated life expectancy, goals of treatment, and preferences of care. Optimal treatment may be complex and may require multimodality treatment strategies.

6.1 Analgesia

Patients with bone metastases will suffer from significant bone pain at some point of the disease course. Initially, for mild to moderate pain, nonopioid analgesic drugs, such as acetaminophen and nonsteroidal anti-inflammatory drugs (NSAIDs), may be used alone, but for moderate to severe pain, opioids should be the therapy of choice, according to the WHO "analgesic ladder" approach [19, 20].

Glucocorticoids may be helpful for selected patients as well as other adjuncts, like antidepressants and antiepileptics such as gabapentin [21, 22]. Actually, for patients with neurologic deficits or pain associated with spinal cord compression, high-dose glucocorticoid therapy is part of the standard treatment - a typical dose is 10 mg dexamethasone intravenously followed by 16 mg daily orally in divided doses, until definite treatment [23].

Multidisciplinary management with a palliative care specialist should be considered for patients whose pain is refractory to analgesia or who develop significant side effects.

6.2 Osteoclast inhibitors

For patients with metastatic bone disease, osteoclast inhibitors, like bisphosphonates and denosumab, may prevent SREs as they slow down or reverse the progression of skeletal metastases and may even improve pain and quality of life. For patients in whom SREs are unlikely (those with minimal bone tumor burden) or those with a limited expected survival, treatment with osteoclast inhibitors should be decided case by case.

Bisphosphonates are analogs of pyrophosphate, a natural inhibitor of bone demineralization. Bisphosphonates bind avidly to exposed bone mineral around resorbing osteoclast, and this leads to very high local concentrations of products in the resorption lacunae. Then, they are internalized by the osteoclast, causing disruption of the chemical process involved in bone resorption [2, 7, 8]. This way, bisphosphonates decrease bone resorption and increase mineralization [5].

There are two classes of bisphosphonates: nonnitrogen containing, such as etidronate, clodronate, and tiludronate, and nitrogen containing, such as pamidronate, alendronate, ibandronate, risedronate, and zoledronic acid, which are more potent osteoclast inhibitors [19]. When a bisphosphonate is chosen, zoledronic acid is suggested over other bisphosphonates.

Zoledronic acid is the most potent bisphosphonate available and has been the bisphosphonate of choice in most clinical settings and healthcare systems [7]. Trials showed zoledronic acid has effectively decreased the risk of SREs in women with bone metastases from breast cancer, men with bone metastases from castration-resistant prostate cancer, and patients with bone metastases from other solid tumors [24–29]. The approved dose and schedule of administration is 4 mg every 4 weeks, with the dose adjusted for creatinine clearance.

If zoledronic acid is not available, **pamidronate** is a reasonable alternative [25, 29]. Other bisphosphonates that have demonstrated efficacy in reducing SREs were **ibandronate** and **clodronate** [30, 31]. The dosage and interval of administration are described in **Table 2**.

In terms of tolerance, nephrotoxicity is one of the most important side effects, which is both dose and infusion time dependent [5, 32]. Other common adverse effects include acute-phase reactions (with pyrexia and flu-like symptoms), gastrointestinal effects, and the most concerning, osteonecrosis of the jaw [5, 33].

Denosumab is a monoclonal antibody that inhibits the RANKL, a key component in the pathway for osteoclast formation and activation [5, 8]. By binding to RANKL, denosumab prevents osteoclast formation, leading to decreased bone resorption and increased bone mass, thus preventing SREs [19]. Several phase III trials have shown a superiority of denosumab when compared to zoledronic acid [34–36]. A combined analysis of these three phase III trials concluded that denosumab was superior to

Bisphosphonates	Dosing	Interval
Zoledronic acid	4 mg	28/28 days
Pamidronate	90 mg	28/28 days
Ibandronate	6 mg	28/28 days
Clodronate	1600 mg	daily

Table 2.
Dosing and interval of bisphosphonates.

zoledronic acid in reducing the risk of a first SRE (hazard ratio [HR] 0.83, 95% CI 0.76–0.90) and in delaying the time to a first SRE (median 26.6 versus 19.4 months), with no difference in survival outcomes [37]. The recommended dose and schedule of administration is 120 mg every 4 weeks. Most common adverse events are similar to those of zoledronic acid, with the benefit of not requiring monitorization of renal function or dose adjustments for patients with renal insufficiency [37].

6.3 Systemic anticancer therapy

Chemotherapy, targeted therapies, and hormone therapy may contribute to pain relief by reducing tumor bulk and/or by modulating pain signaling pathways [38]. In selecting systemic anticancer treatment for metastatic bone disease, the pathological type of the tumor is the most important [2].

6.4 Radiation therapy

Radiation therapy is commonly used in the management of bone metastases, both for pain relief and for the prevention of morbidity and disease progression [5].

External beam radiation therapy (EBRT) is a standard approach for symptomatic skeletal metastases, as it can provide significant palliation of painful bone metastases in 50–80% of patients, with up to one-third of patients achieving complete pain relief at the treated site [39]. For uncomplicated bone metastases, a single fraction of 8 Gy to the involved area has been shown to provide equivalent pain palliation and may be more cost-effective and convenient compared with fractionated regimens, although retreatment is needed more frequently [13, 40].

Stereotactic body radiation therapy (SBRT) utilizes precisely targeted radiation to a tumor while minimizing radiation to adjacent normal tissue, allowing the treatment of small or moderate-sized tumors in either a single or a limited number of dose fractions. This approach should be reserved mostly for patients who have a reasonable life expectancy (superior to 6 months) and persistent or recurrent bone pain after a standard course of EBRT, which requires reirradiation [40]. Additionally, SBRT may be preferred over EBRT in the definitive treatment of patients with symptomatic bone metastases from relatively radioresistant neoplasms (such as renal cell cancer, melanoma, and sarcoma), especially in the setting of vertebral metastases with epidural extension and in patients with oligometastatic disease who have a relatively long life expectancy [41, 42].

6.5 Bone-targeting radiopharmaceutical therapy

Bone-targeted radiopharmaceuticals are radioactive bone-seeking molecules that show efficacy for pain control in patients with osteoblastic bone metastases, such as samarium-153, strontium-89, rhenium-186, and radium-223 [5].

Radium-223 is approved for the treatment of male patients with castration-resistant prostate cancer, with symptomatic bone metastases and no known visceral metastases, as it shows benefit in overall survival (median 14.9 versus 11.3 months, HR 0.70, 95% CI 0.58–0.83) and time to first symptomatic SRE (median 15.6 versus 9.8 months, HR 0.66, 95% CI 0.52–0.83) on a phase III trial, compared to placebo [43]. Its combination with systemic anticancer therapy is being studied; however, the benefit of the combination has not yet been established.

6.6 Surgery

Surgical management of bone metastases is typically reserved for lesions with a complete or impending pathologic fracture or spine metastases that cause mechanical instability or spinal cord compression [5, 44]. Nonetheless, for highly selected patients with advanced cancer who present with or develop a bone lesion as the only focus of cancer beyond the primary site, resection of the bone metastasis may optimize local tumor control, provide durable pain relief, and possibly prolong survival.

6.7 Thermal ablation

For patients who have persistent or recurrent pain due to one or a few skeletal sites with small volume disease after palliative radiation therapy, and who are not candidates for surgery or reirradiation, local thermal ablation is an important therapeutic option. Radiofrequency ablation, microwave ablation, and cryoablation are effective ablative treatments for the palliation of symptomatic skeletal metastases [45–48]. There are no randomized trials comparing these procedures, so the choice of ablation technique should take into account availability, patient preference, and local expertise.

7. Conclusion

Bone metastases are a common manifestation of distant relapse from many types of solid cancers, a significant source of morbidity, and a major contributor to the deterioration of the quality of life. Prompt diagnosis is essential for optimal treatment, which may consist of controlling pain and other symptoms, preserving and restoring function, minimizing the risk of SREs, stabilizing the skeleton, and enhancing local tumor control. This way, a multidisciplinary approach is essential to achieve the best outcome possible.

Author details

Joana Monteiro* and Nuno Bonito
Portuguese Oncology Institute of Coimbra, Coimbra, Portugal

*Address all correspondence to: joanacruzmonteiro@gmail.com

References

[1] Tubiana-Hulin M. Incidence, prevalence and distribution of bone metastases. Bone. 1991;**12**(SUPPL. 1):S9

[2] Coleman RE. Metastatic bone disease: Clinical features, pathophysiology and treatment strategies. Cancer Treatment Reviews. 2001;**27**(3):165-176

[3] Coleman RE, Roodman S, Body S, Vessella. Clinical features of metastatic bone disease and risk of skeletal morbidity. Clinical Cancer Research. 2006;**12**(20 PART 2):6243-6249

[4] Krishnamurthy GT, Tubis M, Hiss J, Blahd WH. Distribution pattern of metastatic bone disease: A need for Total Body skeletal image. JAMA The Journal of the American Medical Association. 1977;**237**(23):2504-2506

[5] Gralow JR, Biermann JS, Farooki A, Fornier MN, Gagel RF, Kumar RN, et al. NCCN task force report: Bone health in Cancer care. Journal of the National Comprehensive Cancer Network. 2009;**7**:S1-S35

[6] Schulman KL, Kohles J. Economic burden of metastatic bone disease in the U.S. Cancer. 2007;**109**(11):2334-2342

[7] Clézardin P, Coleman R, Puppo M, Ottewell P, Bonnelye E, Paycha F, et al. Bone metastasis: Mechanisms, therapies, and biomarkers. Physiological Reviews. 2021;**101**(3):797-855

[8] Macedo F, Ladeira K, Pinho F, Saraiva N, Bonito N, Pinto L, et al. Bone metastases: An overview. Oncology Reviews. 2017;**11**:1

[9] Clohisy DR, Mantyh PW. Bone cancer pain. Cancer. 2003;**97** (3 SUPPL):866-873

[10] Selvaggi G, Scagliotti GV. Management of bone metastases in cancer: A review. Critical Reviews in Oncology/Hematology. 2005;**56**(3): 365-378

[11] Helweg-Larsen S, Sørensen PS. Symptoms and signs in metastatic spinal cord compression: A study of progression from first symptom until diagnosis in 153 patients. European Journal of Cancer. 1994;**30**(3):396-398

[12] Maisano R, Pergolizzi S, Cascinu S. Novel therapeutic approaches to cancer patients with bone metastasis. Critical Reviews in Oncology/Hematology. 2001;**40**(3):239-250

[13] Coleman R, Hadji P, Body JJ, Santini D, Chow E, Terpos E, et al. Bone health in cancer: ESMO clinical practice guidelines. Annals of Oncology. 2020;**31**(12):1650-1663

[14] Hamaoka T, Madewell JE, Podoloff DA, Hortobagyi GN, Ueno NT. Bone imaging in metastatic breast cancer. Journal of Clinical Oncology. 2004;**22**(14):2942-2953

[15] Yang HL, Liu T, Wang XM, Xu Y, Deng SM. Diagnosis of bone metastases: A meta-analysis comparing 18FDG PET, CT, MRI and bone scintigraphy. European Radiology. 2011;**21**(12):2604-2617

[16] Liu T, Wang S, Liu H, Meng B, Zhou F, He F, et al. Detection of vertebral metastases: A meta-analysis comparing MRI, CT, PET, BS and BS with SPECT. Journal of Cancer Research and Clinical Oncology. 2017;**143**(3):457-465

[17] Algra PR, Bloem JL, Tissing H, Falke TH, Arndt JW, Verboom LJ. Detection

of vertebral metastases: Comparison between MR imaging and bone scintigraphy. Radiographics. 1991;**11**(2): 219-232

[18] Monfardini L, Preda L, Aurilio G, Rizzo S, Bagnardi V, Renne G, et al. CT-guided bone biopsy in cancer patients with suspected bone metastases: Retrospective review of 308 procedures. La Radiologia Medica. 2014;**119**(11):852-860

[19] Buga S, Sarria JE. The management of pain in metastatic bone disease. Cancer Control. 2012;**19**(2):154-166

[20] Portenoy RK, Lesage P. Management of cancer pain. Lancet. 1999;**353**(9165):1695-1700

[21] Hardy JR, Jenkins-Marsh S, Pinkerton E, Rickett K, Good P. Corticosteroids for the management of cancer-related pain in adults. Cochrane Database of Systematic Reviews. 2013;**2013**(10):1-42

[22] Portenoy RK. A practical approach to using adjuvant analgesics in older adults. Journal of the American Geriatrics Society. 2020;**68**(4):691-698

[23] Kumar A, Weber MH, Gokaslan Z, Wolinsky JP, Schmidt M, Rhines L, et al. Metastatic spinal cord compression and steroid treatment: A systematic review. Clinical Spine Surgery. 2017;**30**(4):156-163

[24] Kohno N, Aogi K, Minami H, Nakamura S, Asaga T, Iino Y, et al. Zoledronic acid significantly reduces skeletal complications compared with placebo in Japanese women with bone metastases from breast cancer: A randomized, placebo-controlled trial. Journal of Clinical Oncology. 2005;**23**(15):3314-3321

[25] Berenson JR, Rosen LS, Howell A, Porter L, Coleman RE, Morley W, et al. Zoledronic acid reduces skeletal-related events in patients with osteolytic metastases: A double-blind, randomized dose-response study. Cancer. 2001;**91**(7): 1191-1200

[26] Tu SM, Lin SH, Logothetis C, Saad F. A randomized, placebo-controlled trial of zoledronic acid in patients with hormone-refractory metastatic prostate carcinoma. Journal of the National Cancer Institute. 2003;**95**(15):1174-1175

[27] Rosen LS, Gordon D, Tchekmedyian NS, Yanagihara R, Hirsh V, Krzakowski M, et al. Long-term efficacy and safety of zoledronic acid in the treatment of skeletal metastases in patients with nonsmall cell lung carcinoma and other solid tumors: A randomized, phase III, double-blind, placebo-controlled trial. Cancer. 2004;**100**(12):2613-2621

[28] Hatoum HT, Lin SJ, Smith MR, Barghout V, Lipton A. Zoledronic acid and skeletal complications in patients with solid tumors and bone metastases. Cancer. 2008;**113**(6):1438-1445

[29] Rosen LS, Gordon D, Tchekmedyian S, Yanagihara R, Hirsh V, Krzakowski M, et al. Zoledronic acid versus placebo in the treatment of skeletal metastases in patients with lung cancer and other solid tumors: A phase III, double-blind, randomized trial - the zoledronic acid lung cancer and other solid tumors study group. Journal of Clinical Oncology. 2003;**21**(16):3150-3157

[30] Kristensen B, Ejlertsen B, Groenvold M, Hein S, Loft H, Mouridsen HT. Oral clodronate in breast cancer patients with bone metastases: A randomized study. Journal of Internal Medicine. 1999;**246**(1):67-74

[31] Body JJ, Diel IJ, Liehinitzer M, Lazarev A, Pecherstorfer M, Bell R, et al. Oral ibandronate reduces the risk of

skeletal complications in breast cancer patients with metastatic bone disease: Results from two randomised, placebo-controlled phase III studies. British Journal of Cancer. 2004;**90**(6):1133-1137

[32] Perazella MA, Markowitz GS. Bisphosphonate nephrotoxicity. Kidney International. 2008;**74**(11):1385-1393

[33] Diel IJ, Bergner R, Grötz KA. Adverse effects of bisphosphonates: Current issues. The Journal of Supportive Oncology. 2007;**5**(10):475-482

[34] Stopeck AT, Lipton A, Body JJ, Steger GG, Tonkin K, De Boer RH, et al. Denosumab compared with zoledronic acid for the treatment of bone metastases in patients with advanced breast cancer: A randomized, double-blind study. Journal of Clinical Oncology. 2010;**28**(35):5132-5139

[35] Fizazi K, Carducci M, Smith M, Damião R, Brown J, Karsh L, et al. Denosumab versus zoledronic acid for treatment of bone metastases in men with castration-resistant prostate cancer: A randomised, double-blind study. Lancet. 2011;**377**(9768):813-822

[36] Henry DH, Costa L, Goldwasser F, Hirsh V, Hungria V, Prausova J, et al. Randomized, double-blind study of denosumab versus zoledronic acid in the treatment of bone metastases in patients with advanced cancer (excluding breast and prostate cancer) or multiple myeloma. Journal of Clinical Oncology. 2011;**29**(9):1125-1132

[37] Lipton A, Fizazi K, Stopeck AT, Henry DH, Brown JE, Yardley DA, et al. Superiority of denosumab to zoledronic acid for prevention of skeletal-related events: A combined analysis of 3 pivotal, randomised, phase 3 trials. European Journal of Cancer. 2012;**48**(16):3082-3092

[38] Gough N, Miah AB, Linch M. Nonsurgical oncological management of cancer pain. Current Opinion in Supportive and Palliative Care. 2014;**8**(2):102-111

[39] Chow E, Harris K, Fan G, Tsao M, Sze WM. Palliative radiotherapy trials for bone metastases: A systematic review. Journal of Clinical Oncology. 2007;**25**(11):1423-1436

[40] Lutz S, Berk L, Chang E, Chow E, Hahn C, Hoskin P, et al. Palliative radiotherapy for bone metastases: An ASTRO evidence-based guideline. International Journal of Radiation Oncology, Biology, Physics. 2011;**79**(4):965-976

[41] Gerszten PC, Burton SA, Ozhasoglu C, Welch WC. Radiosurgery for spinal metastases: Clinical experience in 500 cases from a single institution. Spine (Phila Pa 1976). 2007;**32**(2):193-199

[42] Palma DA, Olson R, Harrow S, Gaede S, Louie AV, Haasbeek C, et al. Stereotactic ablative radiotherapy versus standard of care palliative treatment in patients with oligometastatic cancers (SABR-COMET): A randomised, phase 2, open-label trial. Lancet. 2019;**393**(10185):2051-2058

[43] Sartor O, Coleman R, Nilsson S, Heinrich D, Helle SI, O'Sullivan JM, et al. Effect of radium-223 dichloride on symptomatic skeletal events in patients with castration-resistant prostate cancer and bone metastases: Results from a phase 3, double-blind, randomised trial. The Lancet Oncology. 2014;**15**(7):738-746

[44] Wood TJ, Racano A, Yeung H, Farrokhyar F, Ghert M, Deheshi BM. Surgical Management of Bone Metastases: Quality of evidence and systematic

review. Annals of Surgical Oncology. 2014;**21**(13):4081-4089

[45] McMenomy BP, Kurup AN, Johnson GB, Carter RE, McWilliams RR, Markovic SN, et al. Percutaneous cryoablation of musculoskeletal oligometastatic disease for complete remission. Journal of Vascular and Interventional Radiology. 2013;**24**(2):207-213

[46] Tomasian A, Wallace A, Northrup B, Hillen TJ, Jennings JW. Spine cryoablation: Pain palliation and local tumor control for vertebral metastases. American Journal of Neuroradiology. 2016;**37**(1):189-195

[47] Deschamps F, Farouil G, Ternes N, Gaudin A, Hakime A, Tselikas L, et al. Thermal ablation techniques: A curative treatment of bone metastases in selected patients? European Radiology. 2014;**24**(8):1971-1980

[48] Winkelmann MT, Clasen S, Pereira PL, Hoffmann R. Local treatment of oligometastatic disease: Current role. The British Journal of Radiology. 2019;**92**(1100):1-10

Section 2

Carcinoma of Breast

Chapter 2

Perspective Chapter: Breast-Tumor-Derived Bone Pre-Metastatic Disease – Interplay between Immune and Bone Cells within Bone Marrow Microenvironment

Ana Carolina Monteiro and Adriana Bonomo

Abstract

The bone marrow is a dynamic organ where osteogenesis and bone remodeling take place side by side with hematopoiesis and the maintenance of immunological memory. It provides a unique microenvironment favoring the colonization and outgrowth of breast cancer cells. The outcome of breast-cancer-derived bone metastases depends on the formation of a pre-metastatic niche, which is initiated through "education" of non-tumoral cells present in the primary cancerous niche. Among other participants, immune cells and their secreted factors can boost the successful seeding of the distant disease. In this chapter, we discuss the reciprocal interplay between bone and T and B cells, particularly in pathological contexts. In the first part, we are exploring the knowledge brought by the osteoimmunology field, especially from the best studied disease in this area, rheumatoid arthritis. In the second part, we summarize the latest findings on underlying cellular and molecular mechanisms for breast-cancer-derived bone pre-metastatic niche formation. In addition, we explore the concept that breast-tumor-primed T and B cells function as messengers from the periphery to the bone marrow, alter bone turnover homeostasis in favor of osteoclasts, before tumor colonization, leading to a pre-metastatic niche formation to further the development of bone metastases.

Keywords: bone metastases, T cells, B cells, dendritic cells, osteoclasts, osteoblasts, breast tumor and pre-metastatic niche

1. Introduction

1.1 Bone marrow: an overview

Bones provide both skeletal scaffolding and a unique microenvironment for hematopoiesis and B cell ontogenesis, osteogenesis, and also function as an immunological memory reservoir, in its marrow [1–3]. The bone marrow (BM) is a complex and dynamic structure composed of different and distinct compartments or niches, which accommodate a multitude of cell types, which functionally create an interactive network, critical for BM/bone integrity [2, 4–8]. These niches are composed of different stromal cell types—osteoblasts (OBs), osteocytes, reticular and perivascular cells, endothelial cells, mesenchymal cells (MSCs), smooth muscle cells, macrophages, and dendritic cells (DCs). Disruptions in these compartments can lead to aberrant pathological processes [2, 8–11].

At least three niches can be identified in the BM: (i) the endosteal/subendosteal niche that supports self-renewal and differentiation of hematopoietic stem cells (HSC); (ii) the central niche for multipotent progenitors (MPP); and (iii) the perisinusoidal niche that guarantees the differentiation to the lineage committed progenitors and hematopoietic cells full commitment [4, 11–14]. The endosteal/subendosteal niche contains OBs, bone-forming cells, and osteoclasts (OCs), bone-resorbing cells, as well MSCs, all collaborating to regulate hematopoietic homeostasis and osteogenesis [13]. The central and perisinusoidal niches recruit MSCs, as well as endothelial cells and their progenitors, to promote HSCs proliferation, mobilization, and differentiation,—(i) myelopoiesis, the process in which innate immune cells, such as granulocytes and monocytes, develop from a myeloid progenitor cell; and (ii) lymphopoiesis, the process in which adaptive and innate lymphocytes develop from a lymphoid progenitor cell [5, 15].

More recently, the anatomy of myelopoiesis in the BM was partially mapped *in situ* and the clonal relationships between myeloid progenitors and surrounding cells were assessed [16]. It was demonstrated that colony stimulating factor 1 (CSF1), also known as macrophage colony-stimulating factor (M-CSF), produced by perisinusoidal vessels provides a unique niche that regulates, spatially organizes, and controls myeloid differentiation [16]. This type of study provides valuable information on the organization of the various niches inside the BM. Dissection of these processes will allow a better understanding of their influence on bone and/or BM and vice versa, during homeostasis and local and/or systemic diseases, which directly or indirectly affect bone/BM homeostasis.

1.2 Bone metabolism and its central players

Bone tissues in adults are classified as: (i) cortical (long and compact bone) and (ii) trabecular (flat and spongy or cancellous bone) [17, 18]. During fetal development, long bones are modeled by endochondral ossification, in which the cartilage formed by chondrocytes—cells of mesenchymal origin, essential for formation and maintenance of cartilage—is replaced by bone at the edge of the growth plate [19, 20]. The cortical bone is mostly structural, supporting the stability and movement of the body, made up of compactly packed osteons—its key structural unit, formed by layers called lamellae, surrounding the Harvesian canal, which contain small blood vessels responsible for blood supply to osteocytes, former OBs embedded in the bone matrix as differentiated cells [21, 22]. The trabecular bone is highly porous and vascularized and harbors red and white bone marrow [17]. Bone matrix is composed of an organic segment, formed by type I collagen secreted by OBs, and a variety of non-collagenous proteins, such as osteocalcin and osteopontin; and an inorganic segment, also known as bone mineral, formed by calcium, phosphorus, and magnesium, which originates the hydroxyapatite [$Ca_{10}(PO_4)_6(OH)_2$] [17].

Even after the modeling phase, bone tissue is constantly renewed by a process called bone remodeling. Bone homeostasis is achieved by the performance of bone remodeling system, which is conducted by the synchronized activities of OBs, OCs, and osteocytes [23–25]. Osteocytes are the most abundant cells in bone tissue and play an essential role in bone homeostasis [26]. They translate mechanical—pressure and tension—low oxygen, matrix mineralization, and hormonal stimuli into biochemical signals, due to their extensive long cytoplasmic extensions. The complex network formed by osteocytes in the bone matrix, enables direct communication among them and other effector cells in the bone/BM, including OBs and OCs [21, 22, 26–29]. OBs, derived from mesenchymal progenitors, promote mineralization and bone formation by secreting matrix vesicles containing type I collagen, alkaline phosphatase, and osteocalcin [22]. OCs, derived from myelomonocytic progenitors, otherwise, dissolve and absorb bone matrix by releasing hydrogen ions that acidify the bone interface and secrete lysosomal enzymes—such as tartrate-resistant acid phosphatase and cathepsin K [30–34].

The receptor activator of nuclear factor-κB (RANK)/receptor activator of nuclear factor-κB ligand (RANKL)/osteoprotegerin (OPG) molecular system is the most important pathway activated during bone remodeling process [35–38]. Notably, BM stromal cells are responsible to initiate osteoclastogenesis, being the main sources of M-CSF and RANKL [39]. Osteocytes first release M-CSF causing myelomonocytic progenitors to commit to the OC line [26, 39]. M-CSF stimulates RANK expression in the late stages of OCs development, which interact with RANKL expressed on or secreted by OBs and osteocytes [26]. This interaction leads to the activation of mitogen-activated protein kinase (MAPK) and nuclear factor-κB (NF-κB) pathways, through tumor necrosis factor receptor–associated factor 6 (TRAF-6) and c-Fos molecules [30, 31, 33, 34, 40], giving rise to large multinucleated differentiated mature OCs [40]. RANKL activation also induces the expression of nuclear factor of activated T cells c1 (NFATc1), the master transcription factor for osteoclastogenesis [41]. B-lymphocyte-induced maturation protein 1 (Blimp1), which can be induced by NFATc1, downregulates the expression of the transcriptional factors interferon (IFN) regulatory factor 8 (IRF-8) [42, 43] and B-cell lymphoma 6 (Bcl6), in turn promoting osteoclastogenesis [43].

Notably, mice that lack RANKL or its receptor RANK develop severe osteopetrosis accompanied by a defect in tooth eruption due to a complete lack of OCs [42, 43]. Conditional deletion of RANKL in chondrocytes [44, 45] and OBs led to a severe osteopetrosis [22, 43, 45–47], whereas osteocytes-specific RANKL-deficient mice displayed a high bone mass phenotype at the adult stage [43, 45]. Thus, chondrocytes and OBs are the major source of RANKL in supporting osteoclastogenesis during skeletal development, whereas osteocyte-derived RANKL contributes to bone remodeling at the adult stage [44, 45] . In humans, loss-of-function mutations in *Tnfrsf11a* (gene encoding RANK) and *Tnfsf11* (gene encoding RANKL) genes cause autosomal recessive osteopetrosis with a complete lack of OCs [43, 48].

OBs and osteocytes also settle the termination of osteoclastogenesis [21, 27, 29, 49]. This step initiates through the secretion of OPG—the RANKL decoy receptor, the main counter-regulator of osteoclastogenesis, which attenuates bone resorption by binding to RANKL with higher affinity than RANK and blocking RANKL osteoclastogenic effects [50]. Of note, mice lacking *Tnfrsf11b* (gene encoding OPG) exhibited severe osteoporosis due to an increased OC number and severe bone resorption [43, 50–52]. The same cells control the beginning of osteoblastogenesis, and several molecules regulate this next step, including parathyroid hormone (PTH), the RUNX Family Transcription Factor 2 (RUNX2), osterix transcription factor, bone morphogenetic protein (BMP), and the Wnt pathway [40, 53]. The Wnt signaling pathway is the most important player in osteoblastogenesis, preventing apoptosis of OBs and accelerating its cell cycle progression and proliferation, leading to inhibition of adipogenesis [54]. Wnt molecules activate G-protein-coupled receptors and coreceptors of the low-density lipoprotein receptor (Lrp) family, resulting in β-catenin activation, effectively upregulating aerobic glycolysis, β oxidation, and other anabolic mechanisms, through activation of the RUNX2 gene [54]. Moreover, binding of BMP to BMP receptors leads to their dimerization followed by phosphorylation of Smad proteins (main signal transducers for receptors of the TGF-β superfamily), which in turn also activate RUNX2, upregulating OB activity and differentiation [54, 55].

More recently, leucine-rich repeat-containing G-protein-coupled receptor 4 (LGR4) was reported to be another receptor for RANKL, which negatively regulates osteoclastogenesis by not only competing with RANK for RANKL binding, but also inhibiting NFATc1 activation via Gq protein alpha subunit (Gαq) [56]. Interestingly, OCs can also regulate the activity of OBs, by secreting bone morphogenetic protein-6 and sphingosine-1-phosphate, which function as coupling factors promoting OBs proliferation and bone formation [57]. Finally, osteocytes negatively regulate osteoblastogenesis by secretion of Dickkopf-1 (DKK-1) and sclerostin molecules, both antagonists of the Wnt pathway [58, 59]. Sclerostin is a marker for mature osteocytes, and its expression increases with age [60, 61], and mice deficient in this molecule show an increase in osteoblastogenesis and a decrease in the shape of BM cavities, resulting in impairment of hematopoiesis and B cells ontogenesis [62].

Taking together, we conclude that intra and intercellular and molecular interactions between osteocytes, OBs, OCs, and chondrocytes are crucial for maintaining the BM/bone niches, under physiological conditions. Currently, we know that bone remodeling process is also regulated by immune cells, residing at, or migrating to BM, such as T and B cells, innate lymphoid cells, macrophages, DCs, and other hematopoietic cells [63]. Any imbalance in one of these connections can lead to several bone pathologies, including, among others, breast-cancer-derived bone metastases [64].

2. Reciprocal interplay between bone and immune cells

2.1 An overview of the "osteoimmunology" field

The relationship between bone and immune systems has been suggested by pioneering studies reported in the early 1970s and showed that molecules secreted from immune cells were capable to induce OC activation and differentiation [65, 66]. Moreover, early studies in the immunology field, using genetically deficient mice in various immunomodulatory molecules, showed unexpected phenotypes in the skeletal systems under physiological conditions [40, 63, 67, 68]. Actually, we know that bone and immune systems share a variety of molecules, including cytokines, chemokines, transcription factors, and signaling molecules [67]. By interacting with each other in the BM, the bone and immune cells cooperatively conduct a series of bone and immune system functions [67]. Studies conducted on bone and immune phenotypes are revealing the physiological significance of the mechanisms shared by both systems [67], and the interdisciplinary field "osteoimmunology" was created to explore these mechanistic interactions, under physiological or pathological conditions [69].

The RANK/RANKL/OPG molecular system is considered the most important pathway explicitly linking immune and bone tissues [35, 38, 43, 70, 71]. Indeed, several studies are showing that RANK and RANKL, besides being the master regulatory via inducing osteoclastogenesis, also play multiple roles in the immune system, including: (i) differentiation of medullary thymic epithelial cells (mTECs) [72–75]—that act as mediators of the central tolerance process, which self-reactive T cells are eliminated while regulatory T cells are generated; (ii) secondary lymphoid tissue organogenesis—the organization of the microarchitecture of lymph nodes (LNs) [42], formation of germinal centers in gut isolated lymphoid follicles [42] and Peyer's patches [42]; and (iii) fine-tuner of adaptive immune response—enhancement of DCs longevity and survival [76], maintenance of immunological memory [77] and B cells ontogenesis [78, 79]. Of note, these molecules are expressed by cells from both systems [63]. OPG, for example, is expressed by mature B cells (accounting alone for almost 40% of OPG produced in BM. Their essential role for bone homeostasis was shown *in vivo*, since B-cell-deficient mice have low bone mass density associated and a marked deficit in BM OPG [80]. This homeostatic balance is achieved by B and T cells interaction, via CD40-CD40L molecules, since mice depleted of CD40 or CD40L co-stimulatory molecules presented a decline in OPG production by B cells and an increase in bone resorption and low bone mass density [80]. Also, mice depleted from T cells showed a complete suppression of OPG production by B cells followed by an increase in osteoclastogenesis and bone loss [80]. Moreover, Cytotoxic T-Lymphocyte Associated Protein 4 (CTLA-4)—a molecule expressed by T cells that helps keep immune responses in check—binds to CD80/CD86 co-stimulatory molecules expressed by OCs, leading to inhibition of osteoclastogenesis mediated by RANKL or TNF-α [81]. CTLA-4 binding to CD80/CD86 in OCs' precursor cells induces the expression of indoleamine 2,3 dioxygenase (IDO), which in turn degrades tryptophan and leads to OCs apoptosis [82]. Consequently, mice deficient in CD80, CD86, or IDO have increased osteoclastogenesis rates and osteopenic phenotypes [82, 83] demonstrating that CTLA-4 plays important roles in the physiological regulation of bone mass preservation [81–83].

We should be aware that most of these findings were conducted in animal models; however, new indications are emerging to support the reciprocal roles of both systems in human diseases aspects [47, 67, 84]. Despite the more recent observations about the impact of immune cells for bone tissue homeostatic integrity, and vice versa, the interplay between both systems is first spotlighted by studies on bone disorders, triggered by abnormal immune responses activation, like the ones seen in rheumatoid arthritis (RA), post-menopausal osteoporosis, chronic periodontitis, multiple myeloma, fractures, HIV chronic infection, and bone metastases [67].

2.2 Role of T and B cells in bone disorders

T and B cells are derived from the same lymphoid progenitor cell during hematopoiesis and are the main cellular representatives of the adaptive immune system, so called because they do not mount an immediate response to an antigen (Ag).

The Ags are recognized by specific receptors—T cell receptor (TCR) and B cell receptor (BCR), which are diverse at the population level and clonal and unique at individual cellular level. TCRs and BCRs are not conserved and are generated by gene rearrangements during T and B cell ontogenesis. T cells ontogenesis takes place in the thymus, while B cells ontogenesis is in BM—both are primary lymphoid organs.

After maturation inside BM or thymus, B and T cells gain the peripheral blood circulation and enter the secondary lymphoid organs. In lymphoid organs, as LNs and spleen, activated/educated by dendritic cells (DCs), the professional Ag-presenting cell (APC) are found. Through their ability to sense changes in their local environment and respond appropriately, DCs activate T cells by the expression of the Major Histocompatibility Molecules (MHC), in complex with linear, short, peptides Ags (9–20 amino acids long). This complex is recognized by T cells via TCR and CD3 ε and δ, ζ chains accessory molecules and their categorized cluster of differentiation (CD) surface expressed molecules, CD4 or CD8. In addition, T cells concomitantly recognize co-stimulatory molecules and cytokines, which will define their functional differentiation fates, in terms of their expression of master transcription factors and functional cytokines [85]. $CD4^+$ helper T cells are divided into specialized subsets, known as: (i) T helper 1 (Th1), expressing T bet transcription factor and IFN-γ; (ii) T helper 2 (Th2), expressing GATA-3 transcription factor and IL-4, IL-5, and IL-13; (iii) T helper 17 (Th17), expressing ROR γT transcription factor and IL-17A, IL-17F, IL-22, and IL-26; (iv) T helper 22 (Th22), expressing Runx1 and RORγt transcription factors and IL-22; T follicular (Tfh), expressing B cell lymphoma 6 (Bcl6) transcription factor and IL-21; and (v) T regulatory (Treg) cells, expressing FoxP3 transcription factor and TGF-β and IL-10; while $CD8^+$ T cells fall into subpopulations, known as: (i) Cytotoxic Type 1 $CD8^+$ T cells (Tc1), expressing T bet and BLIMP-1 transcription factors, IFN-γ, granzyme, and perforin; (ii) Type 2 $CD8^+$ T cells (Tc2), expressing GATA-3 transcription factor and IL-4, IL-5 and IL-13; (iii) Type 17 $CD8^+$ T cells (Tc17), expressing ROR γT and ROR α transcription factors and IL-17A, IL-17F and IL-22 and T reg $CD8^+$ T cells, expressing IL-10 [85].

B cells are also activated in secondary lymphoid organs, but, in contrast to T cells, they do not need APCs to present their cognate Ags, which will be freely recognized in linear or structural forms. At the beginning of immune responses, B cells secrete immunoglobulins M (IgM) independently of T helper cells. The T-cell-independent response is short-lived and does not result in the production of memory B cells, which will not result in a secondary response to subsequent exposures to the same Ags. However, to induce stronger B cell responses and to generate immunological memory, B cells need help from T follicular $CD4^+$ T cells (Tfh). Indeed, to enable homing to B cell follicles, Tfh expresses abundant C-X-chemokine receptor type 5 (CXCR5). Another characteristic of Tfh is the expression of CD40 ligand (CD40L), inducible T cell costimulator (ICOS), programmed death-1 (PD-1), and B and T lymphocyte attenuator (BTLA). Tfh cells colocalize with Ag-specific B cells within germinal centers (GCs), which are transient structures located within B cell follicles, in secondary lymphoid tissues, in which somatic hypermutation of immunoglobulin (Ig) variable region genes and selection of high-affinity B cell clones occur. Immunoglobulin class switch (IgA, IgE, and IgG) will be defined by cytokines produced by these different specialized Tfh, at the moment of B cells activation.

It is clear now that the identity of T cell subsets is critical in guiding their role on bone remodeling system, during homeostasis or in pathological conditions [67]. In particular, Th1, Th2, Th17, Th22, and T reg $CD4^+$ and $CD8^+$ cells have been shown to influence bone metabolism [67, 86–89]. In the RA scenario—the best studied human disease in osteoimmunology—the importance of Th17 $CD4^+$ T cells is evident, beginning by their infiltration into the synovium and the association of disease susceptibility with specific variants of T-cells-related genes, such as HLA-DR (MHC class II cell surface receptor encoded by the human leukocyte Ag gene complex), Protein Tyrosine Phosphatase Non-Receptor Type 22 (PTPN22), and C-C Motif Chemokine Receptor 6 (CCR6) [40, 63]. Moreover, studies performed aiming to confirm the role of T cells showed that T cell deficient mice are protected from arthritis, and clinical trials performed to inhibit effector T cells activities demonstrate the improvement of clinical symptoms [46, 90, 91]. IL-17A, one of the cytokines secreted by Th17 $CD4^+$ T cells, amplifies local inflammation and the production of TNF-α and IL-6, which in turn promote RANKL expression by induction of an intense osteoclastogenesis [37]. Th17 $CD4^+$ T cells also express RANKL, but this molecule only stimulates an additive effect and is not sufficient to induce osteoclastogenesis, independently, in this disease scenario [37, 43, 46]. It was also reported that these cells stimulate the recruitment of OCs progenitors via increasing chemokine production by BM MSCs [40]. Recently, it was shown that IL-22, produced by the Th22 $CD4^+$ T cells, promotes osteoclastogenesis and enhances bone destruction in arthritic mice [46, 92]. Disease severity is shown to be markedly reduced in collagen-induced arthritic mice deficient in IL-22 [92], and elevated IL-22 in serum is also associated with disease activity in patients with RA [92].

Interestingly, it has been found that a particular type of Th17 $CD4^+$ T cells, derived from $FoxP3^+$ Treg $CD4^+$ T cells (called exFoxP3 Th17 T cells), have a much stronger pro-osteoclastogenic activity than conventional Th17 $CD4^+$ T cells [86, 93]. Under arthritic conditions induced in mice model, $FoxP3^+$ Treg $CD4^+$ T cells lose FoxP3 by the action of IL-6 produced by synovial fibroblasts [46, 83, 94]. Indeed, $FoxP3^+$ $IL\text{-}17^+$ $CD4^+$ T cells—a transition state during the conversion to exFoxP3 Th17 T cells—are frequently observed in synovial tissues of patients with active RA, as compared with those with inactive RA, suggesting a pathogenic role for this subset in this pathological condition [46, 95]. Equally important is the fact that $Foxp3^+$ $IL\text{-}17^+$ $CD4^+$ T cells were also observed in periodontal tissues of patients with severe periodontal disease [96, 97]. Notably, in a ligature-induced periodontitis mouse model, it was recently shown that Th17 $CD4^+$ T cells eradicate the bacteria while also inducing bone degradation and tooth loss, which is crucial for the termination of oral infection, avoiding bacterial systemic dissemination [98]. Taken together, it was concluded that Th17 $CD4^+$ T cells orchestrate the host defense against oral microbiota by regulating both osteoclastic bone resorption and antimicrobial immunity [98].

It was reported that IL-4 produced by Th2 T cells inhibits OCs formation and function *in vitro* [86, 99, 100]; nonetheless, no functional activity has been reported *in vivo*. On the other hand, Th1 $CD4^+$ T cells, which counter regulate Th2 cells, are found in the synovium fluid of patients with active RA [101], although it has been demonstrated that the secretion of IFN-γ by this T cell subset strongly inhibits osteoclastogenesis and protects against bone tissue degradation by OCs [102]. IFN-γ induces a strong inhibition of the RANKL-induced activation of the NF-κB, via a rapid degradation of TRAF6 [102]. In arthritic synovium, Th1 CD4⁺ T cells are not considered to be activated but often display an exhausted phenotype and express low levels of IFN-γ [86–89].

It is already known that FoxP3⁺ Treg CD4⁺ cells play an indispensable role in maintaining immune homeostasis, but also exert a strict anti-osteoclastogenic activity [68, 103–106]. In rheumatic patients, the number of FoxP3⁺ Treg CD4⁺ T cells is inversely related to osteoclastogenic markers and disease severity [68, 105, 107]. These results accompany findings in which mice deficient in FoxP3⁺ Treg CD4⁺ T cells were prone to arthritis, showing joint destruction and generalized bone loss, supported by higher number of OCs in joints [105]. The reintroduction of FoxP3⁺ Treg CD4⁺ T cells into these mice significantly reduced arthritic clinical symptoms [105]. As discussed in previous section, OCs express the co-stimulatory molecules CD80 and CD86, and osteoclastogenesis can be regulated via CTLA-4, promoting OCs apoptosis, and thus suppressing bone destruction [81]. Notably, BM resident FoxP3⁺ Treg CD4⁺ T cells express higher levels of CTLA-4, than peripheral FoxP3⁺ Treg CD4⁺ T cells [82]. These resident FoxP3⁺ Treg CD4⁺ T cells remove CD80/CD86 from the surface of OCs precursor cells by CTLA-4 mediated trans-endocytosis, potentially leading to reduced co-stimulation by OCs [82]. Therefore, the interaction between OCs expressing CD80/CD86 and FoxP3⁺ Treg CD4⁺ T cells expressing CTLA-4 is suggested as important player for the cross talk between these cells to support bone homeostasis [81, 82].

More recently, the term immunoporosis—a subarea under osteoimmunology' umbrella—was proposed for the field that studies the importance of immune system for osteoporosis establishment [108]. Osteoporosis—defined by a loss of bone mass and microarchitecture, has a multifactorial etiology but endocrine factors such as hyperparathyroidism, vitamin D deficiency, and menopause are primarily implicated [109]. The disease stems mainly from the cessation of ovarian function, where declining estrogen levels result in the stimulation of bone resorption, leading to a period of rapid bone loss [109]. At the cellular level, the central mechanism by which sex steroid deficiency induces bone loss is via an increase in OC formation and life span [110].

Estrogen exhibits the potential to stimulate the differentiation and survival of regulatory T cells, which in turn suppress the expression of proinflammatory cytokines from Th17 T cells and inhibit bone resorption. In addition, many genetic and non-genetic factors intensify the negative impact of estrogen deficiency on the skeleton, including gut microbiota profile [109]. Indeed, sex steroid deficiency increases gut permeability, allowing intestinal microbiota to activate and expand Th17 and TNF-α⁺ T cells [111]. These expanded T cells increase S1PR1 (sphingosine-1-phosphate receptor 1) expression, which promotes their egress from intestine and influx into BM through CXCR3 and CCL20-mediated mechanisms [111, 112]. Additionally, this steroid deficiency-associated bone loss was prevented by probiotics administration [111, 112]. In this regard, several studies demonstrated that *Lactobacillus species* alleviates gut inflammation and improved barrier function of intestine [113]. Moreover, it was shown that *Lactobacillus rhamnosus* administration enhances bone mass in eugonadal mice [112, 114, 115], inhibits osteoclastogenesis, and skews balance of Th17 T cells to regulatory T cells, under *in vitro* and *in vivo* conditions [112, 115]. Collectively, these studies highlight the osteoprotective role of this probiotic, thereby opening novel avenues in the management and treatment of postmenopausal osteoporosis.

Finally, the effect of B cells in bone is more bidirectional, as compared with T cells, as B cells require the endosteal BM surface to their ontogenesis [78]. Indeed, B cell transcription and growth factors that control B cell differentiation play important roles in bone homeostasis, indicating the tight interaction between this immune cell lineage and bone [116]. In RA, the autoimmune process starts with the presentation of auto-Ags to $CD4^+$ Th T cells, which help B cells to differentiate into plasma cells that produce auto-Abs, such as rheumatoid factor and anti-cyclic citrullinated peptide (anti-CCP), trademarks of this disease [106, 117, 118]. Of note, the substantial number of Tfh cells in the synovial tissue correlates with disease severity [119, 120]. Auto Abs and immune complexes promote bone erosion through FcRγ signaling in OC precursor cells or innate immune cells [121, 122]. More recently, it was demonstrated that plasma B cell numbers increased in BM region near the inflammatory joints during arthritis [119], due to enrichment of plasma B cells survival factors such as IL-6, BAFF, and APRIL [119]. Locally, plasma B cells provide RANKL, TNF-α, IL-17, and Ab-mediated costimulatory signals that cooperate to powerfully promote osteoclastogenesis [119]. Genetic ablation of RANKL in B cells resulted in amelioration of periarticular bone loss, but not of articular erosion or systemic bone loss, in RA [123], and was slightly but significantly protective of ovariectomy-induced bone loss [124].

After reviewing the progress on the central roles of adaptive immunity in the establishment of some bone disorders, we will now explore the knowledge behind the participation of tumor-primed T and B cells in the development of bone pre-metastatic niche, which will lead in turn to the establishment of breast-cancer-derived bone metastases.

3. Breast-cancer-derived bone metastases: molecular interactions within the BM

3.1 Preclinical and clinical implications

Breast cancer is the most frequent cancer in women, with increasing incidence and high mortality rates [125]. Breast-cancer-induced bone metastases are a frequent complication of advanced disease, with up to 70% of incidence, associated with skeletal complications, including pain, osteopenia and bone loss, pathological fracture, hypercalcemia spinal cord compression, BM aplasia, demanding surgery, and radiotherapy for bone complications, and change of antineoplastic therapy for bone pain [126–129]. Collectively, these comorbidities are defined as skeletal-related events (SREs) that dramatically impair the patient's quality of life and reduce overall survival [127, 128, 130].

The preservation of bone mass has been achieved using bone anti-resorptive bisphosphonates, such as zoledronic acid, and denosumab, an anti-RANKL monoclonal antibody, which block OC-mediated bone resorption and are approved for use in patients with cancer metastatic to bone [128]. However, these drugs only alleviate SREs complications, the development of bone metastases remains an incurable condition, and mortality rates are kept at elevated level [131]. Meta-analyses studies showed a statistically significant overall survival benefit with women treated with bisphosphonates [132–134]. It is not surprising, however, that bone-targeted therapies also display systemic immunological effects, regarding the interactions between immune and bone cells, which can partially cause eliminatory anti-tumor effects. Indeed, zoledronic acid and denosumab can modulate immune cells activity, such as γδ T cells, macrophages, and $CD4^+$ Tregs, in many different types of cancer, including breast cancer, leading to an increase in T-cell-mediated anti-tumor cytotoxic effects [135]. Moreover, the knowledge about how current treatments affect the immune landscape in bone metastatic microenvironment is scarcely known. This fact could be due to our limited understanding of osteoimmunological interactions for tumor growth, the low availability of biopsies from bone metastases, and appropriate metastatic models for preclinical studies.

The risk factors for predicting breast-cancer-derived bone metastases are still controversial. In a recent study, a total of 2133 patients, including 327 with bone metastases (15.33%) and 1806 without bone metastases (84.67%), were retrospectively reviewed and showed that the spine is the most common site for bone metastases, including thoracic spine (63.61%) and lumbar spine (53.82%), followed by ribs (57.5%), pelvis (54.1%), and sternum (44.3%) [136]. The results also indicated that combined axillary LN metastases, high serum concentrations of cancer Ag 15-3 (CA15-3), alkaline phosphatase (ALP), and low level of hemoglobin have the highest predictive accuracy for bone metastases in breast cancer [136].

Breast-cancer-derived bone metastases give rise predominantly to most aggressive osteolytic lesions, although 15–20% of clinical cases present an osteoblastic pattern, resulting in a dysregulated bone deposition [126, 128, 137]. Notably, it has been shown that breast cancer osteolytic lesions may also lead to skeletal muscle atrophy and weakness, through bone-muscle cross talk, which in turn leads to a feed-forward cycle of musculoskeletal degradation [138, 139]. Osteoclastic bone resorption releases transforming growth factor-β (TGF-β), which causes oxidative stress and skeletal muscle Ca^{2+} leak and weakness, via the TGFβ-Nox4-RyR1 axis, inducing a muscle atrophy program [138, 139]. Interestingly, the same pattern was shown in both immunodeficient and immunocompetent mice, suggesting that adaptive immune system may be excluded from this pathological aspect [140, 141]. Moreover, it has been suggested that muscle dysfunction occurs prior to the loss of muscle mass—cachexia [142]. In addition, experimental strategies are being analyzed for skeletal muscle mass preservation, including: (i) the blocking of myostatin signaling [143, 144]; and (ii) antagonizing the growth hormone secretagogue receptor (GHSR)-1a [145, 146]. Both strategies showed improved survival in mice with cancer cachexia [147].

Recently, it was reported that breast cancer cell lines and human breast cancer tissue express sclerostin, suggesting that breast cancer cells impair bone formation while promoting bone resorption [140]. In a mouse model of bone metastases, the pharmacological inhibition of sclerostin by setrusumab—an anti-sclerostin monoclonal antibody, reduced bone metastatic burden and destruction, without increasing metastases at other sites [140]. Moreover, this treatment protected from induction of muscle atrophy and loss of function, leading to prolonged life span [148]. Accordingly, the expanding and maintenance of OBs functional properties were then proposed as an approach to restore bone and muscle integrity, in the context of metastases-induced osteolytic disease [140]. In parallel, it was reported that homeodomain protein TG-interacting factor-1 (Tgif1)—an inducer of osteoblastogenesis acting at Wnt and PTH1R-dependent signaling pathways, is increased in OBs upon stimulation by metastatic breast cancer cells [141]. High levels of Tgif1 were associated with poor patient survival in breast cancer [147]. The lack of Tgif1 in

OBs increases Semaphorin 3E (Sema3E) expression and attenuates breast cancer cell migration as well as metastases formation, indicating that Tgif1 plays a role during the early stages of bone metastases establishment [141]. Therefore, the mechanisms driving the early steps of bone metastatic process are still not sufficiently understood and the induction of osteoblastogenesis should be analyzed with caution, since OBs and their molecules seem to play contradictory roles in breast-cancer-derived bone disease.

Finally, preclinical studies suggested that non-coding RNAs (ncRNAs) such as long ncRNAs, microRNAs, and circular RNAs are crucial regulators of breast-cancer-induced bone metastases [149–151]. Indeed, unique miRNA expression patterns were reported in different breast cancer subtypes, displaying both pro- and anti-tumorigenic functional properties [150]. In fact, lower levels of miR-34a were observed in patients suffering from later stages of breast cancer in comparison to benign breast disease and healthy controls [131], while higher expression of miR10b was observed in breast cancer patients with LN and bone metastases [148, 152]. Furthermore, lower levels of miR-124 in primary breast cancer correlate with shorter bone-metastases-free survival [153], and miR-218 serum levels are higher in patients with breast cancer bone metastases when compared with patients without metastases [154]. Currently, since altered expression of miRNAs has been associated with disease progression and clinical outcome, these molecules are emerging as potential therapeutic targets and prognostic biomarkers in the context of bone metastases.

3.2 "The vicious cycle"

Bone metastases are not established randomly, instead they request a complex reciprocal interplay between primary cancer cells and BM microenvironment stroma. Indeed, BM stroma provides an advantageous architecture for bone colonization, playing critical roles for breast cancer cells initial seeding, dormancy, and outgrowth [137]. Circulating breast cancer cells enter BM by the sinusoids—small blood vessels lined with fenestrated endothelial cells, more permissive than other types of capillaries [155, 156]. After extravasation into BM, they migrate to the perisinusoidal or to the endosteal/subendosteal niche, where OBs and other stromal cells secrete a variety of chemo-attracting factors, such as CXCL12, RANKL, osteopontin, and BMPs [155, 156]. Breast cancer cells express high levels of CXCR4—the receptor for CXCL12, which increase their ability to survive in BM and the establishment of overt metastases in this microenvironment [155, 156]. Moreover, CXCL12 stimulates PI3K-AKT signaling pathway and Src activity, which enhance cancer cell survival in challenging environments [41]. These results obtained from animal model studies were validated in clinical datasets, in which Src and CXCR4 expression in tumor cells was associated with breast cancer bone relapse [155]. In BM niches, metastatic cells adapt, survive, and reside for a prolonged period of time—possibly years or even decades [137].

When invading breast cancer cells escape from dormancy, they disrupt the normal bone remodeling process in order to promote their outgrowth, eventually leading to the development of overt bone metastases [137]. Metastatic breast tumor cells express and secrete a series of molecules, such as parathyroid hormone-related protein (PTHrP), IL-11, and TNF-α, vascular cell adhesion molecule 1 (VCAM1), intercellular adhesion molecule 1 (ICAM1), lysyl oxidase (LOX), RANK, RANKL, and IL-6, which in turn mobilize and activate OCs to resorb bone matrix and release chemotactic stimuli and additional growth factors attached to the bone matrix [126, 130, 157]. Bone matrix degradation by the hyperactivated OCs releases TGF-β, which in turn is activated due to pH changes in the local environment and proteolytic cleavage from latent peptides [128]. In sequence, this molecule triggers the production of osteolytic factors, such as PTHrP, IL-11, IL-1β, and Jagged1 from breast cancer cells [156, 158– 165]. Jagged1 promotes osteoclastogenesis via Notch signaling in pre-OCs, while PTHrP induces the production of RANKL by OBs [32]. Activated OCs then degrade the bone matrix on cortical and trabecular surfaces, leading to the release of numerous growth factors, including more TGF-β [158]. Consequently, TGF-β-induced Jagged1 enhances a vicious cycle between bone and tumor cells, by stimulating the expression of IL-6 from stromal cells and OBs, promoting tumor growth [158]. VCAM1 also stimulates the outgrowth of metastases, through the recruitment of OCs progenitors via expression of integrin α4β1 [166]. Importantly, several therapies using denosumab—monoclonal antibody against RANKL [167]; and monoclonal against human Jagged1 [168] or small-molecule inhibitors—have already been approved for clinical use or are under development to treat osteolytic bone metastases, by preventing progression of the vicious cycle [169, 170].

In the last few years, accumulating evidences suggest that breast cancer bone colonization is preceded by changes in BM microenvironment [171–173]. In this context, a pre-metastatic niche is established by cellular and molecular mechanisms, mostly educated by the primary breast cancer cells [64, 171, 174]. Therefore, tumor cells prepare BM microenvironment to host them, before "switching homes" and moving to bone [171]. Importantly, the pre-metastatic niche formation also leads to the disruption of bone remodeling system, in favor of osteoclastogenesis and bone consumption, but prior to metastatic cells arrival [64, 157, 174]. Accordingly, the pre-metastatic osteolytic lesions facilitate subsequent bone tumor colonization [175].

3.3 Bone pre-metastatic niche formation

3.3.1 The "seed and soil" in bone tissue adaptation

Breast cancer cells migration to bone is innately related to the molecular and cellular components provided by the pre-metastatic niche, in sequential and distinct phases [137, 172, 176]. In fact, in the nineteenth century, Stephen Paget proposed that tumor cells ("seeds") only grow in specific and permissive microenvironments ("fertile soil") [177]. Of note, BM is a fertile microenvironment, composed of hematopoietic cells, MSCs, endothelial cells, OBs, OCs, molecules secreted by breast primary tumor, either as soluble or contained in extracellular vesicles (EVs) or exosomes, and immune migrating cells [137, 175]. However, how and when these factors, produced locally or systemically, regulate the crucial mechanisms behind the establishment of this site remains less clear [175].

Recent studies suggest that bone pre-metastatic niche exists prior to metastatic colonization; however, disseminated breast cancer cells are detectable in BM prior to clinically detectable bone metastases [175, 178]. Interestingly, patients without any metastases harbored disseminated breast cancer cells with less genetic heterogeneity compared with the primary tumor or those disseminated cells isolated from bone metastatic patients [175, 178]. Of note, less than 0.1% of disseminated breast cancer cells survive during circulation and homing [179–181]. Based on these findings, we can speculate that bone/BM stromal cellular and molecular components probably play roles in supporting these mutations, for further licensing and selection of the best "seeds" to adapt in the pre-metastatic niche, until their overt bone colonization.

Additionally, a recent study identified LOX-derived by hypoxia condition, a factor significantly associated with bone tropism and relapse. LOX induces an intense osteoclastogenesis, through NFATc1, before, and independent of breast tumor cells arrival at BM [174]. Therefore, this study identified a previous step in bone metastases development, triggered by these osteolytic lesions, opening new opportunities for therapeutic intervention [174]. In fact, in a previous study using an intracardiac mouse model of breast-cancer-derived bone metastases, animals treated with a nonspecific LOX inhibitor—β-aminopropionitrile—reduce bone colonization when administered at the time of tumor inoculation [182].

As mentioned in the last section, recent evidence suggests that breast-cancer-derived miRNAs play key roles in tumor development and progression via exosomes transfer, regulating the outgrowth and metastases of breast cancer [183, 184]. Of note, it was described that miR-21, a highly conserved oncomicro RNA, is expressed in serum of breast cancer patients, significantly higher as compared with healthy controls [185]. Moreover, it was demonstrated that miR-21 induces OCs differentiation, by directly binding programmed cell death 4 (PDCD4), upregulation of NFATc1, and suppression of c-Fos transactivation [186, 187]. Indeed, it was showed that breast cancer cell–secreted exosomes containing miR-21 lead to an exacerbated osteoclastogenesis, which contributes to the generation of a pre-metastatic niche and further enhancing bone metastases development [188]. Importantly, the expression level of miR-21 was detected at higher level in serum exosomes of breast cancer patients with bone metastases, as compared with patients without bone metastases [188].

Almost 20 years ago, a pioneer study challenged the molecular basis for bone metastases. Using human breast cancer cell lines with elevated metastatic activity, it was determined a breast-cancer-derived bone metastases gene signature, which included genes involved in: (i) BM homing (CXCR4); (ii) extracellular matrix alteration (Matrix Metallopeptidase 1 (MMP1), ADAM metallopeptidase with thrombospondin type 1 motif 1 (ADAMTS1), and proteoglycan-1); (iii) angiogenesis (Fibroblast growth factor 5 (FGF5), and Connective tissue growth factor (CTGF); and osteoclastogenesis (IL-11) [189]. Moreover, the overexpression of this gene set is superimposed on a poor prognosis already present in the parental breast cancer population, suggesting that metastases require a set of functions beyond those underlying the emergence of the primary tumor [189]. Thereafter, several other bone metastases gene signatures were proposed, such as Src-dependent [190] or Irf7-regulated genes [191]. To date, it remains unclear the clinical significance and applicability of these gene signatures described, either by tumor heterogeneity in primary and secondary sites or by differences in tumor sources.

3.3.2 Role of breast-tumor-primed T and B cells in bone pre-metastatic niche formation

Primary breast cancer has been shown to "prepare" distant organs for tumor cell colonization even before their arrival [171, 192, 193]. Immune cells such as macrophages [194, 195], DCs [196], neutrophils [197], and T cells [64, 195, 198, 199] are associated with the formation of the pre-metastatic niches, highlighting the importance of basic mechanisms responsible for tumor cells distant establishment [171, 200]. Accordingly, it has been found that cells of the immune system acting as pro-tumor cells are enriched in the pre-metastatic niches and support cancer cell seeding via paracrine signaling and/or by suppressing anti-tumor immune cells [171, 172, 200, 201].

Particularly, our group previously showed that spontaneous bone metastases development, originated from 4 T1 triple negative breast tumor model, depends on RANKL production by tumor primed $CD3^+$ T cells [64]. This conclusion was achieved by adoptive T cell transference to nude mice, which shows that 4 T1 primed T cells, in the total absence of tumor cells, induce a pre-metastatic osteolytic disease [64]. Moreover, inhibition of RANKL production (using shRNA) in fresh tumor-primed T cells does not generate osteolytic disease and the associated bone pre-metastatic niche. Consequently, development of bone metastases is completely absent. Taking together, we proposed an extra step to Mundy's vicious cycle where initial bone consumption, mediated by pre-metastatic $CD3^+$ T cells, generates a rich microenvironment that license further colonization of the bone cavity by the metastatic clones [64]. Once the initial seeding of the bone tissue is achieved, tumor cells shall continue the osteolytic process on their own, feeding themselves through the vicious cycle established within the bone microenvironment [64].

As pre-metastatic osteolytic disease happens much before metastatic colonization, it is not known how the tumor Ag would get to the BM to be recognized by T cells. This is important because T cells' effector functions depend on peptide recognition complexed to MHC molecule, a function better exerted by DCs. Since DCs can carry Ag from peripheral tissues via lymphatics to LNs, and also travel from the peripheral tissue into the blood and to the BM [202, 203], we envisage at least two nonexclusive possibilities for Ag presentation and recognition: (i) cancer-derived exosomes could travel to the bone cavity and provide tumor Ags to be processed and presented by local resident DCs [204, 205] and/or (ii) DCs loaded with tumor Ags at the primary tumor or at the tumor draining LNs, can migrate to the BM where Ag presentation would take place [203, 206]. Moreover, it is already known that BM can prime naive T cells and recruit effector T cells, also serving as a site for $CD4^+$ and $CD8^+$ T cells proliferation [202].

In addition, DCs display a high developmental and functional plasticity depending on local factors and stimuli encountered during their differentiation and maturation, providing a multitude of necessary signals for shaping immune responses [207–210]. Plasticity can also allow DCs to develop into other cell types, among them OCs (DC-OC), what is not unexpected considering their same origin from common myelopoietic stem cell progenitors [211–213]. Indeed, for the last 15 years, it has been reported that immature DCs can develop into OCs *in vitro* and *in vivo*, when cultured with osteoclastogenic factors, M-CSF and RANKL or RA synovial fluids containing pro-osteoclastogenic cytokines [212, 214, 215]. Independently of the presence of DCs at bone resorptive sites during inflammatory conditions [211, 216–221], their direct contribution to bone resorption, either as APCs, keeping osteoclastogenic Th17 T cells locally activated, or overcoming their own phenotype differentiating into OCs mature functional phenotype, has yet to be solved. Indeed, it has been confirmed that multinucleated giant cells expressing markers of DCs and OCs are located next to the bone in inflammatory bone disease [222].

In fact, we recently addressed the role of DCs in breast-tumor-derived bone metastases context [223, 224]. We showed that DC-OC differentiation is induced by

RANKL, either recombinant or produced by specific-tumor T cells [224], and they can act as both an APC for 4 T1 tumor-specific T cells and as an OC-like cell (DC-OC), amplifying the osteolytic phenomena before bone tumor colonization [224]. Furthermore, it is already known that the pretreatment of DCs with high levels of RANKL leads to enhancement of [76] and augments their ability to stimulate T cell proliferation [225–227]. Therefore, we can suppose that RANKL-enriched environment setup by osteoclastogenic $CD3^+$ T cells located inside the BM probably contributes to a higher DC survival ratio, which in turn would support T cells' activities in promoting the pre-metastatic niche formation [224]. Additionally, DC-OCs, but not BM-OCs, are incredibly good in activating T cell proliferation and cytokine secretion [224], and secrete high amounts of IL-23, which in turn boosts IL-17 and RANKL production by T cells, feeding the positive osteoclastogenic loop of adaptive T cell immunity [224]. This positive loop has IL-23 as one limiting step since blocking IL-23 with monoclonal antibody inhibits T cell IL-17 and RANKL production [224]. Adding more information to our work, recent data published [228] showed that monocyte-derived macrophages, rather than bone-residing macrophages, are critical for breast-carcinoma-derived bone metastases outgrowth *in vivo*, in IL-4R and CCR2-dependent manners [228].

More recently, we described that 67NR non-metastatic tumor cells—an *in situ* breast carcinoma sibling of 4 T1 tumor cell line, can modify distant sites promoting bone physiological alterations, increasing in trabecular bone mass on day 11 post-tumor implant [229]. This observation was associated with an expansion of the osteoblastic lineage cells accompanied by a reduction of OCs numbers [229]. Moreover, $CD8^+$ T cells express an anti-osteoclastogenic cytokine milieu enriched by IFN-γ, IL-10 and low levels of RANKL, and the frequency of BM-derived $CD8^+$ $FoxP3^+$ regulatory T cells, as defined as potent suppressors of osteoclastogenesis, was also increased in such animals [229]. This milieu was capable to suppress 4 T1 tumor-specific $CD4^+$ T cells phenotype *in vivo* and *in vitro* and strongly inhibited bone metastases establishment, restoring trabecular bone mass volume [229]. We concluded that the $67NR^+$ tumor derived $CD8^+$ T cells phenotypes, either contributing to bone homeostasis and/or control of 4 T1 breast tumor pre-metastatic disease, interfere with OCs and OBs activities inside BM. Our study highlights the opposing roles of subverted tumor $CD4^+$ and $CD8^+$ T cell subtypes in directing breast cancer progression and bone metastases establishment. Furthermore, this likely reflects the fact that modification of the distant bone site by 67NR breast tumor disfavors pre-metastatic bone niche formation [229].

4. Conclusions and perspectives

Altogether, we assume that the set of our studies are revealing the cellular and molecular dynamic interactions behind breast-cancer-derived pre-metastatic bone niche formation (**Figure 1**). There are still many questions about the factors that determine the chemotaxis of cells, which Ags or ligands are needed, as well as the modulating elements of this distant system. So far, we know, that the immune system is central. Multiple cues need to be investigated to translate our current knowledge toward clinical impact. If these immunophenotypes patterns are confirmed in human disease, this complex network can be used either as prognostic tools or even as therapeutic targets.

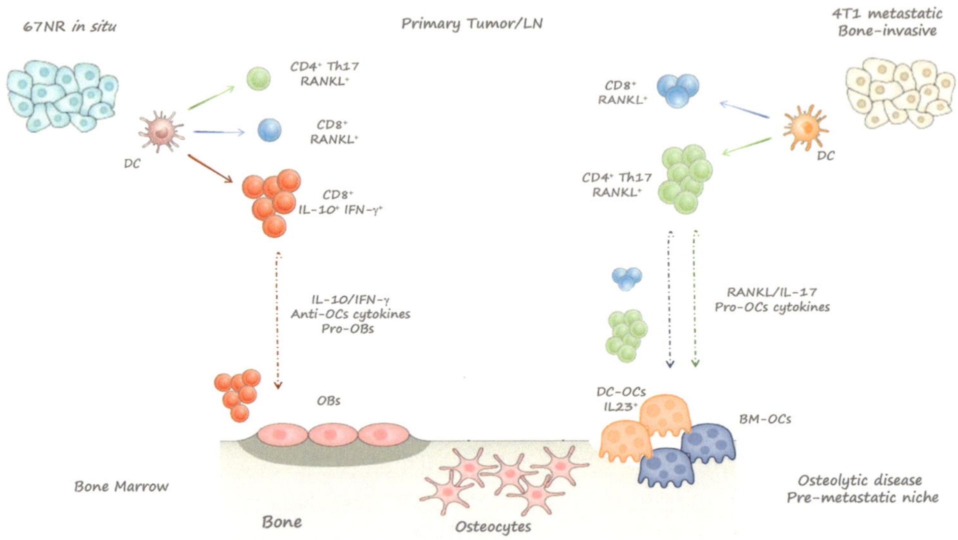

Figure 1.
Left panel: anti-osteoclastogenic cytokines produced by $67NR^+$ $CD8^+$ T cells keep bone homeostasis mediated by OBs and OCs cross talk. Right panel: BM pre-metastatic niche formation by 4T1 Th17 $RANKL^+$ $CD4^+$ T cells and $RANKL^+$ $CD8^+$ T cells activities. DCs loaded with tumor Ags from primary tumor growth site prime naïve $CD4^+$ and $CD8^+$ T cells into draining LNs to differentiate into tumor-activated T cells producing RANKL and IL-17F, which in turn migrate to BM before tumor bone colonization. Migrating DCs can now activate the maintenance of tumor $RANKL^+$ $CD4^+$ Th17 T cells inside BM microenvironment dependent on IL-23 production. Dysregulation of bone homeostasis by an intense activation of BM-OCs by RANKL and M-CSF under breast tumor pre-metastatic osteolytic conditions induced by $RANKL^+$ $CD4^+$ Th17 T cells and $RANKL^+$ $CD8^+$ T cells. Both T cells activities support their osteoclastogenic potential in the establishment of the pre-metastatic niche. Left panel: Bone marrow scenario after subcutaneously 67NR non-metastatic tumor cells challenge. Production of anti-osteoclastogenic cytokines, IFN-γ^+, IL-10, and anabolic levels of RANKL expressed by $CD8^+$ T cells keep bone homeostasis mediated by OCs and OBs cross talk.

Funding

This work was supported by funds from Faperj (Foundation for Research Support of the State of Rio de Janeiro, E-26/203.056/2017, E-26/010.001925/2015, E-26/311.264/2021, SEI-260003/002756/2022; Fopesq 2021/UFF; CNPq (National Research Council, 309611/2018-0); and FOCEM (Fundo para a Convergência Estrutural do MERCOSUL).

Author details

Ana Carolina Monteiro[1,2*] and Adriana Bonomo[2,3,4,5,6]

1 Osteo and Tumor Immunology Laboratory (LOIT), Biology Institute (EGB), Fluminense Federal University (UFF), Brazil

2 Laboratory on Thymus Research, Brazil

3 National Institute of Science and Technology on Neuroimmunomodulation (INCT-NIM), Brazil

4 Research Network on Neuroinflammation (RENEURIN), Oswaldo Cruz Institute, FIOCRUZ, Brazil

5 FIOCANCER Program, Brazil

6 FIOMUCOSA Program, VPPCB, FIOCRUZ, Rio de Janeiro, Brazil

*Address all correspondence to: anacarolinadossantosmonteiro@id.uff.br

References

[1] Zhao E, Xu H, Wang L, Kryczek I, Wu K, Hu Y, et al. Bone marrow and the control of immunity. Cellular and Molecular Immunology. 2012;**9**:11-19. DOI: 10.1038/cmi.2011.47

[2] Morrison SJ, Scadden DT. The bone marrow niche for haematopoietic stem cells. Nature. 2014;**505**:327-334. DOI: 10.1038/nature12984

[3] Lucas D. Structural organization of the bone marrow and its role in hematopoiesis. Current Opinion in Hematology. 2021;**28**:36-42. DOI: 10.1097/MOH.0000000000000621

[4] Balduino A, Hurtado SP, Frazão P, Takiya CM, Alves LM, Nasciutti LE, et al. Bone marrow subendosteal microenvironment harbours functionally distinct haemosupportive stromal cell populations. Cell and Tissue Research. 2005;**319**:255-266. DOI: 10.1007/s00441-004-1006-3

[5] Kandarakov O, Belyavsky A, Semenova E. Bone marrow niches of hematopoietic stem and progenitor cells. International Journal of Molecular Sciences. 2022;**23**(8):4462. DOI: 10.3390/ijms23084462

[6] Comazzetto S, Shen B, Morrison SJ. Niches that regulate stem cells and hematopoiesis in adult bone marrow. Developmental Cell. 2021;**56**:1848-1860. DOI: 10.1016/j.devcel.2021.05.018

[7] Ding L, Morrison SJ. Haematopoietic stem cells and early lymphoid progenitors occupy distinct bone marrow niches. Nature. 2013;**495**:231-235. DOI: 10.1038/nature11885

[8] Méndez-Ferrer S, Michurina TV, Ferraro F, Mazloom AR, MacArthur BD, Lira SA, et al. Mesenchymal and haematopoietic stem cells form a unique bone marrow niche. Nature. 2010;**466**:829-834. DOI: 10.1038/nature09262

[9] Méndez-Ferrer S, Bonnet D, Steensma DP, Hasserjian RP, Ghobrial IM, Gribben JG, et al. Bone marrow niches in haematological malignancies. Nature Reviews Cancer. 2020;**20**:285-298. DOI: 10.1038/s41568-020-0245-2

[10] Chantrain CF, Feron O, Marbaix E, Declerck YA. Bone marrow microenvironment and tumor progression. Cancer Microenvironment. 2008;**1**:23-35. DOI: 10.1007/s12307-008-0010-7

[11] Taichman RS, Emerson SG. Human Osteoblasts Support Hematopoiesis through the Production of Granulocyte Colony-stimulating Factor. Journal of Experimental Medicine. 1994;**179**(5):1677-1682. DOI: 10.1084/jem.179.5.1677

[12] Jung Y, Wang J, Schneider A, Sun YX, Koh-Paige AJ, Osman NI, et al. Regulation of SDF-1 (CXCL12) production by osteoblasts; a possible mechanism for stem cell homing. Bone. 2006;**38**:497-508. DOI: 10.1016/j.bone.2005.10.003

[13] Bonomo A, Monteiro AC, Gonçalves-Silva T, Cordeiro-Spinetti E, Galvani RG, Balduino A. A T cell view of the bone marrow. Frontiers in Immunology. 2016;**7**:184. DOI: 10.3389/fimmu.2016.00184

[14] Zhang J, Niu C, Ye L, Huang H, He X, Tong WG, et al. Identification of the haematopoietic stem cell niche and control of the niche size. Nature. 2003;**425**:836-841. DOI: 10.1038/nature02041

[15] Saçma M, Pospiech J, Bogeska R, de Back W, Mallm JP, Sakk V,

et al. Haematopoietic stem cells in perisinusoidal niches are protected from ageing. Nature Cell Biology. 2019;**21**:1309-1320. DOI: 10.1038/s41556-019-0418-y

[16] Zhang J, Wu Q, Johnson CB, Pham G, Kinder JM, Olsson A, et al. In situ mapping identifies distinct vascular niches for myelopoiesis. Nature. 2021;**590**:457-462. DOI: 10.1038/s41586-021-03201-2

[17] Noble D. Regulation of bone metabolism. Progress in Biophysics and Molecular Biology. 2016;**122**:83-84. DOI: 10.1016/j.pbiomolbio.2016.10.001

[18] Datta HK, Ng WF, Walker JA, Tuck SP, Varanasi SS. The cell biology of bone metabolism. Journal of Clinical Pathology. 2008;**61**:577-587. DOI: 10.1136/jcp.2007.048868

[19] Alliston T, Derynck R. Medicine: Interfering with bone remodelling. Nature. 2002;**416**:686-687. DOI: 10.1038/416686a

[20] Periosteal stem cells control growth plate stem cells during postnatal skeletal growth. Nature Communications. 2022;**13**(1):4166. DOI: 10.1038/s41467-022-31592-x

[21] Prideaux M, Findlay DM, Atkins GJ. Osteocytes: The master cells in bone remodelling. Current Opinion in Pharmacology. 2016;**28**:24-30. DOI: 10.1016/j.coph.2016.02.003

[22] Sims NA, Vrahnas C. Regulation of cortical and trabecular bone mass by communication between osteoblasts, osteocytes and osteoclasts. Archives of Biochemistry and Biophysics. 2014;**561**:22-28. DOI: 10.1016/j.abb.2014.05.015

[23] Chen H, Senda T, Kubo KY. The osteocyte plays multiple roles in bone remodeling and mineral homeostasis. Medical Molecular Morphology. 2015;**48**:61-68. DOI: 10.1007/s00795-015-0099-y

[24] Henriksen K, Neutzsky-Wulff AV, Bonewald LF, Karsdal MA. Local communication on and within bone controls bone remodeling. Bone. 2009;**44**:1026-1033. DOI: 10.1016/j.bone.2009.03.671

[25] Raggatt LJ, Partridge NC. Cellular and molecular mechanisms of bone remodeling. Journal of Biological Chemistry. 2010;**285**:25103-25108. DOI: 10.1074/jbc.R109.041087

[26] Delgado-Calle J, Bellido T. The osteocyte as a signaling cell. Physiological Reviews. 2022;**102**:379-410. DOI: 10.1152/physrev.00043.2020

[27] Intemann J, de Gorter DJJ, Naylor AJ, Dankbar B, Wehmeyer C. Importance of osteocyte-mediated regulation of bone remodelling in inflammatory bone disease. Swiss Medical Weekly. 2020;**150**:w20187. DOI: 10.4414/smw.2020.20187

[28] Franz-Odendaal TA, Hall BK, Witten PE. Buried alive: How osteoblasts become osteocytes. Developmental Dynamics. 2006;**235**:176-190. DOI: 10.1002/dvdy.20603

[29] O'Brien CA, Nakashima T, Takayanagi H. Osteocyte control of osteoclastogenesis. Bone. 2013;**54**:258-263. DOI: 10.1016/j.bone.2012.08.121

[30] Arnett TR, Orriss IR. Metabolic properties of the osteoclast. Bone. 2018;**115**:25-30. DOI: 10.1016/j.bone.2017.12.021

[31] Chambers TJ. The birth of the osteoclast. Annals of the New York Academy of Sciences. 2010;**1192**:19-26. DOI: 10.1111/j.1749-6632.2009.05224.x

[32] Asagiri M, Takayanagi H. The molecular understanding of osteoclast

differentiation. Bone. 2007;**40**:251-264. DOI: 10.1016/j.bone.2006.09.023

[33] Tsukasaki M, Huynh NCN, Okamoto K, Muro R, Terashima A, Kurikawa Y, et al. Stepwise cell fate decision pathways during osteoclastogenesis at single-cell resolution. Nature Metabolism. 2020;**2**:1382-1390. DOI: 10.1038/s42255-020-00318-y

[34] Lorenzo J, Lorenzo J. The many ways of osteoclast activation find the latest version: The many ways of osteoclast activation. The Journal of Clinical Investigation. 2017;**127**:2530-2532

[35] Walsh MC, Choi Y. Biology of the RANKL-RANK-OPG system in immunity, bone, and beyond. Frontiers in Immunology. 2014;5:1-11. DOI: 10.3389/fimmu.2014.00511

[36] Liu C, Walter TS, Huang P, Zhang S, Zhu X, Wu Y, et al. Structural and functional insights of RANKL-RANK interaction and Signaling. The Journal of Immunology. 2010;**184**:6910-6919. DOI: 10.4049/jimmunol.0904033

[37] Takayanagi H. RANKL as the master regulator of osteoclast differentiation. Journal of Bone and Mineral Metabolism. 2021;**39**:13-18. DOI: 10.1007/s00774-020-01191-1

[38] Takegahara N, Kim H, Choi Y. RANKL biology. Bone. 2022;**159**:116353. DOI: 10.1016/j.bone.2022.116353

[39] Nakashima T, Hayashi M, Fukunaga T, Kurata K, Oh-hora M, Feng JQ, et al. Evidence for osteocyte regulation of bone homeostasis through RANKL expression. Nature Medicine. 2011;**17**:1231-1234. DOI: 10.1038/nm.2452

[40] Okamoto K, Takayanagi H. Osteoimmunology. Cold Spring Harbor Perspectives in Medicine. 2019;**9**(1):a031245. DOI: 10.1101/cshperspect.a031245

[41] Kim JH, Kim N. Regulation of NFATc1 in osteoclast differentiation. Journal of Bone Metabolism. 2014;**21**:233. DOI: 10.11005/jbm.2014.21.4.233

[42] Yun Kong Y, Yoshida H, Boyle WJ, Penniger JM. OPGL is a key regulator of osteoclastogenesis, lymphocyte development and lymph-node organogenesis. Nature. 1999:**397**(6717):315-323

[43] Walsh MC, Choi Y. Regulation of T cell-associated tissues and T cell activation by RANKL-RANK-OPG. Journal of Bone and Mineral Metabolism. 2021;**39**:54-63. DOI: 10.1007/s00774-020-01178-y

[44] Takeshita A, Nishida K, Yoshida A, Nasu Y, Nakahara R, Kaneda D, et al. RANKL expression in chondrocytes and its promotion by lymphotoxin-α in the course of cartilage destruction during rheumatoid arthritis. PLoS One. 2021;**16**(17):e0254268. DOI: 10.1371/journal.pone.0254268

[45] Kartsogiannis V, Zhou H, Horwood NJ, Thomas RJ, Hards DK, Quinn JMW, et al. Localization of RANKL (receptor activator of NFB ligand) mRNA and protein in skeletal and extraskeletal tissues. Bone. 1999;**25**(5):525-534

[46] Mechanisms of joint destruction in rheumatoid arthritis—immune cell–fibroblast–bone interactions . Nature Reviews Rheumatology. 2022;**18**(7):415-429. DOI: 10.1038/s41584-022-00793-5

[47] Zhou A, Wu B, Yu H, Tang Y, Liu J, Jia Y, et al. Current understanding of osteoimmunology in certain osteoimmune diseases. Frontiers in Cell and Developmental Biology. 2021;**9**:698068. DOI: 10.3389/fcell.2021.698068

[48] Kim N, Odgren PR, Kim DK, Marks SC, Choi Y. Diverse roles of the tumor necrosis factor family member TRANCE in skeletal physiology revealed by TRANCE deficiency and partial rescue by a lymphocyte-expressed TRANCE transgene. Proceedings of the National Academy of Sciences of the United States of America. 2000;**97**:10905-10910. DOI: 10.1073/pnas.200294797

[49] Metzger CE, Anand Narayanan S. The role of osteocytes in inflammatory bone loss. Frontiers in Endocrinology. 2019;**10**:285. DOI: 10.3389/fendo.2019.00285

[50] Udagawa N, Koide M, Nakamura M, Nakamichi Y, Yamashita T, Uehara S, et al. Osteoclast differentiation by RANKL and OPG signaling pathways. Journal of Bone and Mineral Metabolism. 2021;**39**:19-26. DOI: 10.1007/s00774-020-01162-6

[51] Tsukasaki M, Asano T, Muro R, Huynh NCN, Komatsu N, Okamoto K, et al. OPG production matters where it happened. Cell Reports. 2020;**32**:(10):108124. DOI: 10.1016/j.celrep.2020.108124

[52] Bucay N, Sarosi I, Dunstan CR, Morony S, Tarpley J, Capparelli C, et al. Osteoprotegerin-deficient mice develop early onset osteoporosis and arterial calcification. Genes and Development. 1998;**12**:1260-1268. DOI: 10.1101/gad.12.9.1260

[53] Terashima A, Takayanagi H. Overview of osteoimmunology. Calcified Tissue International. 2018;**102**:503-511. DOI: 10.1007/s00223-018-0417-1

[54] Liu J, Xiao Q, Xiao J, Niu C, Li Y, Zhang X, et al. Wnt/β-catenin signalling: Function, biological mechanisms, and therapeutic opportunities. Signal Transduction and Targeted Therapy. 2022;**7**(1):3. DOI: 10.1038/s41392-021-00762-6

[55] Negishi-Koga T, Takayanagi H. Bone cell communication factors and semaphorins. BoneKEy Reports. 2012;**1**:183. DOI: 10.1038/bonekey.2012.183

[56] Cong F, Wu N, Tian X, Fan J, Liu J, Song T, et al. MicroRNA-34c promotes osteoclast differentiation through targeting LGR4. Gene. 2017;**610**:1-8. DOI: 10.1016/j.gene.2017.01.028

[57] Sims NA, Martin TJ. Coupling signals between the osteoclast and osteoblast: How are messages transmitted between these temporary visitors to the bone surface? Frontiers in Endocrinology. 2015;**6**:41. DOI: 10.3389/fendo.2015.00041

[58] Atkinson EG, Delgado-Calle J. The emerging role of osteocytes in cancer in bone. JBMR Plus. 2019;**3**(3):e10186. DOI: 10.1002/jbm4.10186

[59] Capulli M, Paone R, Rucci N. Osteoblast and osteocyte: Games without frontiers. Archives of Biochemistry and Biophysics. 2014;**561**:3-12. DOI: 10.1016/j.abb.2014.05.003

[60] Rauch F, Adachi R. Sclerostin: More than a bone formation brake. Science Translational Medicine. 2016;**8**:1-4. DOI: 10.1126/scitranslmed.aaf4628

[61] Wehmeyer C, Frank S, Beckmann D, Böttcher M, Cromme C, König U, et al. Sclerostin inhibition promotes TNF-dependent inflammatory joint destruction. Science Translational Medicine. 2016;**8**:1-12. DOI: 10.1126/scitranslmed.aac4351

[62] Cain CJ, Rueda R, McLelland B, Collette NM, Loots GG, Manilay JO. Absence of sclerostin adversely affects B-cell survival. Journal of Bone and

Mineral Research. 2012;**27**:1451-1461. DOI: 10.1002/jbmr.1608

[63] Tsukasaki M, Takayanagi H. Osteoimmunology: Evolving concepts in bone–immune interactions in health and disease. Nature Reviews Immunology. 2019;**19**:626-642. DOI: 10.1038/s41577-019-0178-8

[64] Monteiro AC, Leal AC, Gonçalves-Silva T, Mercadante ACT, Kestelman F, Chaves SB, et al. T cells induce pre-metastatic osteolytic disease and help bone metastases establishment in a mouse model of metastatic breast Cancer. PLoS One. 2013;**8**:1-13. DOI: 10.1371/journal.pone.0068171

[65] Horton JE, Raisz LG, Simmons HA, Oppenheim JJ, Mergenhagen SE. Bone resorbing activity in supernatants fluid from cultured human peripheral blood leukocytes. Science. 1979;**177**(1972):793-795

[66] Mundy GR, Raisz LG, Cooper RA, Schechter GP, Salmon SE. Evidence for the secretion of an osteoclast stimulating factor in myeloma. The New England Journal of Medicine. 1974;**291**(20):1041-1046. DOI: 10.1056/NEJM197411142912001

[67] Takayanagi H. Osteoimmunology as an intrinsic part of immunology. International Immunology. 2021;**33**:673-678. DOI: 10.1093/intimm/dxab057

[68] Schett G, Takayanagi H. Editorial overview: Osteoimmunology. Bone. 2022;**162**:116466. DOI: 10.1016/j.bone.2022.116466

[69] Arron JR, Choi Y. Bone versus immune system. Nature. 2000;**408**:535-536. DOI: 10.1038/35046196

[70] Hosokawa H, Rothenberg EV. How transcription factors drive choice of the T cell fate. Nature Reviews Immunology. 2021;**21**(3):162-176. DOI: 10.1038/s41577-020-00426-6.

[71] Walsh MC, Takegahara N, Kim H, Choi Y. Updating osteoimmunology: Regulation of bone cells by innate and adaptive immunity. Nature Reviews Rheumatology. 2018;**14**:146-156. DOI: 10.1038/nrrheum.2017.213

[72] Sobacchi C, Menale C, Villa A. The RANKL-RANK axis: A bone to thymus round trip. Frontiers in Immunology. 2019;**10**:629. DOI: 10.3389/fimmu.2019.00629

[73] Irla M. RANK signaling in the differentiation and regeneration of thymic epithelial cells. Frontiers in Immunology. 2021;**11**:623265. DOI: 10.3389/fimmu.2020.623265

[74] Otero DC, Baker DP, David M. IRF7-dependent IFN-β production in response to RANKL promotes medullary thymic epithelial cell development. The Journal of Immunology. 2013;**190**:3289-3298. DOI: 10.4049/jimmunol.1203086

[75] Hikosaka Y, Nitta T, Ohigashi I, Yano K, Ishimaru N, Hayashi Y, et al. The cytokine RANKL produced by positively selected thymocytes fosters medullary thymic epithelial cells that express autoimmune regulator. Immunity. 2008;**29**(3):438-450. DOI: 10.1016/j.immuni.2008.06.018

[76] Josien R, Li HL, Ingulli E, Sarma S, Wong BR, Vologodskaia M, et al. TRANCE, a tumor necrosis factor family member, enhances the longevity and adjuvant properties of dendritic cells in vivo. Journal of Experimental Medicine. 2000;**191**:495-501. DOI: 10.1084/jem.191.3.495

[77] Josien R, Wong BR, Li HL, Steinman RM, Choi Y. TRANCE, a

TNF family member, is differentially expressed on T cell subsets and induces cytokine production in dendritic cells. Journal of Immunology. 1999;**162**:2562-2568. Available from: http://www.ncbi.nlm.nih.gov/pubmed/10072496

[78] Mansour A, Anginot A, Mancini SJC, Schiff C, Carle GF, Wakkach A, et al. Osteoclast activity modulates B-cell development in the bone marrow. Cell Research. 2011;**21**:1102-1115. DOI: 10.1038/cr.2011.21

[79] Horowitz MC, Fretz JA, Lorenzo JA. How B cells influence bone biology in health and disease. Bone. 2010;**47**:472-479. DOI: 10.1016/j.bone.2010.06.011

[80] Li Y, Toraldo G, Li A, Yang X, Zhang H. B cells and T cells are critical for the preservation of bone homeostasis and attainment of peak bone mass in vivo. Blood. 2007;**109**:3839-3849. DOI: 10.1182/blood-2006-07-037994

[81] Axmann R, Herman S, Zaiss M, Franz S, Polzer K, Zwerina J, et al. CTLA-4 directly inhibits osteoclast formation. Annals of the Rheumatic Diseases. 2008;**67**:1603-1609. DOI: 10.1136/ard.2007.080713

[82] Bozec A, Zaiss MM, Kagwiria R, Voll R, Rauh M, Chen Z, et al. T cell costimulation molecules CD80/86 inhibit osteoclast differentiation by inducing the IDO/tryptophan pathway. n.d. Available from: www.ScienceTranslationalMedicine.org

[83] Weitzmann MN, Ofotokun I. Physiological and pathophysiological bone turnover-role of the immune system. Nature Reviews Endocrinology. 2016;**12**:518-532. DOI: 10.1038/nrendo.2016.91

[84] Srivastava RK, Schmidt-Bleek K, Chattopadhyay N, de Martinis M, Mishra PK. Editorial: Recent advances in basic and translational osteoimmunology. Frontiers in Immunology. 2021;**12**:800508. DOI: 10.3389/fimmu.2021.800508

[85] Tuzlak S, Dejean AS, Iannacone M, Quintana FJ, Waisman A, Ginhoux F, et al. Repositioning TH cell polarization from single cytokines to complex help. Nature Immunology. 2021;**22**:1210-1217. DOI: 10.1038/s41590-021-01009-w

[86] Yamada H. Adaptive immunity in the joint of rheumatoid arthritis. Immunol Med. 2022;**45**(1):1-11. DOI: 10.1080/25785826.2021.1930371

[87] Alzabin S, Williams RO. Effector T cells in rheumatoid arthritis: lessons from animal models. FEBS Letters. 2011;**585**(23):3649-3659. DOI: 10.1016/j.febslet.2011.04.034

[88] Takeshita M, Suzuki K, Kondo Y, Morita R, Okuzono Y, et al. Multi-dimensional analysis identified rheumatoid arthritis driving pathway in human T cell. Annals of the Rheumatic Diseases. 2019;**78**(10):1346-1356. DOI: 10.1136/annrheumdis-2018-214885

[89] Ponchel F, Vital E, Kingsbury SR, El-Sherbiny YM. CD4 + T-cell subsets in rheumatoid arthritis. International Journal of Clinical Rheumatology. 2012;**7**:37-53. DOI: 10.2217/ijr.11.69

[90] Santos LL, Dacumos A, Yamana J, Sharma L, Morand EF. Reduced arthritis in MIF deficient mice is associated with reduced T cell activation: Down-regulation of ERK MAP kinase phosphorylation. Clinical and Experimental Immunology. 2008;**152**:372-380. DOI: 10.1111/j.1365-2249.2008.03639.x

[91] Schurigt U, Eilenstein R, Gajda M, Leipner C, Sevenich L, Reinheckel T, et al. Decreased arthritis severity in cathepsin L-deficient mice is attributed to

an impaired T helper cell compartment. Inflammation Research. 2012;**61**:1021-1029. DOI: 10.1007/s00011-012-0495-x

[92] Miyazaki Y, Nakayamada S, Kubo S, Nakano K, Iwata S, Miyagawa I, et al. Th22 cells promote osteoclast differentiation via production of IL-22 in rheumatoid arthritis. Frontiers in Immunology. 2018;**9**:2901. DOI: 10.3389/fimmu.2018.02901

[93] Komatsu N, Okamoto K, Sawa S, Nakashima T, Oh-Hora M, Kodama T, et al. Pathogenic conversion of Foxp3 + T cells into TH17 cells in autoimmune arthritis. Nature Medicine. 2014;**20**:62-68. DOI: 10.1038/nm.3432

[94] Danks L, Komatsu N, Guerrini MM, Sawa S, Armaka M, Kollias G, et al. RANKL expressed on synovial fibroblasts is primarily responsible for bone erosions during joint inflammation. Annals of the Rheumatic Diseases. 2016;**75**:1187-1195. DOI: 10.1136/annrheumdis-2014-207137

[95] Catrina AI, Svensson CI, Malmström V, Schett G, Klareskog L. Mechanisms leading from systemic autoimmunity to joint-specific disease in rheumatoid arthritis. Nature Reviews Rheumatology. 2017;**13**:79-86. DOI: 10.1038/nrrheum.2016.200

[96] Okui T, Aoki Y, Ito H, Honda T, Yamazaki K. The presence of IL-17+/FOXP3+ double-positive cells in periodontitis. Journal of Dental Research. 2012;**91**:574-579. DOI: 10.1177/0022034512446341

[97] Bittner-Eddy PD, Fischer LA, Costalonga M. Transient expression of IL-17A in Foxp3 fate-tracked cells in *Porphyromonas gingivalis*-mediated oral dysbiosis. Frontiers in Immunology. 2020;**11**:677. DOI: 10.3389/fimmu.2020.00677

[98] Tsukasaki M, Komatsu N, Nagashima K, Nitta T, Pluemsakunthai W, Shukunami C, et al. Host defense against oral microbiota by bone-damaging T cells. Nature Communications. 2018;**9**(1):701. DOI: 10.1038/s41467-018-03147-6

[99] Hiasa M, Abe M, Nakano A, Oda A, Amou H, Kido S, et al. GM-CSF and IL-4 induce dendritic cell differentiation and disrupt osteoclastogenesis through M-CSF receptor shedding by up-regulation of TNF-α converting enzyme (TACE). Blood. 2009;**114**(20):4517-4526. DOI: 10.1182/blood-2009-04-215020

[100] Palmqvist P, Lundberg P, Persson E, Johansson A, Lundgren I, Lie A, et al. Inhibition of hormone and cytokine-stimulated osteoclastogenesis and bone resorption by interleukin-4 and interleukin-13 is associated with increased osteoprotegerin and decreased RANKL and RANK in a STAT6-dependent pathway. Journal of Biological Chemistry. 2006;**281**:2414-2429. DOI: 10.1074/jbc.M510160200

[101] Sato K, Suematsu A, Okamoto K, Yamaguchi A, Morishita Y, Kadono Y, et al. Th17 functions as an osteoclastogenic helper T cell subset that links T cell activation and bone destruction. Journal of Experimental Medicine. 2006;**203**:2673-2682. DOI: 10.1084/jem.20061775

[102] Takayanagi H, Ogasawara K, Hida S, Chiba T, Murata S, Sato K, et al. T-cell-mediated regulation of osteoclastogenesis by signalling cross-talk between RANKL and IFN-γ. Nature. 2000;**408**:600-605. DOI: 10.1038/35046102

[103] Schett G. Osteoimmunology in rheumatic diseases. Arthritis Research & Therapy. 2009;**11**(1):210. DOI: 10.1186/ar2571

[104] Schett G. Review: Immune cells and mediators of inflammatory arthritis.

Autoimmunity. 2008;**41**:224-229. DOI: 10.1080/08916930701694717

[105] Schett G, David JP. The multiple faces of autoimmune-mediated bone loss. Nature Reviews Endocrinology. 2010;**6**:698-706. DOI: 10.1038/nrendo.2010.190

[106] McInnes IB, Schett G. Mechanism of disease the pathogenesis of rheumatoid arthritis. New England Journal of Medicine. 2011;**365**:2205-2219

[107] Massalska M, Radzikowska A, Kuca-Warnawin E, Plebanczyk M, Prochorec-Sobieszek M, Skalska U, et al. CD4+FOXP3+ T cells in rheumatoid arthritis bone marrow are partially impaired. Cell. 2020;**9**(3):549. DOI: 10.3390/cells9030549

[108] Srivastava RK, Dar HY, Mishra PK. Immunoporosis: Immunology of osteoporosis-role of T cells. Frontiers in Immunology. 2018;**9**:657. DOI: 10.3389/fimmu.2018.00657

[109] Drake MT, Clarke BL, Lewiecki EM. The pathophysiology and treatment of osteoporosis. Clinical Therapeutics. 2015;**37**:1837-1850. DOI: 10.1016/j.clinthera.2015.06.006

[110] Föger-Samwald U, Dovjak P, Azizi-Semrad U, Kerschan-Schindl K, Pietschmann P. Osteoporosis: Pathophysiology and therapeutic options. EXCLI Journal. 2020;**19**:1017-1037. DOI: 10.17179/excli2020-2591

[111] Li JY, Chassaing B, Tyagi AM, Vaccaro C, Luo T, Adams J, et al. Sex steroid deficiency-associated bone loss is microbiota dependent and prevented by probiotics. Journal of Clinical Investigation. 2016;**126**:2049-2063. DOI: 10.1172/JCI86062

[112] Sapra L, Dar HY, Bhardwaj A, Pandey A, Kumari S, Azam Z, et al. Lactobacillus rhamnosus attenuates bone loss and maintains bone health by skewing Treg-Th17 cell balance in Ovx mice. Scientific Reports. 2021;**11**:1-18. DOI: 10.1038/s41598-020-80536-2

[113] Yousefi B, Eslami M, Ghasemian A, Kokhaei P, Salek Farrokhi A, Darabi N. Probiotics importance and their immunomodulatory properties. Journal of Cellular Physiology. 2019;**234**:8008-8018. DOI: 10.1002/jcp.27559

[114] Yu M, Malik Tyagi A, Li JY, Adams J, Denning TL, Weitzmann MN, et al. PTH induces bone loss via microbial-dependent expansion of intestinal TNF+ T cells and Th17 cells. Nature Communications. 2020;**11**:1-17. DOI: 10.1038/s41467-019-14148-4

[115] Tyagi AM, Yu M, Darby TM, Vaccaro C, Li JY, Owens JA, et al. The microbial metabolite butyrate stimulates bone formation via T regulatory cell-mediated regulation of WNT10B expression. Immunity. 2018;**49**:1116-1131.e7. DOI: 10.1016/j.immuni.2018.10.013

[116] Dauba A, Braikia FZ, Oudinet C, Khamlichi AA. Interleukin 7 regulates switch transcription in developing B cells. Cellular and Molecular Immunology. 2021;**18**(3):776-778. DOI: 10.1038/s41423-020-0430-y

[117] Rheumatoid arthritis. Nature Reviews Disease Primers. 2018;**4**:18001. DOI: 10.1038/nrdp.2018.2

[118] Lucas C, Perdriger A, Amé P. Definition of B cell helper T cells in rheumatoid arthritis and their behavior during treatment. Seminars in Arthritis and Rheumatism. 2020;**50**:867-872. DOI: 10.1016/j.semarthrit.2020.06.021

[119] Weyand CM, Goronzy JJ. The immunology of rheumatoid arthritis.

Nature Immunology. 2021;**22**:10-18. DOI: 10.1038/s41590-020-00816-x

[120] Auréal M, Machuca-Gayet I, Coury F. Rheumatoid arthritis in the view of osteoimmunology. Biomolecules. 2021;**11**:1-18. DOI: 10.3390/biom11010048

[121] Negishi-Koga T, Gober HJ, Sumiya E, Komatsu N, Okamoto K, Sawa S, et al. Immune complexes regulate bone metabolism through FcRγ signalling. Nature Communications. 2015;**6**:6637. DOI: 10.1038/ncomms7637

[122] di Ceglie I, Kruisbergen NNL, van den Bosch MHJ, van Lent PLEM. Fc-gamma receptors and S100A8/A9 cause bone erosion during rheumatoid arthritis. Do they act as partners in crime? Rheumatology (United Kingdom). 2019;**58**:1331-1343. DOI: 10.1093/rheumatology/kez218

[123] Komatsu N, Win S, Yan M, Cong-Nhat Huynh N, Sawa S, Tsukasaki M, et al. Plasma cells promote osteoclastogenesis and periarticular bone loss in autoimmune arthritis. Journal of Clinical Investigation. 2021;**131**(6):e143060. DOI: 10.1172/JCI143060

[124] Onal M, Xiong J, Chen X, Thostenson JD, Almeida M, Manolagas SC, et al. Receptor activator of nuclear factor κB ligand (RANKL) protein expression by B lymphocytes contributes to ovariectomy-induced bone loss. Journal of Biological Chemistry. 2012;**287**:29851-29860. DOI: 10.1074/jbc.M112.377945

[125] Harbeck N, Penault-Llorca F, Cortes J, Gnant M, Houssami N, Poortmans P, et al. Breast cancer. Nature Reviews Disease Primers. 2019;**5**(1):66. DOI: 10.1038/s41572-019-0111-2

[126] Coleman RE, Croucher PI, Padhani AR, Clézardin P, Chow E, Fallon M, et al. Bone metastases. Nature Reviews Disease Primers. 2020;**6**(1):83. DOI: 10.1038/s41572-020-00216-3

[127] David Roodman G, Silbermann R. Mechanisms of osteolytic and osteoblastic skeletal lesions. BoneKEy Reports. 2015;**4**:1-7. DOI: 10.1038/bonekey.2015.122

[128] Esposito M, Guise T, Kang Y. The biology of bone metastasis. Cold Spring Harbor Perspectives in Medicine. 2018;**8**(6):a031252. DOI: 10.1101/cshperspect.a031252

[129] Mathis F, Penault-Llorca J, Cortes M, Gnant N, Houssami P, Poortmans K, et al. Breast Cancer. Nature Review Disease Primers. 2019;**5**(1):66. DOI: 10.1038/s41572-019-0111-2

[130] Roodman GD. Mechanisms of bone metastasis. New England Journal of Medicine. 2004;**350**:1655-1664. DOI: 10.1056/NEJMra030831

[131] Zaleski M, Kobilay M, Schroeder L, Debald M, Semaan A, Hettwer K, Uhlig S, Kuhn W, Hartmann G, Holdenrieder S. Improved sensitivity for detection of breast cancer by combination of miR-34a and tumor markers CA 15--3 or CEA. markers CA 15--3 or CEA. Oncotarget. 2018;**9**(32):22523-22536. DOI: 10.18632/oncotarget.25077

[132] O'Carrigan B, Wong MHF, Willson ML, Stockler MR, Pavlakis N, Goodwin A. Bisphosphonates and other bone agents for breast cancer. Cochrane Database of Systematic Reviews. 2017;**2017**. DOI: 10.1002/14651858.CD003474.pub4

[133] Coleman R, Gray R, Powles T, Paterson A, Gnant M, Bergh J, et al. Adjuvant bisphosphonate treatment in early breast cancer: Meta-analyses of individual patient data from randomised trials. The Lancet. 2015;**386**:1353-1361. DOI: 10.1016/S0140-6736(15)60908-4

[134] Ganesh K, Massagué J. Targeting metastatic cancer. Nature Medicine. 2021;**27**:34-44. DOI: 10.1038/s41591-020-01195-4

[135] Kähkönen TE, Halleen JM, Bernoulli J. Osteoimmuno-oncology: Therapeutic opportunities for targeting immune cells in bone metastasis. Cell. 2021;**10**(6):1529. DOI: 10.3390/cells10061529

[136] Chen WZ, Shen JF, Zhou Y, Chen XY, Liu JM, Liu ZL. Clinical characteristics and risk factors for developing bone metastases in patients with breast cancer. Scientific Reports. 2017;7(1):11325. DOI: 10.1038/s41598-017-11700-4

[137] Chen F, Han Y, Kang Y. Bone marrow niches in the regulation of bone metastasis. British Journal of Cancer. 2021;**124**:1912-1920. DOI: 10.1038/s41416-021-01329-6

[138] Waning DL, Mohammad KS, Reiken S, Xie W, Andersson DC, John S, et al. Excess TGF-β mediates muscle weakness associated with bone metastases in mice. Nature Medicine. 2015;**21**:1262-1271. DOI: 10.1038/nm.3961

[139] Regan JN, Mikesell C, Reiken S, Xu H, Marks AR, Mohammad KS, et al. Osteolytic breast cancer causes skeletal muscle weakness in an immunocompetent syngeneic mouse model. Frontiers in Endocrinology. 2017;**8**:358. DOI: 10.3389/fendo.2017.00358

[140] Hesse E, Schröder S, Brandt D, Pamperin J, Saito H, Taipaleenmäki H. Sclerostin inhibition alleviates breast cancer-induced bone metastases and muscle weakness. JCI Insight. 2019;**5**(9):e125543. DOI: 10.1172/jci.insight.125543

[141] Haider MT, Saito H, Zarrer J, Uzhunnumpuram K, Nagarajan S, Kari V, et al. Breast cancer bone metastases are attenuated in a Tgif1-deficient bone microenvironment. Breast Cancer Research. 2020;**22**(1):34. DOI: 10.1186/s13058-020-01269-8

[142] Hain BA, Xu H, Wilcox JR, Mutua D, Waning DL. Chemotherapy-induced loss of bone and muscle mass in a mouse model of breast cancer bone metastases and cachexia. JCSM Rapid Communications. 2019;**2**(1):e00075

[143] Consitt LA, Saneda A, Saxena G, List EO, Kopchick JJ. Mice overexpressing growth hormone exhibit increased skeletal muscle myostatin and MuRF1 with attenuation of muscle mass. Skeletal Muscle. 2017;7(1):17. DOI: 10.1186/s13395-017-0133-y

[144] Lee S-J, McPherron AC. Regulation of Myostatin Activity and Muscle Growth. Proceedings of the National Academy of Sciences of the United States of America. 2001;**98**(16):9306-9311. DOI: 10.1073/pnas.151270098

[145] Liu H, Zang P, Lee I, Anderson B, Christiani A, Strait-Bodey L, et al. Growth hormone secretagogue receptor-1a mediates ghrelin's effects on attenuating tumour-induced loss of muscle strength but not muscle mass. Journal of Cachexia, Sarcopenia and Muscle. 2021;**12**:1280-1295. DOI: 10.1002/jcsm.12743

[146] Cohen S, Nathan JA, Goldberg AL. Muscle wasting in disease: Molecular mechanisms and promising therapies. Nature Reviews Drug Discovery. 2014;**14**:58-74. DOI: 10.1038/nrd4467

[147] Zhang MZ, Ferrigno O, Wang Z, Ohnishi M, Prunier C, Levy L, et al. TGIF governs a feed-forward network that empowers wnt signaling to drive mammary tumorigenesis. Cancer Cell. 2015;**27**:547-560. DOI: 10.1016/j.ccell.2015.03.002

[148] Chen W, Cai F, Zhang B, Barekati Z, Zhong XY. The level of circulating miRNA-10b and miRNA-373 in detecting lymph node metastasis of breast cancer: Potential biomarkers. Tumor Biology. 2013;**34**:455-462. DOI: 10.1007/s13277-012-0570-5

[149] Puppo M, Taipaleenmäki H, Hesse E, Clzardin P. Non-coding RNAs in bone remodelling and bone metastasis: Mechanisms of action and translational relevance. British Journal of Pharmacology. 2021;**178**(9):1936-1954. DOI: 10.1111/bph.14836

[150] Haider MT, Smit DJ, Taipaleenmäki H. MicroRNAs: Emerging regulators of metastatic bone disease in breast cancer. Cancers (Basel). 2022;**14**(3):729. DOI: 10.3390/cancers14030729

[151] Hesse E, Taipaleenmäki H. MicroRNAs in bone metastasis. Current Osteoporosis Reports. 2019;**17**:122-128. DOI: 10.1007/s11914-019-00510-4

[152] Ma L, Teruya-Feldstein J, Weinberg RA. Tumour invasion and metastasis initiated by microRNA-10b in breast cancer. Nature. 2007;**449**:682-688. DOI: 10.1038/nature06174

[153] Cai WL, Huang WD, Li B, Chen TR, Li ZX, Zhao CL, et al. microRNA-124 inhibits bone metastasis of breast cancer by repressing Interleukin-11. Molecular Cancer. 2018;**17**(1):9. DOI: 10.1186/s12943-017-0746-0

[154] Liu X, Cao M, Palomares M, Wu X, Li A, Yan W, et al. Metastatic breast cancer cells overexpress and secrete miR-218 to regulate type i collagen deposition by osteoblasts. Breast Cancer Research. 2018;**20**(1):127. DOI: 10.1186/s13058-018-1059-y

[155] Obenauf AC, Massagué J. Surviving at a distance: Organ-specific metastasis. Trends in Cancer. 2015;**1**:76-91. DOI: 10.1016/j.trecan.2015.07.009

[156] Massagué J, Obenauf AC. Metastatic colonization by circulating tumour cells. Nature. 2016;**529**:298-306. DOI: 10.1038/nature17038

[157] Mundy GR. Metastasis to bone: Causes, consequences and therapeutic opportunities. Nature Reviews Cancer. 2002;**2**:584-593. DOI: 10.1038/nrc867

[158] Trivedi T, Pagnotti GM, Guise TA, Mohammad KS. The role of tgf-β in bone metastases. Biomolecules. 2021;**11**(11):1643. DOI: 10.3390/biom11111643

[159] Briukhovetska D, Dörr J, Endres S, Libby P, Dinarello CA, Kobold S. Interleukins in cancer: From biology to therapy. Nature Reviews Cancer. 2021;**21**:481-499. DOI: 10.1038/s41568-021-00363-z

[160] Haider MT, Ridlmaier N, Smit DJ, Taipaleenmäki H. Interleukins as mediators of the tumor cell—Bone cell crosstalk during the initiation of breast cancer bone metastasis. International Journal of Molecular Sciences. 2021;**22**:1-18. DOI: 10.3390/ijms22062898

[161] Zarrer J, Haider MT, Smit DJ, Taipaleenmäki H. Pathological crosstalk between metastatic breast cancer cells and the bone microenvironment. Biomolecules. 2020;**10**(2):337. DOI: 10.3390/biom10020337

[162] Liang M, Ma Q, Ding N, Luo F, Bai Y, Kang F, et al. IL-11 is essential in promoting osteolysis in breast cancer bone metastasis via RANKL-independent activation of osteoclastogenesis. Cell Death and Disease. 2019;**10**:1-12. DOI: 10.1038/s41419-019-1594-1

[163] Holen I, Lefley DV, Francis SE, Rennicks S, Bradbury S, Coleman RE,

et al. IL-1 drives breast cancer growth and bone metastasis in vivo. Oncotarget. 2016;7:75571-75584. DOI: 10.18632/oncotarget.12289

[164] Tulotta C, Ottewell P. The role of IL-1B in breast cancer bone metastasis. Endocrine-Related Cancer. 2018;**25**:R421-R434. DOI: 10.1530/ERC-17-0309

[165] EyreR, AlférezDG, Santiago-GómezA, Spence K, McConnell JC, Hart C, et al. Microenvironmental IL1β promotes breast cancer metastatic colonisation in the bone via activation of Wnt signalling. Nature Communications. 2019;**10**:1-15. DOI: 10.1038/s41467-019-12807-0

[166] Lu X, Mu E, Wei Y, Riethdorf S, Yang Q, Yuan M, et al. VCAM-1 promotes osteolytic expansion of indolent bone micrometastasis of breast cancer by engaging α4β1-positive osteoclast progenitors. Cancer Cell. 2011;**20**:701-714. DOI: 10.1016/j.ccr.2011.11.002

[167] Kostenuik PJ, Nguyen HQ, McCabe J, Warmington KS, Kurahara C, Sun N, et al. Denosumab, a fully human monoclonal antibody to RANKL, inhibits bone resorption and increases BMD in knock-in mice that express chimeric (murine/human) RANKL. Journal of Bone and Mineral Research. 2009;**24**:182-195. DOI: 10.1359/jbmr.081112

[168] Masiero M, Li D, Whiteman P, Bentley C, Greig J, Hassanali T, et al. Development of therapeutic anti-Jagged1 antibodies for cancer therapy. Molecular Cancer Therapeutics. 2019;**18**:2030-2042. DOI: 10.1158/1535-7163.MCT-18-1176

[169] Hume DA, Macdonald KPA. Therapeutic applications of macrophage colony-stimulating factor-1 (CSF-1) and antagonists of CSF-1 receptor (CSF-1R) signaling. Blood. 2012;**119**(8):1810-1820. DOI: 10.1182/blood-2011-09-379214.

[170] Zheng H, Bae Y, Kasimir-Bauer S, Tang R, Chen J, Ren G, et al. Therapeutic antibody targeting tumor- and osteoblastic niche-derived Jagged1 sensitizes bone metastasis to chemotherapy. Cancer Cell. 2017;**32**:731-747.e6. DOI: 10.1016/j.ccell.2017.11.002

[171] Peinado H, Zhang H, Matei IR, Costa-Silva B, Hoshino A, Rodrigues G, et al. Pre-metastatic niches: Organ-specific homes for metastases. Nature Reviews Cancer. 2017;**17**:302-317. DOI: 10.1038/nrc.2017.6

[172] Liu Y, Cao X. Characteristics and significance of the pre-metastatic niche. Cancer Cell. 2016;**30**:668-681. DOI: 10.1016/j.ccell.2016.09.011

[173] Psailaa B, Kaplana RN, Port ER, Lydena D. Priming the "soil" for breast cancer metastasis: The pre-metastatic niche. Breast Disease. 2006;**26**:65-74. DOI: 10.3233/bd-2007-26106

[174] Cox TR, Rumney RMH, Schoof EM, Perryman L, Høye AM, Agrawal A, et al. The hypoxic cancer secretome induces pre-metastatic bone lesions through lysyl oxidase. Nature. 2015;**522**:106-110. DOI: 10.1038/nature14492

[175] Sowder ME, Johnson RW. Bone as a preferential site for metastasis. JBMR Plus. 2019;**3**:1-10. DOI: 10.1002/jbm4.10126

[176] Zhang W, Bado IL, Hu J, Wan YW, Wu L, Wang H, et al. The bone microenvironment invigorates metastatic seeds for further dissemination. Cell. 2021;**184**:2471-2486.e20. DOI: 10.1016/j.cell.2021.03.011

[177] Fidler IJ. nrc1098 (2e). Nature Reviews of Cancer. 2003;**3**:1-6

[178] Schmidt-Kittler O, Ragg T, Daskalakis A, Granzow M, Ahr A,

Blankenstein TJF, et al. From latent disseminated cells to overt metastasis: Genetic analysis of systemic breast cancer progression. Proceedings of the National Academy of Sciences of the United States of America. n.d. Available from: www.pnas.orgcgidoi10.1073p nas.1331931100

[179] Wan L, Pantel K, Kang Y. Tumor metastasis: Moving new biological insights into the clinic. Nature Medicine. 2013;**19**:1450-1464. DOI: 10.1038/nm.3391

[180] Muscarella AM, Aguirre S, Hao X, Waldvogel SM, Zhang XHF. Exploiting bone niches: Progression of disseminated tumor cells to metastasis. Journal of Clinical Investigation. 2021;**131**(6):e143764. DOI: 10.1172/ JCI143764

[181] Mohme M, Riethdorf S, Pantel K. Circulating and disseminated tumour cells-mechanisms of immune surveillance and escape. Nature Reviews Clinical Oncology. 2017;**14**:155-167. DOI: 10.1038/nrclinonc.2016.144

[182] Bondavera A, Downey CM, Ayres F, Liu W, Boyd SK, Hallgrimsson B, et al. The lysyl oxidase inhibitor, β-aminopropionitrile, diminishes the metastatic colonization potential of circulating breast cancer cells. PLoS One. 2009;**4**(5):e5620. DOI: 10.1371/journal. pone.0005620

[183] Le MTN, Hamar P, Guo C, Basar E, Perdigão-Henriques R, Balaj L, et al. MiR-200-containing extracellular vesicles promote breast cancer cell metastasis. Journal of Clinical Investigation. 2014;**124**:5109-5128. DOI: 10.1172/JCI75695

[184] Melo SA, Sugimoto H, O'Connell JT, Kato N, Villanueva A, Vidal A, et al. Cancer exosomes perform cell-independent microRNA biogenesis and promote tumorigenesis. Cancer Cell. 2014;**26**:707-721. DOI: 10.1016/j. ccell.2014.09.005

[185] Qian B, Katsaros D, Lu L, Preti M, Durando A, Arisio R, et al. High miR-21 expression in breast cancer associated with poor disease-free survival in early stage disease and high TGF-β1. Breast Cancer Research and Treatment. 2009;**117**:131-140. DOI: 10.1007/ s10549-008-0219-7

[186] Zhao Q, Liu C, Xie Y, Tang M, Luo G, Chen X, et al. Lung cancer cells derived circulating miR-21 promotes differentiation of monocytes into osteoclasts. OncoTargets and Therapy. 2020;**13**:2643-2656. DOI: 10.2147/OTT. S232876

[187] Sugatani T, Vacher J, Hruska KA. A microRNA expression signature of osteoclastogenesis. Blood. 2011;**117**(13):3648-3657. DOI: 10.1182/ blood-2010-10-311415

[188] Yuan X, Qian N, Ling S, Li Y, Sun W, Li J, et al. Breast cancer exosomes contribute to pre-metastatic niche formation and promote bone metastasis of tumor cells. Theranostics. 2021;**11**:1429-1445. DOI: 10.7150/thno.45351

[189] Y. Kang, P.M. Siegel, W. Shu, M. Drobnjak, S.M. Kakonen, C. Cordó N-Cardo, T.A. Guise, and J. Massagué, A Multigenic Program Mediating Breast cancer Metastasis to Bone, n.d. Available from: http://www.cancercell.org/cgi/ content/full/3/6/537/DC1

[190] Zhang XHF, Wang Q, Gerald W, Hudis CA, Norton L, Smid M, et al. Latent bone metastasis in breast cancer tied to Src-dependent survival signals. Cancer Cell. 2009;**16**:67-78. DOI: 10.1016/j.ccr.2009.05.017

[191] Bidwell BN, Slaney CY, Withana NP, Forster S, Cao Y, Loi S, et al. Silencing

of Irf7 pathways in breast cancer cells promotes bone metastasis through immune escape . Nature Medicine. 2012;**18**(8): 1224-1231. DOI: 10.1038/nm.2830

[192] Fidler IJ. The pathogenesis of cancer metastasis: The "seed and soil" hypothesis revisited. Nature Reviews Cancer. 2003;**3**:453-458. DOI: 10.1038/nrc1098

[193] Kaplan RN, Rafii S, Lyden D. Preparing the "soil": The premetastatic niche. Cancer Research. 2006;**66**:11089-11093. DOI: 10.1158/0008-5472.CAN-06-2407

[194] Ali HR, Chlon L, Pharoah PDP, Markowetz F, Caldas C. Patterns of immune infiltration in breast cancer and their clinical implications: A gene-expression-based retrospective study. PLoS Medicine. 2016;**13**:1-24. DOI: 10.1371/journal.pmed.1002194

[195] DeNardo DG, Barreto JB, Andreu P, Vasquez L, Tawfik D, Kolhatkar N, et al. CD4+ T cells regulate pulmonary metastasis of mammary carcinomas by enhancing protumor properties of macrophages. Cancer Cell. 2009;**16**: 91-102. DOI: 10.1016/j.ccr.2009.06.018

[196] Michea P, Noël F, Zakine E, Czerwinska U, Sirven P, Abouzid O, et al. Adjustment of dendritic cells to the breast-cancer microenvironment is subset specific. Nature Immunology. 2018;**19**:885-897. DOI: 10.1038/s41590-018-0145-8

[197] Powell DR, Huttenlocher A. Neutrophils in the tumor microenvironment. Trends in Immunology. 2016;**37**:41-52. DOI: 10.1016/j.it.2015.11.008

[198] Palucka AK, Coussens LM. The basis of oncoimmunology. Cell. 2016;**164**:1233-1247. DOI: 10.1016/j.cell.2016.01.049

[199] DeNardo DG, Johansson M, Coussens LM. Immune cells as mediators of solid tumor metastasis. Cancer and Metastasis Reviews. 2008;**27**:11-18. DOI: 10.1007/s10555-007-9100-0

[200] Xiang L, Gilkes DM. The contribution of the immune system in bone metastasis pathogenesis. International Journal of Molecular Sciences. 2019;**20**(4):999. DOI: 10.3390/ijms20040999

[201] Doglioni G, Parik S, Fendt SM. Interactions in the (pre)metastatic niche support metastasis formation. Frontiers in Oncology. 2019;**9**:1-7. DOI: 10.3389/fonc.2019.00219

[202] Di Rosa F. T-lymphocyte interaction with stromal, bone and hematopoietic cells in the bone marrow. Immunology and Cell Biology. 2009;**87**:20-29. DOI: 10.1038/icb.2008.84

[203] Cavanagh LL, Bonasio R, Mazo IB, Halin C, Cheng G, Van Der Velden AWM, et al. NIH Public Access. 2007;**6**:1029-1037

[204] Feuerer M, Beckhove P, Garbi N, Mahnke Y, Limmer A, Hommel M, et al. Bone marrow as a priming site for T-cell responses to blood-borne antigen. Nature Medicine. 2003;**9**:1151-1157. DOI: 10.1038/nm914

[205] Peinado H, Lavotshkin S, Lyden D. The secreted factors responsible for pre-metastatic niche formation: Old sayings and new thoughts. Seminars in Cancer Biology. 2011;**21**:139-146. DOI: 10.1016/j.semcancer.2011.01.002

[206] Skirecki T, Swacha P, Hoser G, Golab J, Nowis D, Kozłowska E. Bone marrow is the preferred site of memory CD4+T cell proliferation during recovery from sepsis. JCI Insight. 2020;**5**:1-17. DOI: 10.1172/JCI.INSIGHT.134475

[207] Dalod M, Chelbi R, Malissen B, Lawrence T. Dendritic cell maturation: Functional specialization through

signaling specificity and transcriptional programming. EMBO Journal. 2014;**33**:1104-1116. DOI: 10.1002/embj.201488027

[208] Guilliams M, Dutertre CA, Scott CL, McGovern N, Sichien D, Chakarov S, et al. Unsupervised high-dimensional analysis aligns dendritic cells across tissues and species. Immunity. 2016;**45**:669-684. DOI: 10.1016/j.immuni.2016.08.015

[209] Granot T, Senda T, Carpenter DJ, Matsuoka N, Weiner J, Gordon CL, et al. Dendritic cells display subset and tissue-specific maturation dynamics over human life. Immunity. 2017;**46**:504-515. DOI: 10.1016/j.immuni.2017.02.019

[210] Balan S, Saxena M, Bhardwaj N. Dendritic Cell Subsets and Locations. International Review of Cell and Molecular Biology. 2019;**348**:1-68. DOI: 10.1016/bs.ircmb.2019.07.004

[211] Lapérine O, Blin-Wakkach C, Guicheux J, Beck-Cormier S, Lesclous P. Dendritic-cell-derived osteoclasts: A new game changer in bone-resorption-associated diseases. Drug Discovery Today. 2016;**21**:1345-1354. DOI: 10.1016/j.drudis.2016.04.022

[212] Rivollier A, Tebib J, Piperno M, Aitsiselmi T, Rabourdin-combe C, Jurdic P, et al. Immature dendritic cell transdifferentiation into osteoclasts: A novel pathway sustained by the rheumatoid arthritis microenvironment. Blood. 2004;**104**:4029-4037. DOI: 10.1182/blood-2004-01-0041.Supported

[213] Miyamoto T, Ohneda O, Arai F, Iwamoto K, Okada S, Takagi K, et al. Bifurcation of osteoclasts and dendritic cells from common progenitors. Blood. 2001;**98**:2544-2554. DOI: 10.1182/blood.V98.8.2544

[214] Speziani C, Rivollier A, Gallois A, Coury F, Mazzorana M, Azocar O, et al. Murine dendritic cell transdifferentiation into osteoclasts is differentially regulated by innate and adaptive cytokines. European Journal of Immunology. 2007;**37**:747-757. DOI: 10.1002/eji.200636534

[215] Rivollier A, Mazzorana M, Tebib J, Piperno M, Aitsiselmi T, Jurdic P, et al. Immature dendritic cell transdifferentiation into osteoclasts : A novel pathway sustained by the rheumatoid arthritis microenvironment immature dendritic cell transdifferentiation into osteoclasts: A novel pathway sustained by the rheumatoid arthritis mi. Blood. 2013;**104**:4029-4037. DOI: 10.1182/blood-2004-01-0041

[216] Scarlett UK, Rutkowski MR, Rauwerdink AM, Fields J, Escovar-Fadul X, Baird J, et al. Ovarian cancer progression is controlled by phenotypic changes in dendritic cells. The Journal of Experimental Medicine. 2012;**209**:495-506. DOI: 10.1084/jem.20111413

[217] Scrivo R, Vasile M, Bartosiewicz I, Valesini G. Inflammation as "common soil" of the multifactorial diseases. Autoimmunity Reviews. 2011;**10**:369-374. DOI: 10.1016/j.autrev.2010.12.006

[218] Madel MB, Ibáñez L, Wakkach A, De Vries TJ, Teti A, Apparailly F, et al. Immune function and diversity of osteoclasts in normal and pathological conditions. Frontiers in Immunology. 2019;**10**:1-18. DOI: 10.3389/fimmu.2019.01408

[219] Alnaeeli M, Park J, Mahamed D, Penninger JM, Teng YTA. Dendritic cells at the osteo-immune interface: Implications for inflammation-induced bone loss. Journal of Bone and Mineral Research. 2007;**22**:775-780. DOI: 10.1359/jbmr.070314

[220] Takayanagi H. New immune connections in osteoclast formation.

Annals of the New York Academy of Sciences. 2010;**1192**:117-123. DOI: 10.1111/j.1749-6632.2009.05303.x

[221] Tucci M, Stucci S, Strippoli S, Dammacco F, Silvestris F. Dendritic cells and malignant plasma cells: An alliance in multiple myeloma tumor progression? The Oncologist. 2011;**16**:1040-1048. DOI: 10.1634/theoncologist.2010-0327

[222] Chakraborty S, Kloos B, Roetz N, Schmidt S, Eigenbrod T, Kamitani S, et al. Influence of Pasteurella multocida toxin on the differentiation of dendritic cells into osteoclasts. Immunobiology. 2018;**223**:142-150. DOI: 10.1016/j.imbio.2017.09.001

[223] Monteiro AC, Bonomo A. Dendritic cells as double-agents for breast tumor pre-metastatic bone disease establishment. Journal of Clinical and Cellular Immunology. 2021;**12**:1000616

[224] Monteiro AC, Bonomo A. Dendritic cells development into osteoclast-type APCs by 4T1 breast tumor T cells milieu boost bone consumption. Bone. 2021;**143**:115755. DOI: 10.1016/j.bone.2020.115755

[225] Anderson DM, Maraskovsky E, Billingsley WL, Dougall WC, Tometsko ME, Roux ER, et al. A homologue of the TNF receptor and its ligand enhance T-cell growth and dendritic-cell function. Nature. 1997;**390**:175-179. DOI: 10.1038/36593

[226] Wong BR, Rho J, Arron J, Robinson E, Orlinick J, Chao M, et al. TRANCE is a novel ligand of the tumor necrosis factor receptor family that activates c-Jun N-terminal kinase in T cells. Journal of Biological Chemistry. 1997;**272**:25190-25194. DOI: 10.1074/jbc.272.40.25190

[227] Wong BBR, Josien R, Lee SY, Sauter B, Li H, Steinman RM, et al. Activation-induced cytokine, a new TNF family member cell—Specific survival factor. Journal of Experimental Medicine. 1997;**186**:2075-2080

[228] Ma RY, Zhang H, Li XF, Zhang CB, Selli C, Tagliavini G, et al. Monocyte-derived macrophages promote breast cancer bone metastasis outgrowth. Journal of Experimental Medicine. 2020;**217**(11):e20191820. DOI: 10.1084/JEM.20191820

[229] Monteiro AC, Bonomo A. CD8 + T cells from experimental in situ breast carcinoma interfere with bone homeostasis. Bone. 2021;**150**:116014. DOI: 10.1016/j.bone.2021.116014

Chapter 5

Perspective Chapter: Management of Bone Health in Breast Cancer Patients

Marcus Vetter, Diana Chiru and Ewelina Biskup

Abstract

Breast cancer is the most common cancer in the world. There are several implications of bone health in early and late breast cancer cases. In early breast cancer, the therapy might cause reduction of bone mineral density due to early menopause induction or as a side effect of therapy options, such as aromatase inhibitors. In late-stage breast cancer, most common site of metastasis is in the skeletal bone. Early management of bone metastasis needs special focus because of skeletal-related complications such as fractures, pain, hypercalcemia, and surgery. This chapter will focus on most common diagnostic and therapeutic measures of osseous metastasis, in early and advanced breast cancer.

Keywords: bone, osteoporosis, bone health, fracture, skeletal-related events

1. Introduction

Breast cancer is the most common cancer in women with a worldwide annual incidence of 2.3 million cases and 685,000 death per year [1]. There is a clear correlation between bone health and breast cancer [2], as bone mineral density can be severely reduced through early menopause or endocrine therapy, including aromatase inhibitors [3]. Secondly, there is also a clear relationship between osteo-oncologic treatment including densoumab and bisphosphonates and outcome in early breast cancer [4]. Thirdly, in stage IV breast cancer, bone is the most common site of metastasis [5].

Disease-specific events related to bone metastasis include complications, such as spinal cord and nerve compression and pathological fractures, needing surgical interventions and/or radiotherapy. This is therefore a major endpoint in treatment of metastatic breast cancer, since targeted therapy has the potential to significantly improve outcome in early and metastatic breast cancer [6].

This chapter will give you an overview on bone health management and prevention in early and metastatic breast cancer patients.

2. Bone remodeling

Bone remodeling is an important process in maintaining bone health, as approximately 10% of the bone is renewed every year [7]. This is a balanced process coupling bone resorption and bone formation. However, in the absence of bone formation, bone resorption continues to occur normally. This process happens with predilection in the elderly population and with even more affinity in postmenopausal women.

Bone remodeling is characterized by a succession of osteoclastic resorption of already formed bone, followed by de novo bone synthesis by osteoblasts.

Development of bone metastasis refers to a specific interaction between osteoclasts, osteoblasts, and several inflammatory modulators such as Parathyroid PTH, Parathyroid hormone-related protein PTHrP, Cyclooxygenase 2 COX-2/PEG-2, interleukins 1 and 11 (IL-1, IL11), tumor necrosis factors TNF-alpha, TGF-beta [8]. In metastatic breast cancer, osteoblasts secrete macrophage colony stimulating factor (M-CSF), which binds to c-fms, and receptor activator of nuclear factor kappa B ligand (RANKL), which binds to RANK, thus stimulating differentiation of pre-osteoclasts into osteoclasts. RANKL inhibitors can be therefore successfully used to stop osteoclastic activity [9].

3. Management of bone health in early breast cancer

The most common breast cancer subtype is luminal cancer with positive estrogen- and progesterone-receptor (ER/PR) expression. Around 50% of all human epidermal growth factor receptor 2 (HER2)-enriched subtypes also express estrogen ER and progesterone PR [10]. These hormonal receptor (HR)-positive cancers are clearly estrogen-driven malignancies; however, estrogen also has a protective effect on bone, and reduced levels can trigger bone loss. Hormonal therapy with aromatase inhibitors (AI) (usually anastrozole, exemestane, or letrozole) represents standard of care in early postmenopausal and in high-risk pre-menopausal patients. In the latter group they are usually administered in combination with a gonadotropin-releasing-hormone receptor antagonist (GnRH-A).

In the postmenopausal patients, use of aromatase inhibitors is shown to lead to a bone mineral density loss of about 2% per year, while in combination with GnRH analogues, bone mineral density loss can reach even 7% and more [11].

Real world data looked at patterns of bone loss in women with breast cancer [12]. In this particular analysis, bone mineral density of patients was significantly decreased in the lumbar spine (6.8%), followed by femoral neck (4.6%), and hip (3.5%). Bone loss seemed to be greatest in the first year.

Chemotherapy was also associated with bone loss at all sites, and the premenopausal status at moment of diagnosis was significantly associated with bone loss in the lumbar spine. No significant relationship between health behavior status and bone mineral density change could be demonstrated.

Based on different guidelines including National Comprehensive Cancer Network (NCCN), European Society of Medical Oncology (ESMO), and the Swiss SVGO (Swiss Association Against Osteoporosis), patients with early-stage breast cancer should receive comprehensive care measures focusing on bone metastasis prevention. This includes regular bone scans (DEXA Scans), life style modifications, calcium and vitamin D supplementation, and bisphosphonates.

Figure 1 demonstrates general practical guidelines in breast cancer and other cancer subtypes. Our own data [2] showed treatment adherence in only 75% of patients with breast cancer (small single center analysis).

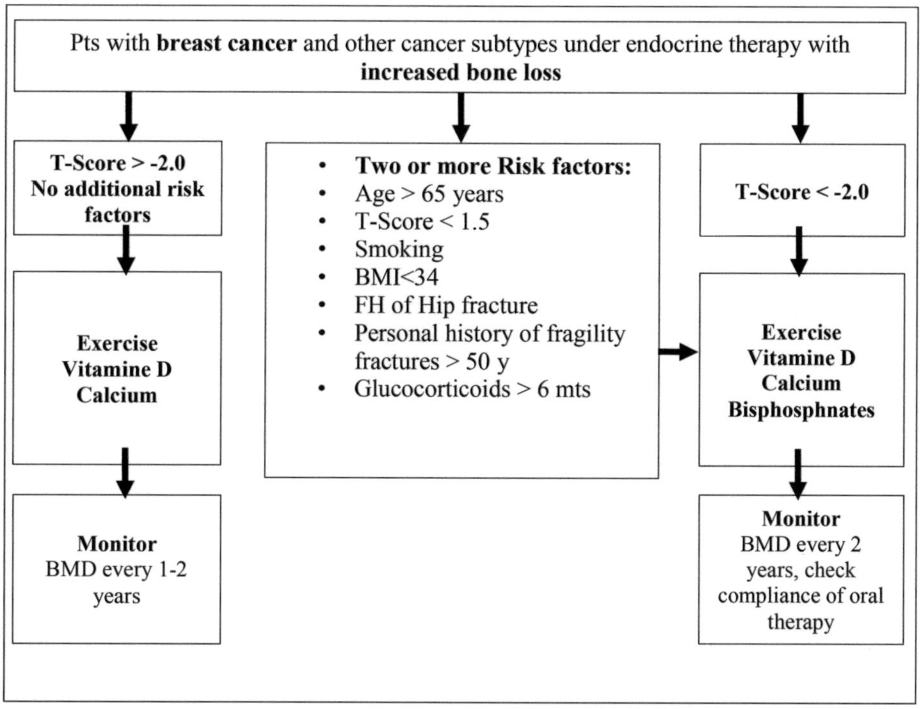

Figure 1.
Treatment recommendation for bone health in cancer patients. Demonstrated bone health guidelines for patients with breast cancer and other cancers, under endocrine therapy. Adapted from Coleman R. [13, 14].

4. Current date and use of bisphosphonates

4.1 Zoledronic acid and mode of action

Zoledronic acid is one of the nitrogen-containing antiresorptive agents, which inhibits osteoclast proliferation. Owing to the chemical similarity to inorganic pyrophosphate, zoledronic acid (and other bisphosphonates) attaches to hydroxyapatite binding sites on the osseous extracellular matrix [2, 15, 16]. The exact mechanism of apoptosis induction in osteoclasts is not fully understood. However, animal experiments have suggested that zoledronic acid inhibits specific transferases, such as geranyl transferase I inhibitor (GGTI-298), leading to loss of protein prenylation in osteoclasts, disrupting their cytoskeleton and inducing programmed death [15, 17, 18]. The main effect is reduced bone resorption, which allows for more time for bone formation and remodeling [9, 19]. It has also been hypothesized that zoledronic acid might stimulate osteoblastic differentiation and bone mineralization. Zoledronic acid seems to have the highest potential among bisphosphonates, because of its high affinity to bone, especially bones undergoing active resorption and increased turnover, such as in malignant processes [20].

4.2 Current guidelines and data on bisphosphonates

Current NCCN guidelines recommend adjuvant bisphosphonate therapy for 3–5 years in the case of menopausal patients with early stages of breast cancer, as well as in patients who recently went through menopause and who are under treatment with GnRH-A and aromatase inhibitors. In daily clinical routine, many oncologists use zoledronic acid [21].

The recently published Southwest Oncology Group (SWOG) S0307 trial was a randomized three-arm trial including more than 6000 patients, aiming to assess differences in zoledronic acid, oral clodronate, and oral ibandronate therapies. No significant difference in disease-free survival and overall survival for the three drugs was found. Authors concluded that oral bisphosphonates could be a valid option with regards to osteo-oncologic treatment [22].

In a 2017 published Cochrane analysis, data collected from more than 37,000 patients were also able to demonstrate the benefits of bisphosphonate therapy. This showed a clear survival benefit with addition of bisphosphonates for postmenopausal patients (HR 0.77, 95% CI 0.66–0.90; p = 0.001; 4 studies; 6048 women; high-quality evidence with no evidence of heterogeneity), but not for premenopausal patients (HR 1.03, 95% CI 0.86–1.22; p = 0.78; 2 studies; 3501 women; high-quality evidence with no heterogeneity) [5].

In conclusion, for women with early breast cancer, bisphosphonates were able to reduce the risk of bone metastases and provide an overall survival benefit compared to the placebo or no bisphosphonates group. There is preliminary evidence suggesting that bisphosphonates provide an overall survival and disease-free survival benefit in postmenopausal women only when compared to placebo or no bisphosphonate.

The Early Breast Cancer Clinical Trials Group (EBCCTG) designed a meta-analysis incorporating data from more than 18,000 women, derived from 26 randomized adjuvant bisphosphonate trials in breast cancer. In postmenopausal patients, there was a statistically significant reductions in the 10 years recurrence rate, (RR = 0.72, 95%, CI = 0.60–0.86, 6.6% vs. 8.8%; two-sided Pp = .0002), as well as in the breast cancer mortality rate (RR = 0.82, 95% CI = 0.73–0.93, 14.7% vs. 18.0%; two-sided p = .002) with the addition of bisphosphonates. The reduction was independent of choice of bisphosphonate therapy, estrogen receptor expression status, axillary lymph node involvement, or use of adjuvant chemotherapy [10].

5. Current data and use of Denosumab

Denosumab is a human recombinant monoclonal antibody against RANKL. Inhibition of RANKL leads to reduced maturation of preosteoclasts into osteoclasts, osteoclast survival, and activity. As a result, diminished bone resorption occurs [20].

In the Austrian Breast and Colorectal Cancer Study Group (ABCSG)-18 Study (ClinicalTrials.gov NCT00556374), 3425 postmenopausal women with early luminal breast cancer and aromatase inhibitor therapy were randomized to receive denosumab 60 mg every 6 months or placebo. The primary endpoint was occurrence of clinically relevant fractures. Secondary endpoints included disease-free survival (DFS), bone-metastasis-free survival (BMFS), and overall survival (OS). In the follow-up presented at American Society of Clinical Oncology (ASCO) 2022 with an 8-year follow-up, all clinical endpoints were positive: fractures were 201 in the denosumab and 255 in the placebo arm (HR 0.76, 95% CI 0.63–0.92, p = 0.004). The absolute 9-year DFS difference is 3.5% (79.4% vs. 75.9%, respectively). No new safety signals were presented at the meeting. The authors concluded that denosumab should be considered in routine practice for patients with early hormonal-receptor positive breast cancer [23].

DOI: http://dx.doi.org/10.5772/intechopen.109030

On the other hand, there is a very huge body of evidence that intravenous bisphosphonates improve outcome in postmenopausal women with early breast cancer. In a vast systematic meta-analysis by the *Early Breast Cancer Trialists Collaborative Group* EBCTCG including more than 18,000 patients, clear benefit was proven in regard to the overall reduction of recurrence (RR 0·94, 95% CI 0·87–1·01; 2p = 0·08), distant recurrence (0·82, 0·74–0·92; 2p = 0·0003), bone recurrence (0·72, 0·60–0·86; 2p = 0·0002), and breast cancer mortality (0·82, 0·73–0·93; 2p = 0·002) [10]. The authors were able to thus clearly demonstrate the advantages of bisphosphonate administration in postmenopausal women. Therefore, it quickly became a worldwide current standard to use bisphosphonates in management of early breast cancer, stages I–III. Current indications, dosage, and toxicity are displayed in **Table 1**.

	Bisphosphonates	**Denosumab**
Indications	Osteoporosis, hypercalcemia of malignancy, Paget's disease of bone, multiple myeloma, skeletal-related events (SRE) associated with metastatic bone disease in breast (and other) cancers, adjuvant therapy for postmenopausal breast cancer patients and potentially also in premenopausal patients	Unresectable giant cell tumor of bone in adults and skeletally mature adolescents; to increase bone mass in patients at high risk for fracture including ADT for non- metastatic prostate cancer or adjuvant AI therapy for breast cancer, prevention of SREs in patients with bone metastases from solid tumors, treatment of postmenopausal women with osteoporosis at high risk for fracture [24]
Dosing	Clodronate 1600 mg p.o. daily for 3–9 mo., Pamidronate 300–360 mg p.o. for 18–2 mo. or 45 mg i.v. until progression, 90 mg iv every 28 d for 12–24 mo. Zoledronic acid 4 mg i.v. every 28 d for 12 mo. Ibandronate 6 mg i.v. every 28 d or 50 mg p.o. daily	60 mg administered as a single subcutaneous injection once every 6 months, for osteoporosis [25]
Side effects	Acute-phase-like reaction, renal toxicity, osteonecrosis of the jaw	Acute-phase-like reaction, renal toxicity, osteonecrosis of the jaw
Supplementation of calcium and vitamin D	Vitamin D and calcium supplements must not be routinely given during bisphosphonate administration (supplementation may increase the bone resorption and decrease the efficacy of bisphosphonates). Consider vitamin D supplementation in people with, or at risk of, vitamin D deficiency. Consider calcium supplements if patient's dietary intake is low.	At least 500 mg calcium and 400 IU vitamin D daily
Monitoring	Serum creatinine prior to each dose, regular dental examinations, electrolytes/hematocrit/ hemoglobin	Electrolytes (incl. Phosphate and magnesium), signs of infections or skin rash, regular dental examinations

SRE = skeletal-related events, ADT = androgen deprivation therapy; AI = aromatase inhibitor; i.v. = intravenous; p.o. = oral; mo = months.

Table 1.
Indication, dosing, and toxicity of bone-targeted agents (adapted from Biskup [1, 20]).

6. Management of metastatic disease in breast cancer

Breast cancer can be in many cases, cured today, but around 20% of patients will experience recurrence in the first 10 years of follow-up. Late recurrence is possible and is depends on many factors such as biology and anatomic stage. Bone metastasis is the most common site of metastasis followed by lung, liver, and lymph nodes, in all breast cancer subtypes.

In advanced breast cancer, 60–80% of patients will develop bone metastasis [5]. Complications are mostly related to skeletal bone and refer mostly to pathological

Regime	N	Outcome	Toxicity	Literature
i.v. pamidronate vs. Placebo q3–4 wks., 2y	382	SRE at 2 years 50 vs. 70% p < 0.001 Median time to SRE 13.9 vs. 7 mo.	Arthralgia, flu-like syndrome	[19, 28, 29]
Clodronate 1/d vs. placebo for 18 mo.	173	SRE 218.6 vs. 304.8 per 100 pts. y, p < 0.001 Vertebral fractures 84 vs. 124 per 100 pts. y, p < 0.025, No OS difference	No difference	[12, 30]
Oral ibandronate vs. placebo up to 96 wks.	564 Pooled Analysis	Number of events per pts. 1.15 vs. 1.85, p = 0.008 Risk reduction for SRE = HR 0.62 (95% CI 0.48–0.79, p < 0.001), Death 20% vs. 15% NS for pain, time to progression	Any AE 94 vs. 95% Drug related AE 26 vs. 17% Hypocalcemia 9.4% vs. 5.1%	[3, 31]
Zoledronic acid vs. i.v. pamidronate for 12 mts (in BC, MM)	1130 (BC)	SRE at 13 mo. 44% vs. 46% Skeletal morbidity rate 1.13 vs. 1.08 events/y/NS	Bone pain 49% vs. 59%	[29, 32]
Ibandronate p.o. vs. zoledronic acid i.v. q 3–4 weeks for 96 weeks	1401	SRE 42% vs. 41% (HR 1.15, 95% CI 0.97–1.62) Median time for SRE 97 vs. 99 wks. Median OS 111 vs. 113 wks.	Dyspepsia 35 vs. 25% Hypocalcemia 11 vs. 11% Renal impairment 24 vs. 32% ONJ 5 vs. 9 events	[25, 33]
SC denosumab and i.v. placebo vs. i.v. zoledronic acid 4 mg and SC placebo q 4 wks.	2046 (BC)	Delay time to SRE HR 0.82 (95% CI 0.71–0.95, p < 0.001) Risk of multiple SRE HR 0.77 (95% CI 0.66–0.89, p < 0.001) OS: HR = 0.95 (95% CI 0.81–1.11, NS) Disease progression: HR = 1.00, (95% CI 0.89–1.11, NS) Quality of life effect: in the denosumab group, 10% more patients had a clinically meaningful improvement	AE leading to discontinuation 9.6 vs. 12.3% Serious AE 44.4 vs. 46.5% Pyrexia 16.7 vs. 24.4% ONJ 2 vs. 1.4%	[1, 24]

BC = breast cancer, i.v. = intravenous, MM = multiple myeloma, mo. = months, NS = Not significant, ONJ = Osteonecrosis of the jaw, AE = adverse effects, OS = Overall survival, pts. = patients, SRE = Skeletal-related events, wks. = weeks, y = years.

Table 2.
Clinical trials of bisphosphonates in the metastatic setting.

fractures, major surgery, radiotherapy, and spinal cord and nerve compression symptoms. This leads to loss of quality of life, pain, and increased health costs.

Hypercalcemia is, among others, a severe manifestation of metastatic disease or para-neoplastic events in breast cancer patients, related to high mortality risk. It is considered oncologic emergency requiring rapid evaluation and treatment.

Bone metastases are diagnosed through imaging, such as CT scan, MRI, PET-CT, and nuclear bone scans [26, 27]. A biopsy is usually required to confirm diagnosis and can help determine the immunohistochemical assay. Analysis of sampled bone biopsy needs more time because of preparation, which includes decalcification of the bone. Therefore, many oncologists will collect biopsies from different organs, e.g., liver, soft tissue, or lung. The receptor conversion rate (estrogen, progesterone and HER2 status) in bone metastases is much lower than in liver metastases. And this should be taken into consideration when deciding treatment options. For patients with breast cancer bone metastasis, this includes HER2-directed, endocrine-directed, and chemotherapy options.

Established as standard of care more than 20 years ago, bisphosphonates still remain a go-to drug for many oncologists in the daily clinical setting. Initial trials demonstrated reduction of skeletal-bone-related events, including, but not limited to, pain, as well as quality of life improvement for oncologic patients (See **Table 2**) [34–37].

Traditionally, standard application of zoledronic acid referred to dosing every 4 weeks, but newer trials showed that a deescalation to a 12 weekly based regime is as feasible and did not worsen outcome.

7. Summary and conclusion

Bone health is an important topic in early and advanced breast cancer. Bisphosphonates have been established in management of metastatic disease since more than 20 years ago and have shown to clearly improve the outcome in patients with bone metastasis. Since 2010, denosumab, an RANKL antibody, was also accepted and adopted as standard of care in patients with metastatic breast cancer and bone metastasis. Both options significantly reduce skeletal-bone-related complications and are important therapeutic agents considered in metastatic breast cancer cases.

In early stages of breast cancer, bisphosphonates should be used in postmenopausal women for improved outcome (recurrence risk and bone health including prevention of osteoporosis) [14].

However, patients should be informed, before treatment initiation with these agents, about possible side effects including osteonecrosis of the jaw (ONJ), pain, and flu-like symptoms.

Nowadays, bisphosphonates and denosumab are internationally recognized as part of standard practice in breast cancer treatment, and every physician should be aware of their indications, therapy regimens, and possible complications.

Author details

Marcus Vetter[1*], Diana Chiru[2] and Ewelina Biskup[3,4]

1 Cancer Center Baselland, Medical University Clinic, Liestal, Switzerland

2 Department of Internal Medicine, Cantonal Hospital Baselland, Medical University Clinic, Liestal, Switzerland

3 Shanghai University of Medicine and Health Sciences Affiliated to Jiaotong University School of Medicine, Shanghai, China

4 University Hospital, Basel, Switzerland

*Address all correspondence to: marcus.vetter@ksbl.ch

References

[1] Biskup E, Cai F, Vetter M. Bone targeted therapies in advanced breast cancer. Swiss Medical Weekly. 2017;**147**:w14440

[2] Bischof E, Schwab FD, Georgescu Margarint EL, Montavon C, Zünti I, Schollbach A, et al. Adherence to bone health guidelines in patients with hormone receptor-positive early breast cancer: Status and clinical impact in a Swiss cohort experience. Bone Reports. 2021;**16**:101160

[3] Body JJ, Diel IJ, Lichinitzer M, Lazarev A, Pecherstorfer M, Bell R, et al. Oral ibandronate reduces the risk of skeletal complications in breast cancer patients with metastatic bone disease: Results from two randomized, placebo-controlled phase III studies. British Journal of Cancer. 2004;**90**(6):1133-1137

[4] Du Y, Cullum I, Illidge TM, Ell PJ. Fusion of metabolic function and morphology: Sequential [18F] fluorodeoxyglucose positron-emission tomography/computed tomography studies yield new insights into the natural history of bone metastases in breast cancer. Journal of Clinical Oncology. 2007;**25**(23):3440-3447. DOI: 10.1200/JCO.2007.11.2854 Epub 2007 Jun 25

[5] Diana A, Carlino F, Giunta EF, Franzese E, Guerrera LP, Di Lauro V, et al. Cancer treatment-induced bone loss (CTIBL): State of the art and proper Management in Breast Cancer Patients on endocrine therapy. Current Treatment Options in Oncology. 2021;**22**(5):45. DOI: 10.1007/s11864-021-00835-2

[6] Early Breast Cancer Trialists' Collaborative Group (EBCTCG)*. Adjuvant bisphosphonate treatment in early breast cancer: meta-analyses of individual patient data from randomized trials, Gnant M, Pfeiler G, Dubsky PC, Hubalek M, Greil R, et al. Adjuvant denosumab in breast cancer (ABCSG-18): A multicentre, randomised, double-blind, placebo-controlled trial. Lancet. 2015;**386**(9992):433-443

[7] Gralow JR, Barlow WE, Paterson AHG, M'iao JL, Lew DL, Stopeck AT, et al. Phase III randomized trial of bisphosphonates as adjuvant therapy in breast cancer: S0307. Journal of the National Cancer Institute. 2020;**112**(7):698-707

[8] Hortobagyi GN, Theriault RL, Lipton A, Porter L, Blayney D, Sinoff C, et al. Long-term prevention of skeletal complications of metastatic breast cancer with pamidronate. Protocol 19 Aredia 9. Breast cancer study group. Journal of Clinical Oncology. 1998;**16**(6):2038-2044

[9] Irelli A, Cocciolone V, Cannita K, Zugaro L, Di Staso M, Lanfiuti Baldi P, et al. Bone targeted therapy for preventing skeletal-related events in metastatic breast cancer. Bone. 2016;**87**:169-175. DOI: 10.1016/j.bone.2016.04.006 Epub 2016 Apr 26

[10] Kim SH, Cho YU, Kim SJ, Han MS. Changes in bone mineral density in women with breast cancer: A prospective cohort study. Cancer Nursing. 2019;**42**(2):164-172

[11] O'Carrigan B, Wong MH, Willson ML, Stockler MR, Pavlakis N, Goodwin A. Bisphosphonates and other bone agents for breast cancer. Cochrane Database of Systematic Reviews. 2017;**10**(10):CD003474

[12] Paterson AH, Powles TJ, Kanis JA, McCloskey E, Han-son J, Ashley S. Double-blind controlled trial of oral clodronate in patients with bone

metastases from breast cancer. Journal of Clinical Oncology. 1993;**11**(1):59-65

[13] Eisen A, Somerfield MR, AccordinoMK,BlanchettePS,ClemonsMJ, Dhesy-Thind S, et al. Use of Adjuvant Bisphosphonates and Other Bone-Modifying Agents in Breast Cancer: ASCO-OH (CCO) Guideline Update. Journal of Clinical Oncology. 2022;**40**(7):787-800. DOI: 10.1200/JCO.21.02647

[14] Coleman R, Body JJ, Aapro M, Hadji P, Herrstedt J. On behalf of the ESMO guidelines working group bone health in cancer patients: ESMO clinical practice guidelines. Annals of Oncology. 2014;**25**(S3):iii124-iiii37. DOI: 10.1093/annonc/mdu103

[15] Scheid V, Buzdar AU, Smith TL, Hortobagyi GN. Clinical course of breast cancer patients with osseous me- tastasis treated with combination chemotherapy. Cancer. 1986;**58**(12):2589-2593

[16] Siegel RL, Miller KD, Fuchs HE, Jemal A. Cancer statistics, 2022. CA: a Cancer Journal for Clinicians. 2022;**72**(1):7-33. DOI: 10.3322/caac.21708

[17] Rachner TD, Coleman R, Hadji P, Hofbauer LC. Bone health during endocrine therapy for cancer. The Lancet Diabetes and Endocrinology. 2018;**6**(11):901-910. DOI: 10.1016/S2213-8587(18)30047-0

[18] Gnant M, Pfeiler G, Dubsky PC, Hubalek M, Greil R, Jakesz R, et al. Austrian breast and colorectal cancer study group. Adjuvant denosumab in breast cancer (ABCSG-18): A multicentre, randomised, double-blind, placebo-controlled trial. Lancet. 2015;**386**(9992):433-443

[19] Siddiqui JA, Partridge NC. Physiological bone remodeling: Systemic regulation and growth factor involvement. Physiology (Bethesda, Md.). 2016;**31**(3):233-245. DOI: 10.1152/physiol.00061.2014

[20] Chen YC, Sosnoski DM, Mastro AM. Breast cancer metastasis to the bone: Mechanisms of bone loss. Breast Cancer Research. 2010;**12**(6):215. DOI: 10.1186/bcr2781

[21] Boyce BF, Xing L. Functions of RANKL/RANK/OPG in bone modeling and remodeling. Archives of Biochemistry and Biophysics. 2008;**473**(2):139-146. DOI: 10.1016/j.abb.2008.03.018

[22] Harbeck N, Gnant M. Breast cancer. Lancet. 2017;**389**(10074):1134-1150. DOI: 10.1016/S0140-6736(16)31891-8

[23] Russell RGG. Bisphosphonates: Mode of action and pharmacology. Pediatrics. 2007;**119**(Suppl. 2):S150-S162. DOI: 10.1542/peds.2006-2023H

[24] Stopeck AT, Lipton A, Body JJ, Steger GG, Tonkin K, de Boer RH, et al. Denosumab compared with zoledronic acid for the treatment of bone metastases in patients with advanced breast cancer: A randomized, double-blind study. Journal of Clinical Oncology. 2010;**28**(35):5132-5139

[25] Barrett-Lee P, Casbard A, Abraham J, Hood K, Coleman R, Simmonds P, et al. Oral ibandronic acid versus intravenous zoledronic acid in treatment of bone metastases from breast cancer: A randomized, open label, non-inferiority phase 3 trial. The Lancet Oncology. 2014;**15**(1):114-122

[26] Rogers MJ, Frith JC, Luckman SP, Coxon FP, Benford HL, Mönkkönen J, et al. Molecular mechanisms of action of bisphosphonates. Bone. 1999;**24** (Suppl. 5):73S-79S. DOI: 10.1016/S8756-3282(99)00070-8

[27] Roelofs AJ, Ebetino FH, Reszka AA, Russell RGG, Rogers MJ. Chapter 81 - Bisphosphonates: Mechanisms of action. Principles of Bone Biology (Third Edition) [Internet]. 2008;**2**:1737-1767. DOI: 10.1016/B978-0-12-373884-4.00095-1

[28] Coxon FP, Helfrich MH, Van't Hof R, Sebti S, Ralston SH, Hamilton A, et al. Protein geranylgeranylation is required for osteoclast formation, function, and survival: Inhibition by bisphosphonates and GGTI-298. Journal of Bone and Mineral Research. 2000;**15**(8):1467-1476. DOI: 10.1359/jbmr.2000.15.8.1467

[29] Rosen LS, Gordon DH, Dugan W Jr, Major P, Eisenberg PD, Provencher L, et al. Zoledronic acid is superior to pamidronate for the treatment of bone metastases in breast carcinoma patients with at least one osteolytic lesion. Cancer. 2004;**100**(1):36-43

[30] Roodman GD. Cell biology of the osteoclast. Experimental Hematology. 1999;**27**(8):1229-1241. DOI: 10.1016/S0301-472X(99)00061-2

[31] Diel IJ. Bisphosphonates in breast cancer patients with bone metastases. Breast Care (Basel). 2010;**5**(5):306-311. DOI: 10.1159/000322043

[32] Green JR. Chemical and biological prerequisites for novel bisphosphonate molecules: Results of comparative preclinical studies. Seminars in Oncology. 2001;**28**(2, Suppl. 6):4-10. DOI: 10.1016/S0093-7754(01)90259-3

[33] Boissier S, Ferreras M, Peyruchaud O, Magnetto S, Ebetino FH, Colombel M, et al. Bisphosphonates inhibit breast and prostate carcinoma cell invasion, an early event in the formation of bone metastases. Cancer Research. 2000;**60**(11):2949-2954

[34] O'Carrigan B, Wong MHF, Wilson ML, Stockler MR, Pavlakis N, Goodwin A. Bisphosphonates and other bone agents for breast cancer. Cochrane Database of Systemic Reviews. 2017;**10**:CD003474. DOI: 10.1002&14651858.CD003474.pub4

[35] Early Breast Cancer Trialists' Collaborative Group (EBCTCG). Adjuvant bisphosphonate treatment in early breast cancer: Meta-analyses of individual patient data from randomised trials. The Lancet. 2015;**386**(10001):1353-1361. DOI: 10.1016/S0140-6736(15)60908-4

[36] Gnant M, Frantal S, Pfeiler G, Steger GG, Egle D, Greil R, et al. Long-term outcomes of adjuvant denosumab in breast cancer: Fracture reduction and survival results from 3,425 patients in the randomised, double-blind, placebo-controlled ABCSG-18 trial. Journal of Clinical Oncology. 2022;**40**(16_suppl):507. DOI: 10.1200/JCO.2022.40.16_suppl.507 507

[37] Hamaoka T, Madewell JE, Podoloff DA, Hortobagyi GN, Ueno NT. Bone imaging in metastatic breast cancer. Journal of Clinical Oncology. 2004;**22**(14):2942-2953. DOI: 10.1200/JCO.2004.08.181

Section 3

Sarcomas and Blastomas

Chapter 6

Perspective Chapter: Osteosarcomas of the Head and Neck

Ingrid Plass

Abstract

Osteosarcomas of the head and neck (HNOS) are an infrequent disease, representing less than 10% of all osteosarcomas and 1% of all head and neck cancers. However, they exhibit a different clinical behavior and natural history than extremities osteosarcomas (OS), therefore requiring a specific study and analysis. Specifically, in head and neck sites, OS have shown a different presentation age, reduced likelihood of distant metastases, and a severely higher local recurrence rates. This may be due to the difficulties in ensuring wide negative margins, given the multiple vital structures surrounding tumors in this particular region. This singular features render HNOS a different prognosis and prognostic factors, becoming a topic that should be assessed independently, as they may need a different treatment approach than osteosarcomas of the trunk or extremities.

Keywords: osteosarcoma, jaw osteosarcoma, head and neck, mandible osteosarcoma, head and neck cancer, head and neck sarcomas, chemotherapy, radiotherapy, oncologic surgery, reconstructive surgery

1. Introduction

Osteosarcomas (OS) are the most frequent primary malignant tumor arising in the bone, formed by neoplastic cells that synthesize and secrete organic components of the bone matrix, which may or may not be mineralized [1]. It usually affects long bones, occurring in the craniofacial area in only 6–10% of cases and accounting for less than 1% of all head and neck cancers [2–5]. However, it has a unique clinical behavior, different from OS in other parts of the body, which grants head and neck osteosarcoma (HNOS) a distinctive prognosis. This makes it a subject that should be reviewed separately. However, given its infrequency, the evidence we have on the subject is scarce, mostly based on retrospective studies and case series, and most of its management approaches are extrapolations of the treatment established for long bones OS.

2. Epidemiology

OS itself is a rare tumor, accounting for less than 1% of all cancers diagnosed annually in the United States [4], and osteosarcomas presenting on the head and neck region are even more uncommon, with incidence approximately of 2–3 per million persons per year [6].

In addition, OSHN has specific demographic characteristics at diagnosis.

While the peak incidence of extremity osteosarcomas occurs during adolescence, HNOS generally presents at a later age, albeit with significant variability. According to different series, HNOS usually presents between the third and fourth decade of life, with a wide range. Kassier et al. [7], for example, in a meta-analysis of non-randomized studies between 1980 and 1994 with 173 patients, report a median age of presentation of 36 years, with a range from 5 to 78 years. Smith et al. [8], in a review of the US National Cancer Database (NCDB) cancer registry, with 496 patients diagnosed with HNOS between 1985 and 1996, describes a median age at presentation of 38 years, with 41% of patients aged 30–60 years, 35% younger than 30 years, and 24% older than 60 years. In this study, it is also noteworthy that the age at presentation was strikingly lower in men than in women (34 vs. 44 years respectively, $p < 0.001$). Finally, in a study conducted by Lee et al. [9], published in 2015, using the Surveillance, Epidemiology and End Results (SEER) cancer registry database to determine the epidemiology and prognostic factors associated with osteosarcoma of the jaw (OSJ), with 541 patients (1973–2011), reported an age at presentation with a median age of 41 years and a range of 0–91 years [9]. Furthermore, the demographic distribution of this study showed 75% where white, 17% African-American, and 8% other races, and in terms of gender as a risk factor, in these two large cohorts, the sex distribution was equal, with a 1:1 ratio [8, 9].

Regarding the clinical subsite, HNOS affects the jaw in more than 80% of cases, with the mandible usually being the most common site [10, 11]. In the mandibular region, it frequently involves the mandibular body and ramus, and in the maxilla, the upper alveolar ridge, maxillary sinus floor, or hard palate. In fact, in a study by Guadagnolo et al. [10] from MD Anderson, with 119 cases of craniofacial OS, they observed 45% mandibular OS, disease in the mandible, 40% maxilla, calvarium 5%; paranasal sinuses 2%, hard palate, 2%; mastoid, 2%; skull base, 1%; zygoma, 1%; infratemporal fossa, 1%; and cervical soft tissues 1%. However, some series report a slightly higher percentage in the skull and facial bones, as in the Smith et al. [8] analysis of the NCDB where the majority of patients (55.6%) had HNOS of the skull and facial bones, and HNOS of the mandible accounted for 38.9%. Approximately 5% of patients had HNOS tumors in the other subsites, which included the soft tissues of the head and neck, parotid gland, the nasopharynx, and the tongue [8]. Likewise, in the SEER series by Lee et al. [9], the distribution of HNOS was 55.6% in the skull or facial bones and 44.4% in the mandible [9].

3. Risk factors

As for the risk factors described, genetic predisposition of young patients with some specific genetic syndromes has been evidenced:

3.1 Syndromes associated with germline mutations in tumor suppressor genes

- Sd. Li-Fraumeni (p53): autosomal dominant disorder involving a germline mutation of the p53 tumor suppressor gene. Affected individuals may suffer from breast cancers, soft-tissue sarcomas, central nervous system malignancies, leukemia, and adrenocortical carcinomas [11]

- Retinoblastoma (Rb1, 13q14 deletion) [11]. Huber et al. in a retrospective analysis of 14 patients between 1974 and 1999, reported four patients (28.6%) with this history, with an average latency of 9 years (range 3–15 years) for OSHN [12].

3.2 Syndromes associated with germline DNA helicase mutations

- Rothmund Thomas Syndrome: a recessive autonomic genodermatoses presenting with characteristic facial erythema (poikiloderma), short stature due to intrauterine and postnatal growth retardation, sparse hair, eyebrows and eyelashes, juvenile cataracts, skeletal anomalies, radial axis defects, premature aging, and predisposition to certain cancers, including OSHN.

- Werner syndrome: a rare autosomal disorder characterized by features of premature aging that appears in the third decade of life. This disorder is known to present with bilateral cataracts, short stature, graying and thinning of scalp hair, characteristic skin disorders, and increased incidence of specific tumors, including HNOS [13, 14].

- Sd. Bloom: a rare disorder associated with prenatal and postnatal growth deficiency, an erythematous telangiectatic rash on the face and other sun-exposed areas, insulin resistance, and predisposition to early-onset and recurrent cancer in multiple organ systems.

3.3 Other risk factors

Association with different bone dysplasias has also been documented: fibrous dysplasia, Paget's dysplasia, and enchondromatosis [11].

- Fibrous dysplasia: a bone embryonic disorder in which normal bone is replaced with a mixture of immature fibrous tissue and small fragments of immature trabecular bone. The fibrous tissue proliferates within the bone marrow, compresses the cortex from the inside, and produces the expansion that characterizes the disease.

- Paget Disease: relatively common metabolic bone disorder characterized by increased rate of bone turnover, with increased bone resorption and deposition, resulting in cortical and trabecular thickening. Clinically it presents as progressive bone deformities, growth problems, fractures, vertebral collapse, increased skull size, and sensorineural hearing loss. The incidence of osteosarcoma secondary to Paget's disease is not known, but it is estimated to be about 1%. This association accounts for about half of the osteosarcomas reported in elderly patients [13].

- Enchondromatosis: also known as Ollier disease, it is a rare sporadic nonhereditary skeletal disorder with development of multiple enchondromas distributed predominantly unilaterally or asymmetrically in the metaphyses of the long bones.

Additionally, HNOS has also been associated with trauma, bone infarcts, and chronic osteomyelitis [13].

Finally, one of the most strongly associated factors is a history of previous radiotherapy. In fact, Patel et al. [15] reported on 44 patients treated at Memorial Sloan-Kettering Cancer Center between 1981 and 1998: six patients (15%) had a history of previous radiotherapy. Different authors describe that this would be mainly for patients who received radiotherapy for leukemia or lymphoma, but no correlation has been found with respect to low-dose radiation received for diagnostic medical tests [13]. In a cohort study from Massachusetts general hospital [16], with 47 patients, prior radiation to the head or neck was documented in 27% of subjects and was statistically associated with decreased overall survival on univariate analysis (p = .01).

In parallel, it is important to consider the epidemiology of the place where we are observing the OS cases. For example, in a Chinese series reported by Luo et al. [17] in 2019, with 37 patients with HNOS, 43% of them had a history of previous radiotherapy for Nasopharyngeal Ca, given that the latter is an endemic disease in that country.

4. Clinical presentation

Clinical signs and symptoms will depend on the location of the tumor, its size, and growth rate. The vast majority of patients, up to 70–75%, present with local swelling, associated with pain in more than one-third of patients. This may be followed by facial dysesthesia in about 30% and loose teeth in about 15% [13, 16]. In fact, in Patel's et al. [15] series, up to 27% had infraorbital nerve paresis (V2). Other manifestations include trismus, nasal obstruction or epistaxis, and/or headache, depending on their subsite.

HNOS are tumors that usually report rapid growth, and on average the time of presentation at consultation is 2–6 months [15].

Physical examination usually identifies a non-painful mass, fixed to the underlying bone, and it is important to note that the mucosa and superficial soft tissue may be normal or with some very slight alteration. The size can be variable, from an initial tumor, as seen in **Figure 1**, showing a patient from our institution who consulted with a relatively small swelling in right maxillary, hard, with bony consistency, in which we can see a slight irritation of the mucosa, to an obvious enlargement and bone

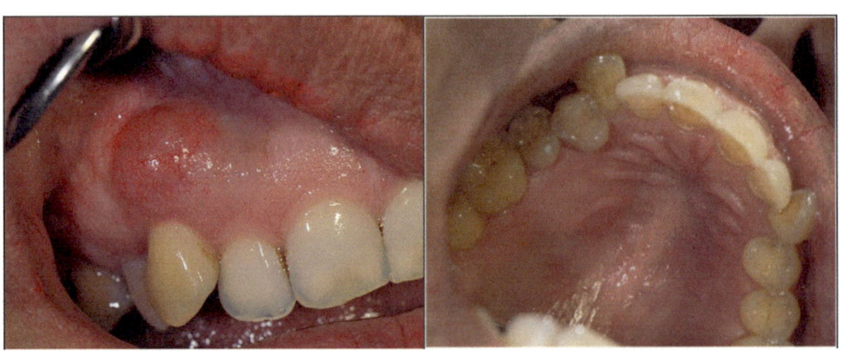

Figure 1.
Initial presentation of a 35-year-old female patient with a maxillary osteosarcoma.

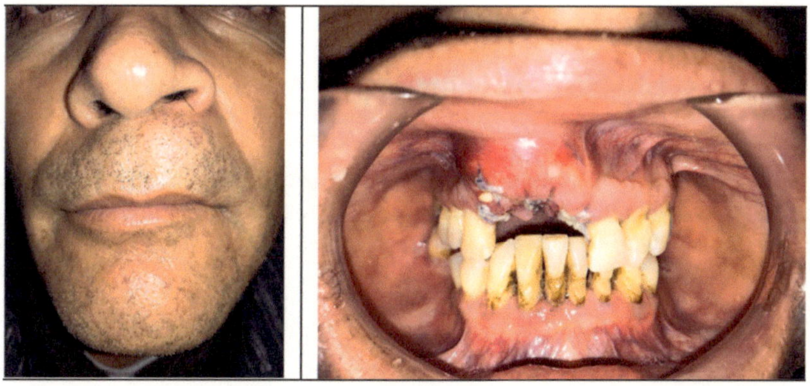

Figure 2.
Locally advanced maxillary osteosarcoma on a 48-year-old male.

destruction, as we see on **Figure 2**, with a patient with significant involvement of the maxillary bone and adjacent soft tissue.

In fact, in Guadagnolo's et al. cohort [10], the median tumor size at presentation was 5.5 cm with a range between 1 and 15 cm. However, large series [8] report tumors smaller than 6 cm in 79%, with the majority being between 3 and 6 cm (41–44%), with no significant differences according to anatomic site. According to Granowski-LeCornu et al. [16], increasing tumor size was associated with decreased overall survival (P = .0167).

In addition, although HNOS patients present normally with tumors in the described size ranges, it is necessary to take into account that they are fast-growing tumors, as we see in **Figure 3** showing mandibular OS of the left retromolar trigone at presentation (**Figure 3a**) and its growth in 3 weeks from the first consultation (**Figure 3b**).

As part of the physical examination, the evaluation of possible cervical adenopathies is mandatory; however, locoregional lymph node involvement in these patients is very unusual [11].

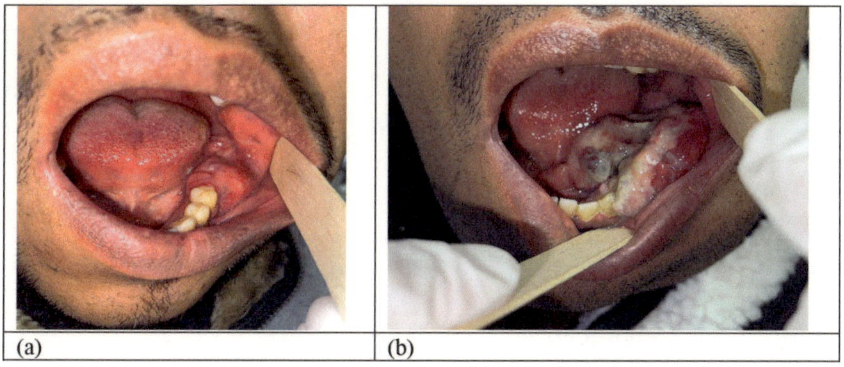

Figure 3.
A 27-year-old male patient with osteosarcoma of the left mandible. (a) Patient on first consult and (b) same patient 3 weeks later.

5. Diagnosis

The diagnosis of HNOS is based on radiological and pathological findings. Most tumors arise within the medullary cavity of the affected bone, with rare examples developing on the bone surface [1].

It constitutes a diagnostic challenge due to its rare occurrence, diverse clinical presentation, and the fact that typical radiological features may not always be present, which can often lead to misinterpretation of lesions or delay in diagnosis.

5.1 Imaging tests

Specific features have been described for these bone tumors on radiographs, CT, and MRI scans.

The effort in the evaluation of HNOS imaging should focus on searching for specific radiological features that may point to the diagnosis of HNOS, assessing bone involvement and destruction, evaluating the extent of adjacent soft tissue involvement, and ensuring the resectability of the tumor. And finally, but most importantly, looking for possible distant disease, especially pulmonary metastases. An initial diagnosis of HNOS should be considered when tumors with matrix mineralization are present early in the fourth decade of life.

The radiologic appearance of HNOS depends on the interplay of three processes: bone formation and mineralization, bone destruction, and periosteal bone formation. On plain radiography, an ill-defined radiolucent lesion is usually seen. Early tumors may show a symmetrical widening of the periodontal membrane space about one or more teeth (**Figure 4**). Indeed, Lindquist et al. reported that the widening of periodontal ligament space and inferior dental canal, together with sunburst effect, is almost pathognomonic of osteosarcoma of jaw bone [17]. **Figure 4** shows X-rays of the patient presented in **Figure 1**.

CT and MRI both have their own superiorities in detecting osteosarcoma, and the combination of CT and MRI has proven to improve the diagnostic accuracy for patients suffering from HNOS. Key points that are important when analyzing a CT and MRI scan for a possible HNOS are summarized below.

On CT, key points include assessing:

- The extent of bone involvement and pattern of bone destruction (lytic/mixed or sclerotic lesions).
- Cortical evaluation and periosteal reaction, which can be aggressive (e.g., lamellar or spiculated) vs. non-aggressive or none.
- Presence of matrix mineralization (identification of high density osteoid matrix).
- Tumor size and tumor margins (well or ill-defined)
- Possible presence of prior bone disease.
- Evaluation of possible distant metastasis (mainly lung).

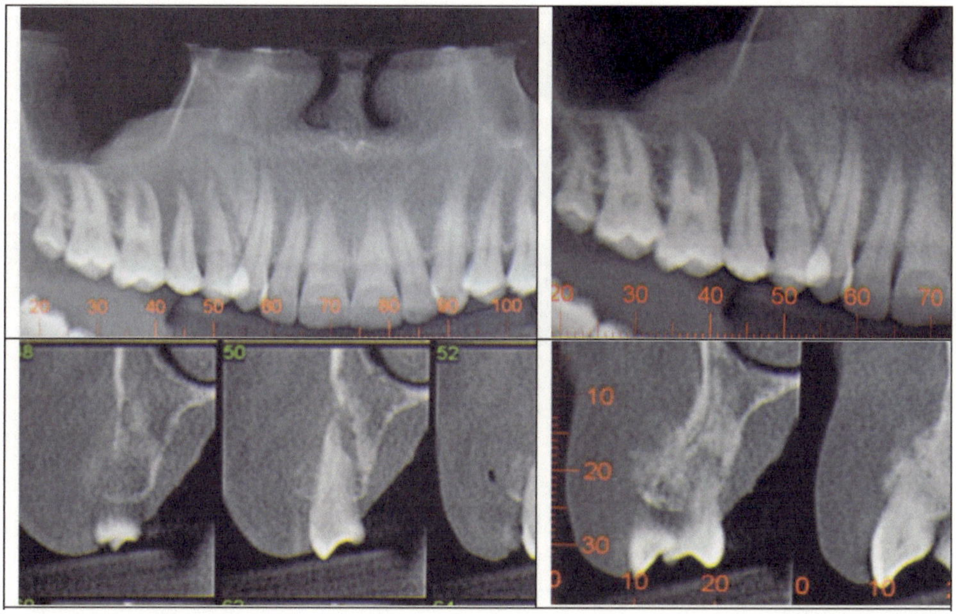

Figure 4.
Radiographic imaging of patient showed in **Figure 1***, a 35-year-old female with a maxillary osteosarcoma.*

HNOS primarily exhibits osteolysis and/or osteoblastic destruction, as well as having an irregular tumor margin on CT imaging. According to Luo et al. [18], in CT, more than 97% of patients have some degree of bone destruction, presenting lytic (43%), sclerotic (19%), or mixed lytic-sclerotic (35%) lesions, with or without soft tissue involvement (**Figure 5**). The mixed and sclerotic radiological pattern in the head and neck region is highly suggestive of osteosarcoma, with differential diagnosis of metastasis, lymphoma, and chondrosarcoma (**Figure 5**). In purely lytic lesions, the diagnosis can be difficult, as osteosarcomas that mimic hollow areas without new bone formation cannot be differentiated from metastatic disease radiographically. For HNOS, primary features are local or patchy high-density shadows in the medullary cavity with varying degrees of bone destruction and matrix mineralization. In the series of Luo et al., matrix mineralization was present in (86.5%), and high-density osteoid matrix is found in 86% of lesions [15].

It is important to evaluate the cortical, as it can be invaded and eroded by the tumor, which extends into the soft tissues, frequently eliciting a periosteal reaction. The pattern of periosteal reaction can be classified as aggressive or non-aggressive according to Rana et al. [19]. Aggressive reactions include laminated, spiculated (hair-on end, sunburst), disorganized, or Codman triangle reaction patterns, while non-aggressive periosteal reactions include thin, solid, thickly irregular, or septated patterns. Up to 70–87% of the cases have an aggressive periostic reaction [1, 15]. However, sometimes, the tumor grows expanding the bone but without violating the cortex, or it can have a homogeneously radiodense surface, well demarcated from the soft tissues, resembling an osteoma, which may hinder diagnostic suspicion. In the extremities, the Codman triangle signifies subperiosteal bone formation. This feature is less frequent in the head and neck, where the classic "sunburst" appearance of malignant osteoid formation is observed, forming radiopaque striations arising from the tumor.

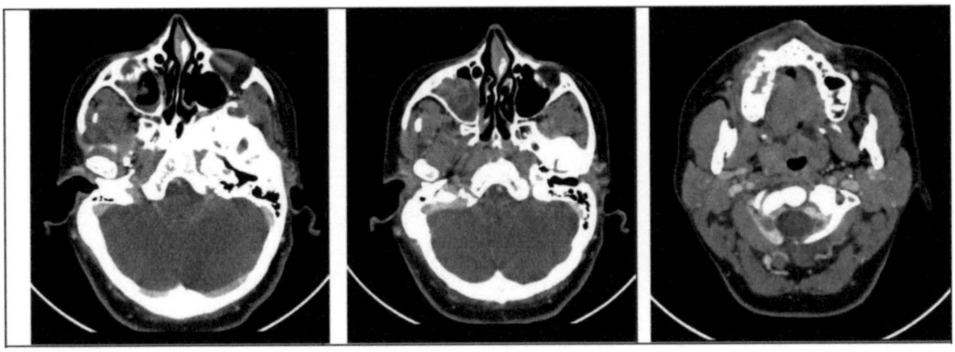

Figure 5.
Computed tomography of patient showed in **Figure 1***, a 35-year-old female with a maxillary osteosarcoma.*

The rest of the regional bone structure should be examined as previous bone diseases are found in up to 8% cases [15].

Figure 5 shows CT imaging of the patient presented in **Figure 1**.

On MRI, key points include assessing:

- Presence of soft tissue involvement.
- Size of the mass (measurement of longest diameter).
- Signal intensities of the mass on T1- and T2-weighted images (classified as low, isointense, or high) compared with those of normal bone marrow
- Contrast-enhanced images (classified as homogeneous, heterogeneous, or with peripheral enhancement).

MRI allows a better evaluation of possible soft tissue involvement and relationship with anatomical structures, including the skull base, being crucial to determine the resectability of a tumor in some subsites.

MRI depicts soft tissues and bone marrow infiltration (medulla) better than CT imaging, showing cortical destruction and expansive masses. HNOS tumors may present with low or heterogeneous signal intensities on T1-weighted images and high or heterogeneous signal intensities on T2-weighted images. However, features of osteoblastic HNOS on MRI scans are nonspecific and often indistinguishable from those of other types of sarcoma with T2 hyperintense signals and heterogeneous post-contrast enhancement. Nevertheless, the peripheral rim enhancement observed on Gd-enhanced MR images supports the diagnosis of chondroblastic HNOS [16].

Also, non-enhanced and Gd-DTPA-enhanced MR also allows to evaluate intra-medullary involvement and to differentiate osteoid matrix and necrotic, hemorrhagic or mucosal content, especially useful in sinonasal subsites. And of course, it also allows to determine the possible neural invasion.

All these features make MRI an important tool that should be considered for the assessment of biopsy taking, preoperative surgical planning, and eventually for adjuvant radiotherapy planning.

Imaging also plays an important role in the evaluation of possible distant metastases, for which the best tool remains PET CT, followed perhaps by a combination of

CT + bone scintigraphy. It is important to note that in HNOS distant disease is less frequent than that observed for OS of long bones, occurring in about 5% of patients at diagnosis and affecting mainly the lung [11].

5.2 Histology, subtypes, and histological grade

The varied radiographic appearance of this lesion highlights the importance of histopathologic analysis in the diagnosis of osteosarcomas.

5.2.1 Cytology

As stated before, diagnosis is based on imaging and tissue histology. However, cytology obtained through a fine needle aspiration (FNA) has been described and could be useful to make a first diagnostic approach to a high-grade sarcoma. On a series reported by Fleshman et al. [20], with 91 patients who had an FNA reporting a high-grade sarcoma, despite only 4% were head and neck tumors, the diagnosis was confirmed by core needle biopsy, open biopsy, or excision with 8% of them being osteosarcoma and an overall diagnostic accuracy of FNA of 91%, an VPP 97%, and sensitivity of 94%. Nonetheless, current practice normally states that FNA biopsy could be used to confirm or rule out local disease recurrence or metastasis in a known sarcoma patient, but never for an initial sarcoma diagnosis or to perform a major resection based on FNA diagnosis.

5.2.2 Histology

The gold standard in the diagnosis of osteosarcoma is tissue histology, from an incisional or open biopsy.

The diagnosis of osteosarcoma is based on recognition of osteoid production by tumor cells [13, 19]. Besides the production of osteoid and immature bone, histological features are the presence of neoplastic cells showing anaplasia with epithelioid, plasmacytoid, or spindle aspects and the growth with a permeative pattern, filling the marrow space surrounding and eroding preexisting trabeculae.

Of note, it is important to highlight that osteoid and immature bone can generate confusion in the differential diagnosis of low-grade carcinomas and other conditions of fibro-osseous lesions that may contain osteoid, such as ossifying fibromas, especially in pediatric patients.

This allows solving sampling errors, histologic heterogeneity, and necrosis that can be often found in a sarcoma sample. Also, it often grants a reliable mitotic count and estimation of the percentage of necrosis, thus permitting accurate grading.

Grossly the tumors are gritty, tan-white, and sometimes myxoid. They destroy the underlying bone with or without soft tissue extension [1].

Histologically, osteosarcomas are matrix-producing tumors that contain neoplastic osteoblasts that produce bone. These osteoblasts are highly pleomorphic and/or may be spindled, epitheloid, plasmacytoid, round, or a mixture of all the above (**Figure 6**). Approximately, half of all osteosarcomas present as high-grade lesions [1].

On small biopsies, it can sometimes be difficult to distinguish osteosarcoma from a fibro-osseous lesion. In those instances, the presence of an infiltrative growth pattern can be helpful as it is seen in osteosarcoma, but not in benign lesions [13]. According to the WHO 2017, immunohistochemistry such as Ki67, Mdm2, and cdk-4 is useful in diagnostic confirmation for inconclusive cases.

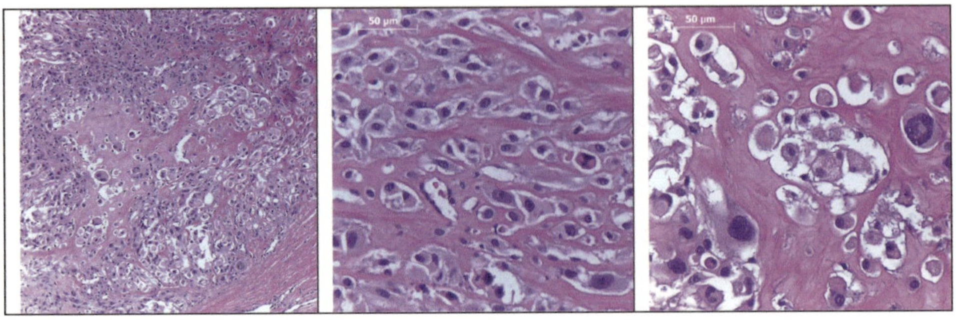

Figure 6.
Histology of patient shown in **Figure 1**, *a 35-year-old female with a maxillary chondroblastic osteosarcoma. Courtesy of Dr. Cristobal Araya.*

5.2.3 Histological subtypes

Histologically, osteosarcoma is divided into the central (intramedullary) and peripheral (surface) subtypes.

5.2.3.1 Central sarcomas

The main type of central osteosarcoma is the conventional osteosarcoma. Conventional osteosarcoma arising in the head and neck region has the same histologic appearance seen in other locations, being composed of malignant neoplastic cells and lace-like deposition of bone.

Depending upon the predominant-type extracellular matrix present (osteoid, cartilage, or collagen fibers produced by the tumor), conventional OSs are classified into osteoblastic, chondroblastic, and fibroblastic subtypes [13]. All of these subtypes of osteosarcomas can occur in the jaw bones [1].

- Osteoblastic OS is microscopically characterized by malignant-appearing osteoblasts arranged on a matrix consisting mainly of compact bone. Large amount of osteoid is identified on the sample.

- Chondroblastic OS has a lobular architecture consisting of a cartilaginous matrix with lacunae surrounded by hypercellular regions in which malignant spindle cells are arranged. It has minimal osteoid component, thus in many chondroblastic osteosarcomas, with minimal bone production, it may be difficult to distinguish between an osteosarcoma and a chondrosarcoma (**Figure 6**).

- Fibroblastic OS is the least common variant. It shows the morphology of a malignant spindle cell neoplasm, in which the only indicator that it is an osteosarcoma is the scarce identifiable osteoid. The tumor usually has a mixed morphology that becomes hard to differentiate from fibrosarcoma [19].

Traditionally, it has been reported that osteoblastic and chondroblastic subtypes are the most common subtypes. Osteoblastic HNOS have been reported to account for up to 75% of the cases, leaving fibroblastic subtype as the least frequent representing 3–15% of the cases [8, 9, 15].

5.2.3.2 Peripheral sarcomas

Peripheral osteosarcomas are represented by parosteal, periosteal, and high-grade surface.

Osteosarcomas occasionally affect the jaw. The most frequent is parosteal (or juxtacortical) osteosarcoma, which represents less than 5% of all osteosarcomas. It is well differentiated and characterized by spindle cell stroma with minimal atypia and rare mitotic figures separating irregular trabeculae of woven bone, arranged in a parallel manner. Even in histopathology, peripheral osteosarcoma could have osteoblastic, fibroblastic, or chondroblastic differentiation.

Approximately 10–25% of parosteal osteosarcomas dedifferentiate into high-grade osteosarcoma with a corresponding worsening of prognosis [13].

Figure 6 shows the histology of the patient presented in **Figure 1**.

5.2.4 Histological grading

Histologic grade is a key part of the microscopic description of a HNOS, as it has been shown to be an independent prognostic factor. Its importance is such that nowadays, it constitutes part of the information required for staging. However, there are still substantial differences in the various expert groups on how to measure and report it.

Some authors report tumors as classified into high and low grade, as others use three categories: high, intermediate, and low. The large series to date report the histologic grade in four levels, with low grade being levels 1 and 2 and high grade, levels 3 and 4 [8, 9]. In addition, apart from different classification groups in terms of grade, there is high interobserver variability, thus making the grading reproducibility poor.

As far as consensus is concerned, cellularity and mitosis are the most important criteria used for histological grading. In general, the more cellular a tumor is, the higher is the grade. With increased cellularity, tumor loses the trabecular bone architecture and more nuclear atypia appears. Irregularity of the nuclear contour, enlargement, and hyperchromasia of the nuclei are correlated with grade.

Some authors state that the majority of HNOS are high grade [6]. Ha et al. reported up to 76.9% high-grade HNOS in a series of 27 patients [21]. Similarly grade was reported on 60 of 119 patients treated at MD Anderson Cancer Center, informing low grade on 22%, intermediate on 15%, and high grade on 63%. However, on larger series, high-grade tumors represent about 30–40% of the cases. On the.

series by Lee et al., analyzing the SEER database on 2011, with 541 HNOS patients, 40.9% of all tumors were diagnosed to be high grade at presentation, 19.6% low grade, and 39.5% were unknown [9]. In Smith et al. analysis of the NCDB database on 1996, with 496 cases, tumor grade was reported for 47.4% of the patients, a proportion that increased from 39.6% in the first years (1985–1991) to 55.9% in the later years (1992–1996), probably as the importance of histologic grading on treatment planning and prognosis became evident. In this study, of the patients with a reported grade, 38.3% had well-differentiated or moderately well-differentiated tumors, 35.7% had poorly differentiated tumors, and 26.0% had undifferentiated tumors. Interestingly, authors also report that the percentage of high-grade tumors increased as tumor size increased. Also, although mandibular tumors were distributed evenly, with 46.9% low-grade tumors (Grade 1–2) and 53.1% high-grade tumors (Grade 3–4), a greater percentage of skull and facial bone tumors were high-grade lesions (67.4% and 70%, respectively) [8].

5.2.5 Immunohistochemistry

Immunohistochemistry (IHC) plays an important role in clarifying the differential diagnoses between low grade sarcomas and fibro-osseous lesions and between chondrosarcoma and chondroblastic OS.

Focal positivity with CD68 suggests fibrohistiocytic nature of the tumors to be one of the variants of OS. Previous studies have analyzed the clinicopathological features and immunohistochemical expression of p53, MDM2, CDK4, PCNA, and Ki67 proteins in head-and-neck OS and found PCNA as one of the most favorable prognostic markers [1].

The immunohistochemistry such as Ki67, MDM2, and CDK4, is useful in diagnostic confirmation for inconclusive cases. Yoshida et al. reported that the combination of MDM2 and CDK4 by immunohistochemical analysis shows 100% sensitivity and 97.5% specificity for the diagnosis of low-grade OS and reliably distinguishes low-grade osteosarcoma from benign lesions [22].

IHC will show chondrosarcoma to be positive for S100 and vimentin and negative for cytokeratin and epithelial membrane antigen (EMA). Chondroblastic OS will be positive for vimentin, EMA, S100, and rarely cytokeratin.

Fibroblastic OS will be positive for vimentin and S100 negative, thus ruling out the neural tumors [1]. Osteonectin and osteocalcin have been widely used to study OS. Osteocalcin is specific for osteoblasts, whereas the osteonectin is not specific for osteoblasts, but consistently immunostained other cell types such as fibroblasts, pericytes, endothelial cells, chondrocytes, basal layer of the skin epithelium, nerves, and osteoclastic giant cells [23].

6. Staging

Unlike the vast majority of cancers, in OS, the staging system must incorporate not only local and distant spread, but also the degree of differentiation, in order to estimate the prognosis of the patient.

The commonly used lymph node metastasis (TNM) staging system is not commonly used for HNOS because they are unlikely to metastasize to lymph nodes. Also, the current version has been tailored for OS long bones, so it is not entirely applicable to the head and neck region, for example, the tumor size for T1 is up to 8 cm, which in this anatomical subsites generally represents a very locally advanced tumor (**Table 1**).

The most commonly system used most often to formally stage bone sarcomas is known as the Musculo-skeletal Tumor Society (MSTS) or Enneking system [13]. It is based on the grade (G) of the tumor, the local extent of the primary tumor (T), and whether or not it has metastasized to regional lymph nodes or other organs (M). The extent of the primary tumor is classified as either intra-compartmental (T1), which refers to the tumor remaining confined to the subsite in which it originated, or extra-compartmental (T2), meaning it has extended into other nearby structures. Tumors that have not spread to the lymph nodes or other organs are considered M0, while those that have spread are M1 (**Table 1**) [25].

Definition of primary tumor (T)		**Definition of regional lymph node (N)**	
T category	**T criteria**	**N category**	**N criteria**
Tx	Primary tumor cannot be assessed	Nx	Regional lymph node cannot be assessed
T1	No evidence of primary tumor	N0	No regional lymph node metastasis
T2	Tumor ≤8 cm in greatest dimension	N1	No regional lymph node metastasis
T3	Tumor >8 cm in greatest dimension		
T4	Discontinuous tumors in the primary bone site		
Histologic grade (G)		**Definition of distant metastasis (M)**	
G	**G definition**	**M category**	**M criteria**
Gx	Grade cannot be assessed	M0	No distant metastasis
G1	Well differentiated, low grade	M1	Distant Metastasis
G2	Moderately differentiated, high grade	M1a	Lung metastasis
G3	Poorly differentiated, high grade	M1b	Bone or other distant sites metastasis

Table 1.
AJCC 8th edition TNM staging for bone sarcomas [24].

In summary, with this staging system, low-grade tumors are defined as stage I, regardless of extend of primary tumor, high-grade tumors as stage II, and metastatic tumors (regardless of grade) as stage III (**Table 2**).

At presentation, Lee et al. describe 18.5% of patients with stage IA disease; 0.7%, stage IB; 24.4%, stage IIA; 2.2%, stage IIB; 10.7%, stage III, stage IVA, or stage IVB (advanced disease); and 43.5%, unknown stage [9]. In Smith's et al. analysis of the NCDB, of the 487 patients with tumors that could be staged, an AJCC stage was recorded for only 56.1%, of which 90.1% of patients with locally confined (Stage I

Stage	Primary tumor (T)	Regional lymph node (N)	Distant metastasis (M)	Histologic grade (G)
IA	T1	N0	M0	G1 or Gx
IB	T2 or T3	N0	M0	G1 or Gx
IIA	T1	N0	M0	G2 or G3
IIB	T2	N0	M0	G2 or G3
III	T3	N0	M0	G2 or G3
IVA	Any T	N0	M1a	Any G
IVB	Any T	N1	Any M	Any G
	Any T	Any N	M1b	Any G

Table 2.
AJCC 8th edition prognostic stage groups for bone stage primary tumor (T) sarcoma in the appendicular skeleton, trunk, skull, and facial bones.

45%, stage II 38.9%, stage III 6.2%, and stage IV 9.9%). Interestingly, in this study, a difference was noted with regard to stage distribution by tumor location, with mandibular tumors being more likely to remain localized than skull/facial bones (92.7 vs. 82.8%, p = .032) and the other craniofacial bony sites showing higher rate of metastases of metastases than mandible (10.5% vs. 3.3) [8].

7. Treatment alternatives

Overall, HNOS are rare tumors that present unique treatment challenges. Due to its infrequency, most studies on the subject are retrospective analyses of small cohorts that utilize multiple treatment modalities, thus most treatment strategies are dictated by the existing knowledge of OS in long bones, and a variety of approaches are being applied without a standardized method of comparing relative outcomes and an answer for which the optimal treatment modality remains inconclusive.

Moreover, as stated before, HNOS has major differences from OS in the rest of the body, which could mean the need for a different treatment approach. HNOS presents at an older age than OS of long bones, has a lower metastatic potential, but a markedly higher rate of local recurrence.

Nevertheless, surgery remains the cornerstone of treatment, and negative margins the main prognostic factor and the only way to ensure locoregional control.

7.1 Surgery

The impact of impact of surgical treatment on 5-year disease-specific survival is dramatic and was evidenced on the analysis of the NCDB [8], where patients who did not undergo surgical therapy had a markedly worse survival. Patients who underwent surgery alone and surgery plus chemotherapy demonstrated similar 5-year survival rates (74.7% and 71.3%, respectively). In comparison, nonsurgical therapy resulted in a 21.7% 5-year survival [8].

However, surgical success in these patients represents a real challenge, as ensuring negative margins can be difficult, because of the anatomical complexity of the region, tumor resections are occasionally incomplete. Local recurrences and intracranial invasion have long been reported as the major causes of treatment failure due to incomplete neoplasm resection.

Furthermore, in addition to the presence of noble structures surrounding the tumor and the significant rate of irresectability that we can find in these fast-growing tumors, the lack of consensus on what we define as "adequate margins," "close margins," or "insufficient margins" also poses a problem. Obtaining disease-free resection margins is of course imperative, to avoid the risk of local recurrence; however, adequate margins of several centimeters, usually required for long bone OS, are often not achievable on HNOS since resecting few millimeters more often means endangering pivotal functional structures, with a noticeable decrease in the patients' quality of life.

Of course, this may vary by tumor subsite, and the rationale and surgical treatment planning will depend on the location. It has been documented that mandibular tumors have a significantly higher chance of achieving a wide negative margin, probably because these tumors are detected earlier than in other bones of the skull/face and because larger resections can be performed with less damage to surrounding noble structures and with better chances of functional reconstruction [7, 16].

On the other hand, while intraoperative determination of resection margins might represent a useful tool in other head and neck malignancies, osteosarcomas do often pose a significant challenge for the surgeon as intraoperative pathological examination does not indeed allow for the assessment of bone margins. Only soft tissue margins can be assessed through the intraoperative consultation, thus the need to wait for final pathology report to assess adequate margins.

Anyhow, surgery should be discussed even though we can only provide a close but negative margin and not a wide free negative margin of safety as desired.

According to Ha et al., a positive margin will mean a drop on overall survival from 75–35% (P = .008) [21]. In a meta-analysis by Smeele et al. [26], in 1998, it was already state clearly that patients benefit on overall and disease-free survival when complete resection was achieved versus incomplete resection (P < .001). The latter group was still better off compared with those who did not undergo resection at all (P < .01). Survival curves show a dramatic drop on overall survival from around 50% at 5 years for complete resection to less that 25% at 3 years for incomplete resection.

When discussing the management of the neck, it is widely agreed that regional spread of osteogenic sarcomas is rare, thus prophylactic dissection of N0 patients is not indicated, regardless of histologic grade or tumor size. Therefore, selective neck dissection is only indicated in patients with clinical/radiologic nodal metastases [5].

Although there is no general consensus, nodal localization should be treated surgically and should be considered an adverse feature when evaluating adjuvant treatments.

Unlike in the management of most other head and neck cancers, prophylactic neck dissection is not advised for high-grade or large osteosarcomas of the head and neck region.

Further research in this regard would be advisable, though, as the only data available on this matter are now old and suggest that prophylactic lymph node dissection has a detrimental effect on patients overall survival [27, 28].

Figure 7 shows the surgical resection, osteo-integrated implants, and reconstruction of patient presented in **Figure 1**, a 35-year-old female with a maxillary chondroblastic osteosarcoma, and **Figure 8** shows the surgery for patient shown in **Figure 3**, a 27-year-old male patient with osteosarcoma of the left mandible.

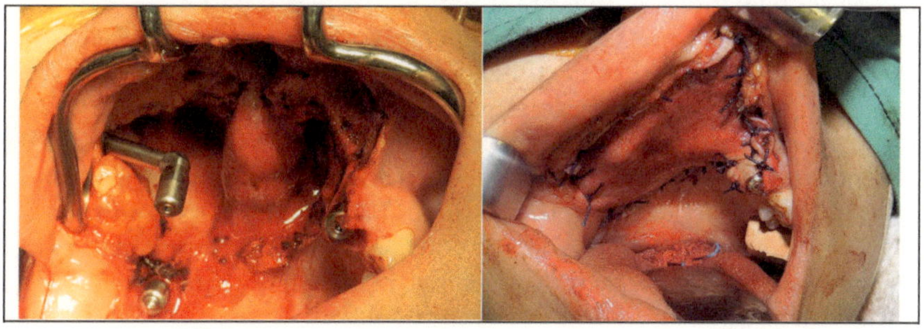

Figure 7.
Surgical resection, osteo-integrated implants and reconstruction of patient presented in **Figure 1**, *a 35-year-old female with a maxillary chondroblastic osteosarcoma.*

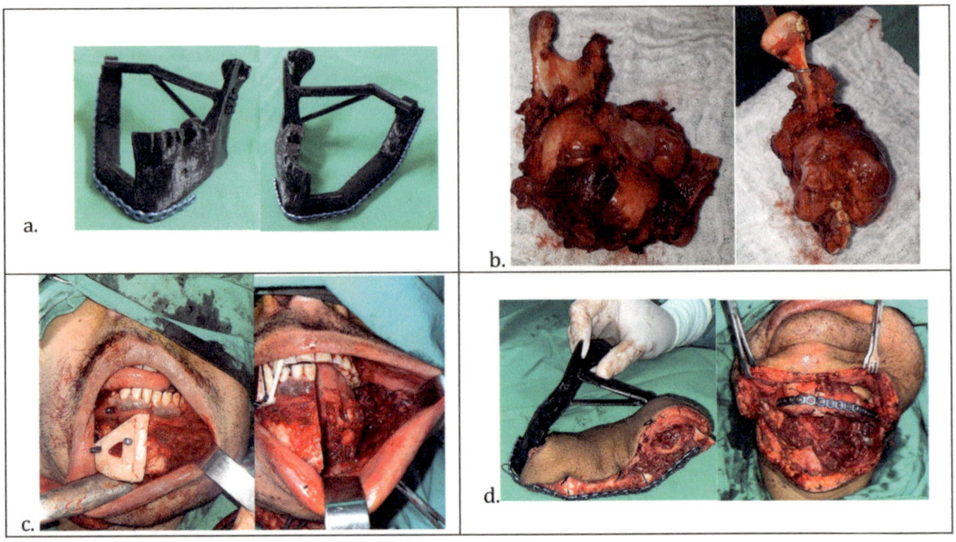

Figure 8.
Surgery for patient shown in **Figure 3**, *a 27-year-old male patient with osteosarcoma of the left mandible. (a) 3D model for preoperative surgical planning. (b) Surgical tumor excised (left mandibulectromy). (c) Mandibule with the cutting guide for medial osteotomy and surgical defect after mandibulectomy. (d) Fibula-free flap harvested for reconstruction according to surgical preoperative planning and flap in-situ on left mandibule defect.*

7.2 Chemotherapy

Surgery still is the main therapeutic modality for cure on HNOS. However, many trials indicate the benefit of adjuvant chemotherapy in improving survival of patients with extremity OS. Treatment approach for this disease had a major shift when several studies evidenced that chemotherapy improved significantly overall and disease-free survival [29]. Link et al. evidenced an improvement on 2 years of disease-free survival from 17 to 66% with the addition of chemotherapy to the treatment of long bones OS [30]. After that, implementation of standardized treatment protocols involving both neoadjuvant and adjuvant chemotherapy has resulted in significantly improved overall survival up to 60–80% for extremity osteosarcomas, compared with 10–20% with surgery alone [31, 32]. Multimodal treatment has also shown to improve disease-free survival, and some trials on the role of neoadjuvant chemotherapy were even successful on facilitating limb preservation in selected patients [33].

However, these trials repeatedly avoided enrolment of head and neck cases because of significant difference in clinical presentation, course of disease, prognosis, and the need for multidisciplinary treatment.

There are few retrospective studies, meta-analyses, or reviews that assess the role of chemotherapy specifically in HNOS; however, they have shown conflicting results [26, 32, 34–38]. In addition, these studies have small samples and use different chemotherapeutic agents or their combinations, which limits the evaluation of chemotherapy as an independent factor impacting treatment outcomes and prognosis. As a result, the benefit of chemotherapy remains unclear.

Guadagnolo et al. studied 119 patients with HNOS and failed to find a survival benefit in patients who received chemotherapy plus surgery versus surgery alone [10]. Chen et al. reported comparable findings in their study of 160 patients with HNOS [39].

On the contrary, Smeele et al. published on 201 patients with HNOS treated between 1974 and 1994 and did found a statistically significant survival benefit in patients who underwent chemotherapy and surgery versus surgery alone, on overall survival and disease-free survival. Moreover, chemotherapy was found to increase survival even in those cases of incomplete surgical resection [26].

In 2017, Boon et al. on a retrospective single-institution study of 77 patients with HNOS, where 30 patients received chemotherapy, reported an improved disease-free survival of 33% vs. 67% with addition of neoadjuvant/adjuvant chemotherapy in HNOS vs. non-chemotherapy treated patients, while the overall survival and disease-free survival were non-significant when all other cofactors were analyzed [34], a similar observation was made by Thariat et al. [35] in mandibular osteosarcomas. Nonetheless, the study by Boon et al. [34] did demonstrate a significant improvement in local recurrence rates among patients with intermediate or high-grade tumors, aged younger than 75 years, who received chemotherapy, in both univariate and multivariable analyses, postulating that the benefit of chemotherapy is thereby likely to depend on individual tumor characteristics, including grade and the presence of positive surgical margins.

While the Cooperative Osteosarcoma Study Group (COSS) protocols (neoadjuvant chemotherapy plus surgery plus adjuvant chemotherapy) have demonstrated significantly better disease-free survival in patients with extremity osteosarcoma, there is no consensus as to whether this treatment approach provides a survival benefit in patients with HNOS and timing of chemotherapy in HNOS continues to be heavily debated [7, 8, 26].

In 2021, a study by Shim et al. [32], using data from the NCDB with HNOS from 2004 to 2016, demonstrated a shift in treatment trends since the last HNOS-specific retrospective NCDB analysis was completed in 2003 [8], which mirrors treatment approach of extremity OS, showing a steady increase in the utilization of neoadjuvant and adjuvant chemotherapy in addition to surgery, with fewer patients being treated with surgery alone. However, interestingly, with no corresponding changes in estimated 2-year and 5-year overall survival, as they did not demonstrate a long-term survival benefit for HNOS patients treated with perioperative chemotherapy or radiation therapy in addition to surgery. Nonetheless, this study, which included 694 HNOS patients for the treatment analysis, found that patients treated with neoadjuvant chemotherapy and surgery plus adjuvant chemotherapy demonstrated significantly improved survival in the first 18 months after treatment compared with patients treated with surgery alone, although there was no difference in OS [32]. This observed trend in early survival could be due, in part, to benefits of neoadjuvant chemotherapy in decreasing the confines of the tumor, allowing for a more complete surgical resection. Anyhow, early increases in survival dissipate beyond 5 years after treatment. This phenomenon is perhaps a result of the tumor's propensity for local recurrence and progression, to which patients eventually succumb.

As explained before, complete resection with negative margins is essential to adequately treating osteosarcoma. While this is relatively straightforward in extremity osteosarcoma, HNOS present unique anatomic challenges to R0 resections. Thus, neoadjuvant chemotherapy could help by shrinking the primary tumor burden, allowing higher rates of negative surgical margins, thereby reducing rates of local recurrence.

On the other hand, for OS, the rationale for adjuvant chemotherapy is treating occult disease and preventing distant metastases, which are common in extremity osteosarcomas (up to 44–49%), 9,15, with pulmonary micro metastases known to be present up to 80%. Unlike long bones OS, HNOS metastasize much less frequently (7–17%), with disease progression or failure more likely due to local recurrence [13].

The study by Shim et al. [32] found only 39 out of 1035 (3.8%) HNOS patients in their cohort with metastatic disease. Given the lower metastases rates in HNOS in comparison to extremity osteosarcoma, caution should be used before extrapolating treatment protocols aimed at preventing distant metastases as adjuvant therapy is associated with several adverse effects, including increased risk of secondary malignancy.

Finally, the moment in which to administer chemotherapy in HNOS remains under discussion. Neoadjuvant chemotherapy reported a poor response (a good response being <10% viable tumor) in the COSS study group in 66% of patients in a subgroup of maxillofacial OS patients (n = 16) [40]. However, it becomes important to assess the results from studies specifically focusing on the use of neoadjuvant chemotherapy on HNOS. Thariat et al. [35] evidenced improvement on disease-free and metastatic-free survival and an increased in clear margins rates from 50% to 68% with the use of neoadjuvant chemotherapy for HNOS. Mücke et al. also evidenced, in 2014, that neoadyuvant chemotherapy improved survival for HNOS versus surgery alone and proved to be an independent factor impacting survival on multivariate analysis [37]. Thus, Neoadyuvante Chemotherapy allows for the determination of percent tumor kill at the time of surgical resection and guides requisite changes in chemotherapeutic regimens after surgery; furthermore, it allows the evaluation of response to chemotherapy, and this may be useful as a prognostic marker or to determine adjuvant treatment [16, 36].

As for the chemotherapeutic agents studied and validated for use, Cisplatin, Doxorubicin, Adriamycin, Ifosfamide, Methotrexate, cyclophosphamide, and leucovorin are described in different combinations and schemes.

In summary, chemotherapy has shown to improve survival when added to surgery as multimodal treatment for selected tumors; however, the moment of administration (adjuvant vs. neoadjuvant) is still debated.

Figure 9 shows the final appearance, 6 months after surgery and chemotherapy, of patient presented in **Figure 1**.

7.3 Radiotherapy

It has been stated that conventional osteosarcoma is relatively resistant to RT; however, RT may have the positive effect of reducing the rate of local recurrence [41, 42].

Generally, radiotherapy (RT) is indicated only in HNOS patients who have close or positive resection margins [6], as the combined treatment of surgery and radiotherapy has shown to have impact on local control and on disease-free survival on HNOS

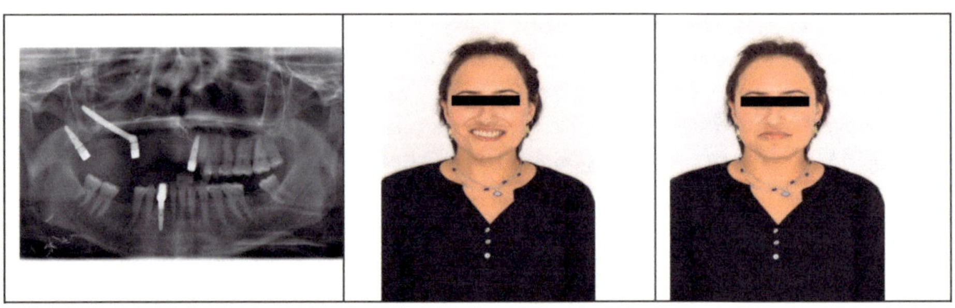

Figure 9.
Appearance 6 months after treatment (surgery and chemotherapy) of patient presented in **Figure 1**, *a 35-year-old female with a maxillary chondroblastic osteosarcoma.*

patients with unknown or close margins [10]. However, its impact on overall survival has evidenced conflicting results [43].

Guadagnolo et al. studied on 119 patients, of which 92 underwent surgery alone and in the other 27 cases surgery was followed by RT [10]. They revealed on a multivariate analysis that only the margin status predicted overall survival. Analysis by resection margin status demonstrated that the combined use of surgery and 55–60 Gy dose radiotherapy was superior to surgery alone and could improve overall survival (80 vs. 31%) and disease-free survival (80 vs. 35%) in patients with positive or uncertain margins. Moreover, the addition of adjuvant RT did not improve local control for those with negative margins but did improve local control for those with positive or uncertain margins, concluding that this high-risk group is inclined to get the best results, while no advantage is expected for patients with negative margins. However, the rates of RT-associated complications were 40% and 47% at 5 years and 10 years, respectively, and severe RT complications were observed in five (19%) of 27 patients.

In addition, while the evidence supports the use of RT in patients with positive or uncertain surgical margins, the role of combined adjuvant chemoradiotherapy is not established [10]. Some experts alternatively offer chemoradiation, typically with concurrent cisplatin as a radiosensitizer [41], extrapolating from the treatment approach used for squamous cell carcinoma of the head and neck. However, since there are limited data to support the use of chemoradiation in HNOS, the decision to use it should be made in a multidisciplinary setting. If both adjuvant chemotherapy and RT are being used, some groups chose to delay RT until the end of adjuvant chemotherapy.

The optimal dose for RT on HNOS is probably similar to that used for carcinomas and is the one commonly reported to be used in different series.

The use of heavy-particle radiation such as proton beam or carbon ion therapy is promising, particularly in patients with unresectable HNOS [44]. Proton therapy may offer some benefit to those with skull base lesions, allowing to reduce the dose to the eye and central nervous system, decreasing the risk of long-term complications [6].

There is also concern for increased risk of long-term complications of adjuvant chemotherapy and radiotherapy, including development of secondary malignancies [5, 10].

In summary, key points in the treatment of HNOS:

- The treatment for HNOS cannot be extrapolated directly from that of OS in extremities, due to substantial differences in its biological behavior.

The rationale of implementing neo/adjuvant chemotherapy is always questioned as it has a notoriously lower rate of distant metastasis, and the need for a complete resection becomes increasingly important as it has greater failure due to local recurrence.

- Surgery remains the cornerstone of treatment.

- Low-grade tumors could be candidates for exclusive surgical treatment.

- Regardless of whether the planned approach is uni or multimodality treatment, the effort must be placed on achieving a complete resection, since positive or close margins have an important impact on survival.

- Controversy persists as to what we define as adequate margin.

- In high-grade and advanced-stage tumors, multimodality treatment using surgery and chemotherapy is accepted as standard and has shown to improve survival outcomes vs. surgery alone. However, the order in which treatments provide the greatest benefit is not yet clearly established. This controversy is especially centered on the management of resectable tumors, since unresectable tumors will probably be approached primarily with chemotherapy, which may also serve as a prognostic marker.

- Controversy persists as to when to indicate chemoradiotherapy, but the indication for adjuvant radiotherapy is fairly well accepted in HNOS patients with close or positive margins.

8. Prognostic factors

Unfortunately, regardless of the treatment regimen, survival of patients afflicted with osteosarcomas of the head and neck remains poor.

While there are several single and multicenter studies reported, population data are scarce and controversial. On a literature review by Mendehall et al. [6] in 2011, overall survival shows a very wide range among the different series, going from 24 to 86% at 5 years. In Smith et al. [8] NCDB study with 496 patients, the 5-year disease-specific survival was reported to be 59.7%, for patients who were diagnosed with HNOS between 1985 and 1991. Similarly, in Lee et al. [9] cohort of the SEER tumor registry, with 541 patients, the 5-year overall and disease-specific survival were 52% and 62%, respectively, and the 10-year overall and disease-specific survival were 35% and 54%, respectively, with a median overall survival of 8 years.

Both of this large series report multiple patient, tumor, and treatment factors that were associated independently with a significantly worse survival. These risk factors included: skull or facial bone sites (vs. mandible); age older than 60 years; tumor size >6 cm; osteoblastic/NOS histology; high histological grade; advanced stage at presentation; nonsurgical initial therapy; and the presence of residual disease after surgical resection [8, 9].

Different series confirm the finding that mandibular tumors appear to have a better prognosis than maxillary tumors, showing significant difference in the metastatic rate and local recurrence [8, 9, 16]. The median overall survival for osteosarcoma of the mandible has been reported to be 10.4 years vs. 6.3 years for osteosarcoma of the skull/facial bones, including the maxilla [9]. This may be due to a greater metastatic potential in more vascularized sites such as the maxilla and skull base and/or to a more economical resection in these areas, compared with the mandible, with smaller oncologic safety margins, given the greater anatomic complexity and proximity to vital structures. Maxillary tumors show greater rate of positive margins [16]. In any case, this observation emphasizes the need for greater therapeutic consideration.

Age is another factor named repeatedly by different authors to impact survival, generally 60 years and older. Advanced age could affect by an age-dependent T-lymphocyte depletion, an intolerance to the cytotoxic effects of chemotherapy, a higher propensity to development of metastatic disease, or differences in management based on age [9].

In addition, a tumor size, histology, and grade have also shown to impact survival. Of note, osteoblastic OS has evidenced worse overall survival [8], and fibroblastic and chondroblastic osteosarcoma had the best prognosis of histological subtypes, while osteosarcoma in Paget disease had a particularly poor outcome with an overall survival not longer than 6 months [9].

Histological Grade has been proved to impact severely on survival, thus is now taken into account for staging [8, 9, 16, 39]. Within the NCDB [8], patients with low-grade HNOS tumors showed a 74% 5-year survival rate, compared with 42% for patients with high-grade tumors. Ha et al. [21] also noted a marked discrepancy in survival for patients with high-grade versus low-grade HNOS tumors, with a difference at 5 years of nearly 60%. However, on the SEER tumor registry [9], the multivariate analysis found that grade was not considered to be and independent significant determinant of survival, which could perhaps be explained by the high percentage of cases defined to be unknown.

On another hand, treatment has shown to impact dramatically patients' outcome, and surgical resection has been found to improve 5-year overall and disease-specific survival [8, 9, 16]. Complete surgical resection with wide margins has been reported as the most significant prognostic factor in HNOS [6, 13, 15]. It is reasonable to state that patients with HNOS who are not candidates for surgical resection because of advanced disease or notable comorbidities at presentation may bias the survival advantage seen in the different cohorts. However, according to Smith et al. [8], patients who did not undergo surgical therapy had a markedly worse survival with a 5-year overall survival of 21.7% compared with 74.7% for patients treated with surgery alone and 71.3% surgery plus chemotherapy.

Finally, prognosis follows a dynamic course that has been and will continue to change as the best treatment approach for these patients becomes clearer. In a study by Granowski-LeCornu et al. [16], where patients with OS of the jaw were treated from 1967 to 1991 where compared with patients treated from 1992 to 2009, this second group had better prognosis than patients in the earlier treatment group (overall 5-yeral survival rate of 77% vs. 52%). They discuss that this could be explained by several factors favoring the latter group, such as better imaging, both CT and MRI, allowing for earlier diagnosis, thus, smaller tumors at diagnosis and better treatment planning. Also, more sophisticated reconstructive techniques allow wider ablative procedures and better chance of achieving clear margins.

For more recent HNOS patients, we now offer improved diagnostic tools, more aggressive treatment, and better surveillance. The role of neoadjuvant chemotherapy remains to be elucidated and may perhaps, added to all this other factors, continue to improve prognosis.

9. Conclusions

HNOS is a rare and complex disease, for which its treatment approach is still under debate. It shows different clinical and oncologic behavior from OS of the extremities, thus requiring specific studies, which are scarce due to its infrequency. Further population-based studies are required to determine the therapeutic approach that will prove most successful. Surgical resection with large, clear margins remains the mainstay of optimal treatment, and adjuvant treatments should be discussed on a case-by-case basis. For the time being, there is consensus in that it should be managed in tertiary centers that concentrate the cases and that can offer the tools to confirm the correct diagnosis and perform the correct staging, evaluate and offer the possibility of adequate ablative and reconstructive surgery, adjuvant treatment if required, and the correct follow-up.

Acknowledgements

Dr. Cristobal Araya, maxillofacial surgeon and pathologist at Instituto Nacional del Cáncer Chile.

Head and Neck Surgery Department at Instituto Nacional del Cáncer Chile, Drs. Rodrigo Montes, Fabio Valdés, Marcelo Veloso, Luis Pizarro, Felipe Bustos, and Katherine Lozano.

Conflict of interest

The author declares no conflict of interest.

Author details

Ingrid Plass
Instituto Nacional del Cancer, Santiago, Chile

*Address all correspondence to: ingrid.plass@incancer.cl

References

[1] Nielsen GP, Rosenberg AE. Update on bone forming tumors of the head and neck. Head and Neck Pathology. 2007;**1**(1):87-93. DOI: 10-1007/s12105-007-0023-4

[2] Hoffman HT, Robinson RA, Spiess JL, Buatti J. Update in management of head and neck sarcoma. Current Opinion in Oncology. 2004;**16**(4):333-341. DOI: 10.1097/01.cco.0000127880.69877.75

[3] Unni KK. In: Tumors D's B, Unni KK, editors. Osteosarcoma—General Aspects and Data on 11,087 Cases. Philadelphia: Lippincott-Raven; 1996. p. 143

[4] Up to date, Osteosarcomas. [Internet]. July 2022. Available from: https://www.uptodate.com/contents/osteosarcoma-epidemiology-pathology-clinical-presentation-and-diagnosis

[5] Sturgis EM, Potter BO. Sarcomas of the head and neck region. Current Opinion in Oncology. 2003;**15**(3):239-252. DOI: 10.1097/00001622-200305000-00011

[6] Mendenhall WM, Fernandes R, Werning JW, Vaysberg M, Malyapa RS, Mendenhall NP. Head and neck osteosarcoma. American Journal of Otolaryngology. 2011;**32**(6):597-600. DOI: 10.1016/j.amjoto.2010.09.002

[7] Kassir RR, Rassekh CH, Kinsella JB, Segas J, Carrau RL, Hokanson JA. Osteosarcoma of the head and neck: Meta-analysis of nonrandomized studies. The Laryngoscope. 1997;**107**(1):56-61. DOI: 10.1097/00005537-199701000-00013

[8] Smith RB, Apostolakis LW, Karnell LH, Koch BB, Robinson RA, Zhen W, et al. National Cancer Data Base report on osteosarcoma of the head and neck. Cancer. 2003;**98**(8):1670-1680. DOI: 10.1002/cncr.11716

[9] Lee RJ, Arshi A, Schwartz HC, Christensen RE. Characteristics and prognostic factors of osteosarcoma of the jaws: A retrospective cohort study. JAMA Otolaryngology. Head & Neck Surgery. 2015;**141**(5):470-477. DOI: 10.1001/jamaoto.2015.0340

[10] Guadagnolo BA, Zagars GK, Raymond AK, Benjamin RS, Sturgis EM. Osteosarcoma of the jaw/craniofacial region: Outcomes after multimodality treatment. Cancer. 2009;**115**(14):3262-3270. DOI: 10.1002/cncr.24297

[11] O'Neill JP. Head and neck sarcomas: Epidemiology, pathology, and management. Neurosurgery Clinics of North America. 2013;**24**(1):67-78. DOI: 10.1016/j.nec.2012.08.010

[12] Huber GF. Head and neck osteosarcoma in adults: The province of Alberta experience over 26 years. Journal of Otolaryngology - Head & Neck Surgery. 2008;**37**(5):738-774

[13] Ferrari D. Osteosarcoma of the jaw: Classification, diagnosis and treatment. In: Moneghini L, editor. Osteosarcoma. Rijeka: IntechOpen; 2017. p. Ch. 12

[14] Capasso M, Montella A, Tirelli M, Maiorino T, Cantalupo S, Iolascon A. Genetic predisposition to solid Pediatric cancers. Frontiers in Oncology. 2020;**10**:590033. DOI: 10.3389/fonc.2020.590033

[15] Patel SG, Meyers P, Huvos AG, Wolden S, Singh B, Shaha AR, et al. Improved outcomes in patients with osteogenic sarcoma of the head and neck. Cancer. 2002;**95**(7):1495-1503. DOI: 10.1002/cncr.10849

[16] Granowski-LeCornu M, Chuang SK, Kaban LB, August M. Osteosarcoma of the jaws: Factors influencing prognosis. Journal of Oral and Maxillofacial Surgery. 2011;**69**(9):2368-2375. DOI: 10.1016/j.joms.2010.10.023

[17] Lindquist C, Teppo L, Sane J, Holmstrom T, Wolf J. Osteosarcoma of mandible: Analysis of 9 cases. Journal of Oral and Maxillofacial Surgery. 1986;**44**:759-764

[18] Luo Z, Chen W, Shen X, Qin G, Yuan J, Hu B, et al. Head and neck osteosarcoma: CT and MR imaging features. Dento Maxillo Facial Radiology. 2020;**49**(2):20190202. DOI: 10.1259/dmfr.20190202

[19] Rana RS, Wu JS, Eisenberg RL. Periosteal reaction. AJR. American Journal of Roentgenology. 2009;**193**(4):W259-W272. DOI: 10.2214/AJR.09.3300

[20] Fleshman R, Mayerson J, Wakely PE Jr. Fine-needle aspiration biopsy of high-grade sarcoma: A report of 107 cases. Cancer. 2007;**111**(6):491-498. DOI: 10.1002/cncr.23122

[21] Ha PK, Eisele DW, Frassica FJ, Zahurak ML, McCarthy EF. Osteosarcoma of the head and neck: A review of the Johns Hopkins experience. The Laryngoscope. 1999;**109**(6):964-969. DOI:10.1097/00005537-199906000-00023

[22] Yoshida A, Ushiku T, Motoi T, Beppu Y, Fukayama M, Tsuda H, et al. MDM2 and CDK4 immunohistochemical coexpression in high-grade osteosarcoma: Correlation with a dedifferentiated subtype. The American Journal of Surgical Pathology. 2012;**36**(3):423-431. DOI: 10.1097/PAS.0b013e31824230d0

[23] Saify F, Jain S. Osteosarcoma of jaws: An insight into literature. International Journal of Orofacial Biology. 2018;**2**:41-46

[24] Amin MB, Edge SB, Greene FL, et al., editors. AJCC Cancer Staging Manual. 8th ed. Switzerland: Springer; 2017

[25] Chaudhary M, Chaudhary SD. Osteosarcoma of jaws. Journal of Oral and Maxillofacial Pathology. 2012;**16**(2):233-238. DOI: 10.4103/0973-029X.99075

[26] Smeele LE, Snow GB, van der Waal I. Osteosarcoma of the head and neck: Meta-analysis of the nonrandomized studies. The Laryngoscope. 1998;**108**(6):946. DOI: 10.1097/00005537-199806000-00030

[27] Goepfert H, Raymond K, Spires JR, et al. Osteosarcoma of the head and neck. Cancer Bulletin. 1990;**42**:347-354

[28] Rao RS, Rao DN. Prognostic significance of the regional lymph nodes in osteosarcoma. Surgical Oncology. 1977;**9**(2):123-130

[29] The ESMO/European Sarcoma Network Working Group. Bone sarcomas: ESMO clinical practice guidelines for diagnosis, treatment and follow-up. Annals of Oncology. 2012;**23**:vii100-vii109

[30] Link MP, Goorin AM, Horowitz M, Meyer WH, Belasco J, Baker A, et al. Adjuvant chemotherapy of high-grade osteosarcoma of the extremity. Updated results of the multi-institutional osteosarcoma study. Clinical Orthopaedics and Related Research. 1991;**270**:8-14

[31] Anninga JK, Gelderblom H, Fiocco M, et al. Chemotherapeutic adjuvant treatment for osteosarcoma: Where do we stand? European Journal of Cancer. 2011;**47**(16):2431-2445

[32] Shim T, Chillakuru Y, Darwish C, Chalif E, Strum D, Benito DA, et al. Head and neck osteosarcomas: Analysis of

treatment trends and survival outcomes in the United States (2004-2016). Head & Neck. 2021;**43**(11):3294-3305. DOI: 10.1002/hed.26817

[33] Bacci G, Ferrari S, Donati D, Longhi A, Bertoni F, Di FM, et al. Neoadjuvant chemotherapy for osteosarcoma of the extremity in patients in the fourth and fifth decade of life. Oncology Reports. 1998;**5**:1259-1263

[34] Boon E, van der Graaf WT, Gelderblom H, Tesselaar ME, van Es RJ, Oosting SF, et al. Impact of chemotherapy on the outcome of osteosarcoma of the head and neck in adults. Head & Neck. 2017;**39**(1):140-146. DOI: 10.1002/hed.24556

[35] Thariat J, Schouman T, Brouchet A, Sarini J, Miller RC, Reychler H, et al. Osteosarcomas of the mandible: Multidisciplinary management of a rare tumor of the young adult a cooperative study of the GSF-GETO, rare cancer network, GETTEC/REFCOR and SFCE. Annals of Oncology. 2013;**24**(3):824-831. DOI: 10.1093/annonc/mds507

[36] Eilber F. Adjuvant chemotherapy for osteosarcoma: A randomized prospective trial. Journal of Clinical Oncology. 1987;**5**(1):21-26

[37] Mücke T, Mitchell DA, Tannapfel A, Wolff KD, Loeffelbein DJ, Kanatas A. Effect of neoadjuvant treatment in the management of osteosarcomas of the head and neck. Journal of Cancer Research and Clinical Oncology. 2014;**140**(1):127-131. DOI: 10.1007/s00432-013-1550-x

[38] Ketabchi A, Kalavrezos N, Newman L. Sarcomas of the head and neck: A 10-year retrospective of 25 patients to evaluate treatment modalities, function and survival. The British Journal of Oral & Maxillofacial Surgery. 2011;**49**(2):116-120. DOI: 10.1016/j.bjoms.2010.02.012

[39] Chen Y, Shen Q, Gokavarapu S, Lin C, Yahiya, Cao W, et al. Osteosarcoma of head and neck: A retrospective study on prognostic factors from a single institute database. Oral Oncology. 2016;**58**:1-7. DOI: 10.1016/j.oraloncology.2016.04.008

[40] Jasnau S, Meyer U, Potratz J, Jundt G, Kevric M, Joos UK, et al. Cooperative osteosarcoma study group COSS. Craniofacial osteosarcoma experience of the cooperative German-Austrian-Swiss osteosarcoma study group. Oral Oncology. 2008;**44**(3):286-294. DOI: 10.1016/j.oraloncology.2007.03.001

[41] Machak GN, Tkachev SI, Solovyev YN, Sinyukov PA, Ivanov SM, Kochergina NV, et al. Neoadjuvant chemotherapy and local radiotherapy for high-grade osteosarcoma of the extremities. Mayo Clinic Proceedings. 2003;**78**(2):147-155. DOI: 10.4065/78.2.147

[42] DeLaney TF, Park L, Goldberg SI, Hug EB, Liebsch NJ, Munzenrider JE, et al. Radiotherapy for local control of osteosarcoma. International Journal of Radiation Oncology, Biology, Physics. 2005;**61**(2):492-498. DOI: 10.1016/j.ijrobp.2004.05.051

[43] Nthumba PM. Osteosarcoma of the jaws: A review of literature and a case report on synchronous multicentric osteosarcomas. World Journal of Surgical Oncology. 2012;**10**:240. DOI: 10.1186/1477-7819-10-240

[44] Kalavrezos N, Sinha D. Head and neck sarcomas in adulthood: Current trends and evolving management concepts. The British Journal of Oral & Maxillofacial Surgery. 2020;**58**(8):890-897. DOI: 10.1016/j.bjoms.2020.05.015. Epub 2020 Jul 4

Chapter 7

Drug Targeting of Chromosomal Translocations in Fusion-Positive Sarcoma

Günther H.S. Richter

Abstract

Sarcomas are heterogeneous cancers of bone or soft tissue. They occur in children, adolescents, and young adults (AYAs). Herein, the subgroup of fusion-positive (FP) sarcomas is characterized by chromosomal rearrangements generating pathognomonic fusion transcripts and oncoproteins. In Ewing sarcoma (EwS), FP-rhabdomyosarcomas (FP-RMS) and synovial sarcomas (SyS), the most common and aggressive forms of sarcomas in childhood and adolescence, the oncogenic rearrangements involve transcription cofactors such as by FET-ETS, PAX3/7-FOXO1 or SS18-SSX fusion oncogenes in EwS, FP-RMS, or SyS, respectively causing widespread epigenetic rewiring and aberrant gene expression. Regardless of these translocations, few recurrent mutations are observed in these sarcomas that may contribute to disease; thus, it is of particular interest to consider the consequences of these translocations for tumor development. Results of current research examining the disease, analyzing, and classifying the role of associated rearrangements of chromatin, and investigating possibilities for tumor-specific intervention such as blocking the transcriptional activity of the fusion protein, or the processes caused by this activity are summarized here and some resulting therapeutic opportunities are presented.

Keywords: fusion-positive sarcoma, epigenetic rewiring, aberrant gene expression, targeted therapy

1. Introduction

Sarcomas are heterogeneous cancers of bone or soft tissue. They occur in children as well as adolescents and young adults (AYAs). They are rare among adult malignancies but account for 12–15% of all pediatric tumors [1]. Despite the introduction and continued optimization of multimodal therapies, approximately one-third of sarcoma patients still die from the disease. Current therapies combine surgery, polychemotherapy, radiation, immunotherapy, and/or targeted therapeutics. Scientific advances have enabled more precise molecular characterization of sarcoma subtypes [2–4] and discovered new therapeutic targets and prognostic biomarkers [5]. Patients with primary metastatic disease or recurrence have a very poor prognosis in both age groups [6].

The pathogenesis of many sarcomas is poorly understood, but research over the past 20 years has identified recurrent, characteristic chromosomal translocations in approximately one-third of sarcomas (including most pediatric, adolescent, and young adult tumors). Chromosomal rearrangements resulting in oncogenic fusion genes are more common in childhood cancers than in adult tumors [7, 8].

The first sarcoma-specific chromosomal translocation was detected in 1982 in patients with alveolar rhabdomyosarcoma [9]. In subsequent years, chromosomal aberrations were identified in additional sarcomas [10]. These translocations are specific to the individual sarcomas and are considered tumor-initiating in those in which they occur [11, 12].

Fusion-positive sarcomas are characterized molecularly by a relatively quiescent genome with recurrent, balanced translocations leading to the formation of novel fusion oncogenes that are key to pathogenesis [13]. In these sarcomas, fusion protein-forming translocations are often the primary driver of disease pathogenesis and are accompanied by very few other mutations [14], although a limited number of recurrent, cooperating mutations have been identified (e.g., STAG2 in Ewing sarcomas and KRAS in synovial sarcomas) [15–19].

With the advent of advanced techniques in molecular genetics and pathology, new translocations in sarcomas are regularly reported, leading to reclassification and adjusted risk stratification. Many sarcomas are now diagnosed and classified or reclassified based on these underlying molecular alterations [2, 4, 20].

The marked tumor specificity, of the individual fusion genes, suggests that their oncogenic roles are specific to a particular cell type and/or developmental stage. Consistent with the consideration that factors related to developmental timing are associated with oncogenesis triggered by the fusion genes, many of these sarcomas occur primarily in children [8].

Unlike other cancers, these diseases contain chimeric and neomorphic proteins that are clonally present, and due to their tumor specificity and demonstrated role in tumorigenesis, these fusion proteins often represent unique and promising targets for therapeutic intervention and robust opportunities to cure these diseases [11, 12, 15, 21].

2. Ewing sarcoma

Ewing sarcoma is a rare, aggressive bone or soft tissue tumor that primarily affects children, adolescents, and young adults (AYAs) with ~1.5 cases per million children and AYAs worldwide. The average age at diagnosis is 15 years. Approximately 20–25% of patients have metastatic disease at diagnosis, which is often unresponsive to intensive therapy [22]. Standard therapy for Ewing sarcoma consists of a multimodality treatment regimen that includes surgical resection and/or local radiation therapy, as well as intensive five-drug chemotherapy and the administration of compressed interval cycles [23].

Most Ewing sarcomas have a chromosomal rearrangement at 22q12 [10]. This led to the identification of the EWSR1 gene, which can be fused to one of several partner genes: FLI1 t(11;22), ERG t(21;22), ETV1 t(7,22), ETV4 t(17,22), or FEV t(2,22). The most common fusion is EWSR1-FLI1, which occurs in ~85% of tumors [24]. In a recent comprehensive study, it was found that in 42% of Ewing sarcomas, the fusion gene results from a loop-like rearrangement, a process known as chromoplexia. These loops always contained the disease-defining fusion at the center, but they interrupted several additional genes and appear to be associated with an aggressive form of Ewing sarcoma [25].

Ewing sarcomas have few other infrequently recurring mutations besides an EWSR1/ETS translocation, including TP53 (5–10%), CDKN2A (10%), and STAG2 (15–20%) [16, 26]. The loss of P53 and STAG2 suggests a rare group of tumors that, together with the translocation, form an aggressive subset of Ewing sarcoma [15, 18]. Furthermore, very little is known about the genetic heterogeneity within the tumor in Ewing sarcoma, its subclonal genetic architecture, and the relationship between these factors and clinical outcome. The majority of pediatric solid tumors, including Ewing sarcoma, express an active DNA transposase, PGBD5, that can promote site-specific genomic rearrangements in human cells and may promote resistance to therapy [27, 28]. However, whether the genomic landscape of Ewing sarcomas differs in relapse from primary disease is unknown [24]. Recent analyses of DNA methylation status in Ewing sarcoma showed that primary tumors from patients with metastatic disease were more heterogeneous than those with localized disease [29]. However, most Ewing sarcomas have very few additional genetic alterations, suggesting that the fusion is likely the primary cause of disease development. Previous findings suggest that either mesenchymal stem cells or neural crest-derived stem cells are the cell of origin of Ewing sarcoma, although this is still a matter of debate [30, 31].

EWSR1 encodes a protein with a function in RNA binding and transcriptional regulation. The amino terminus of the EWSR1 protein functions as a strong transcriptional activator [32]. All Ewing sarcoma fusion partner genes encode related transcription factors, with conserved DNA-binding ETS domain. These ETS domain transcription factors play an important role in biological development [33]. During each fusion, the amino-terminal transactivation domain of EWSR1 is fused to the ETS domain-containing carboxyl terminus of the corresponding fusion partner. The resulting fusion gene functions primarily as an aberrant transcription factor. The dominant EWSR1/ETS translocation EWSR1-FLI1 results in heterogeneous expression profiles that have different biological implications. Therefore, variable expression of EWSR1-FLI1 has recently been proposed as a source of heterogeneity in these tumors. Cells with high EWSR1-FLI1 expression (EWSR1-FLI1^{high}) are highly proliferative, whereas EWSR1-FLI1^{low} cells have a strong propensity to migrate, invade, and metastasize [34].

EWSR1-FLI1 can act as both a transcriptional activator and a transcriptional repressor, depending on the sequence of DNA binding sites and the presence of additional co-factors [35, 36]. EWSR1-FLI1 acts directly or indirectly on many important cellular processes such as cell cycle, apoptosis, angiogenesis, metabolism, and cell migration by binding to these sites [24]. EWSR1-FLI1 binds to DNA either at ETS-like consensus sites with a GGAA core motif or at GGAA microsatellites (GGAA-mSats). EWSR1-FLI1 multimers directly induce open chromatin at GGAA-mSats by recruiting the nucleosome remodeling BRG1/BRM-associated factor complex (BAF) and establishing de novo enhancers that interact with promoters to drive gene expression [35, 37]. Fusion multimers physically interact with BAF complexes, which appear to be critical for EWS-FLI1 function, as BAF complexes are required for activation of EWS-FLI1 target genes. The variable length of GGAA-mSats in the germline may lead to differential activity of these enhancers and is an important determinant of tumor progression [38].

Conversely, EWSR1-FLI binds to canonical ETS recognition sites without repeats and represses wild-type ETS factors, which can lead to suppression of enhancers and downregulation of nearby genes [35]. The chimeric transcription factor can directly repress certain genes such as LOX and TGFBR2 through direct interaction and recruitment of the nucleosome remodeling and deacetylase repressor complex (NuRD), which includes histone deacetylases and the histone demethylase LSD1 [39].

Interestingly, EWSR1-ETS fusion proteins also bind to DEAD/DEADH box RNA helicases and modulate their activity, thus also affecting the transcription and splicing machinery of tumor cells and causing changes in overall transcriptome processing [40, 41].

These data demonstrate that EWSR1-FLI1 utilizes distinct chromatin regulatory mechanisms whose interplay at the right time and in the right cellular context leads to the transformed phenotype of Ewing sarcoma.

3. Rhabdomyosarcoma

Rhabdomyosarcoma (RMS), the most common soft tissue sarcoma in children and adolescents, comprises a diverse group of cancers [42]. There are several subtypes: embryonal, alveolar, and pleomorphic rhabdomyosarcoma. Embryonal RMS occurs in infants and children, and as patients age, the proportion of embryonal RMS decreases. Conversely, the proportion of alveolar and pleomorphic types increases in adolescents and older patients. Currently available multimodal therapy results in an overall survival rate of approximately 65% in children and adolescents diagnosed with RMS [43]. However, cure rates have stagnated since the 1990s. Rhabdomyosarcoma is very sensitive to cytotoxic combination chemotherapy [44]. For low- or intermediate-risk RMS patients (who are mostly pediatric patients with embryonal-type tumors), a high cure rate can be expected with current standard treatment. In adolescents and elderly patients, most of whom have had alveolar or pleomorphic type RMS, the prognosis is poor [6].

Chromosomal translocations are observed in alveolar rhabdomyosarcomas in two translocation patterns: The DNA binding site of PAX, a member of the paired-box family of transcription factors, is fused to a transactivation domain on FOXO1 (FKHR), a member of the forkhead transcription factor family [45, 46]. The t(2;13) translocation results in the fusion of the PAX3 gene with FOXO1, whereas the t(1;13) translocation fuses PAX7 with FOXO1, both of which now serve as important prognostic biomarkers for this disease (Barr et al. 1995). The O subgroup of the FOX family includes four members (FOXO1, FOXO3, FOXO4, and FOXO6). FOXO factors are considered tumor suppressors that are inactivated by the phosphatidylinositol 3-kinase (PI3K)-AKT pathway, which is regulated by several microRNAs [47]. The prevalence of the translocation with PAX3-FOXO1 is higher than that with PAX7-FOXO1 [48].

PAX3-FOXO1 is an aberrant transcription factor that disrupts gene regulatory networks that control myogenic differentiation, proliferation, cell death, and invasiveness [49, 50]. The translocation product overlaps with wild-type PAX3 function while modifying it through changes in abundance, transcriptional activity, target gene recognition, and chromatin regulation [51–56]. Patients with fusion-positive alveolar rhabdomyosarcoma (FP-ARMS) have a strikingly low somatic mutation burden and are also associated with a significantly higher rate of metastasis and lower survival compared to FP-negative RMS [56]. Metastatic FP-RMS remains essentially incurable [57].

PAX3/7:FOXO1-positive RMS (FP-RMS) is associated with alveolar histology [58]. Silencing of PAX3/7:FOXO1 (P3F) *in vitro* has been associated with decreased growth of human FP-RMS cells [59]. The effects of the fusion on tumor induction have been studied by ectopic expression and conditional activation in various cell types [60–62]. The fusion was necessary but not sufficient to induce FP+ myogenic tumors, as the fusion oncoprotein alone did not reliably induce tumor formation [60–62]. When combined with additional oncogenic hits, only those cells that expressed the fusion prior to the introduction of additional events formed tumors [62]. These observations are consistent with genomic subclonality analyses identifying PAX3/7:FOXO1 as a founding event and driver in FP-RMS [63]. Cooperating genetic events in FP-ARMS include amplification of MYCN or CDK4 or loss of CDKN2A, TP53, or ARF [17, 61].

PAX-FOXO1 fusions are thought to contribute to the phenotype and malignancy of ARMS by dysregulating PAX-specific target genes such as the epigenetic regulator JARID2, the receptor tyrosine kinases MET and FGFR4, and IGF2, Hippo and their downstream signaling pathways [64–67]. In addition, rearrangement of the PAX gene is thought to lead to dysregulation and amplification of a shared receptor tyrosine kinase/RAS/PIK3CA signaling axis [17]. PAX-FOXO1 fusion is also thought to affect normal FOXO function and its regulation of TGF-β signaling [68]. Recently, PAX3-FOXO1 was shown to directly establish super-enhancers in cooperation with the master transcription factors MYOG, MYOD, and MYCN to drive a myogenic transcriptional program in ARMS [55]. Thus, as in Ewing sarcoma, both aberrant transcriptional and epigenetic regulation drive the development and maintenance of FP-ARMS.

4. Synovial sarcoma

Synovial sarcoma (SyS) is a rare malignancy of soft tissue near the joints that occurs in patients of all ages but is particularly common in children and young adults. Synovial sarcoma accounts for 10% of soft tissue malignancies diagnosed annually [69]. The incidence of this disease has increased over the past three decades, while survival rates (~56%) have remained stagnant [69, 70]. Treatment of this disease consists of radical surgical resection, radiotherapy, and adjuvant chemotherapy, which offers a chance of cure in localized disease. However, the disease is prone to relapse, and metastases are common and almost always fatal [70].

Synovial sarcoma is associated with the occurrence of a chromosomal rearrangement, t(X;18) [71]. This aberration results in the formation of a fusion gene involving SS18 (also known as SYT) and one of three related genes: SSX1, SSX2, or SSX4. The presence of an SS18-SSX fusion gene is the characteristic genomic abnormality associated with the development of Synovial sarcoma [71–73]. Similar to Ewing sarcoma, Synovial sarcoma is characterized by low somatic mutation rates and no chromosomal aberrations other than the pathognomonic fusion [74, 75]. Some genes are mutated in more than 5% of Synovial sarcoma cases, including TP53, PTEN, CTNNB1, and APC [74]. Histologically, Synovial sarcoma shows a unique pattern with variable mesenchymal and epithelial components [74]. Expression of an SS18-SSX fusion leads to transformation of cultured fibroblasts and development of high-penetrance synovial sarcoma-like disease in mice when expressed in muscle progenitor cells [76, 77]. On the other hand, knockdown of the fusion protein in Synovial sarcoma cells results in the death of these cells [78].

SS18-SSX fusions do not act as transcription factors because neither SS18 nor the SSX proteins contain DNA-binding domains. Instead, they function as transcriptional regulators, aberrant chromatin regulators that drive oncogenesis by deregulating epigenetic processes and gene expression [79, 80]. SS18 is a member of the BAF complex (also known as the SWI/SNF complex) that directly interacts with the catalytic subunit of this nucleosome remodeling complex, BRM [81, 82]. BAF complexes promote gene activation through nucleosome remodeling that opens DNA for access by transcription factors and the transcription machinery. SSX proteins, on the other hand, have been shown to colocalize with Polycomb group proteins, which tend to function as gene repressors [83]. Current models suggest two potentially competing mechanisms of transforming activity in synovial sarcomas: SS18-SSX displaces wild-type SS18 and BAF47 (also known as SMARCB1, SNF5, or INI1) from the BAF complex, which may then drive Sox2-mediated proliferation/differentiation [79]. Alternatively, there is evidence that SS18-SSX can directly recruit Polycomb repressor complex 2 (PRC2) and Histone-Deacetylases (HDAC) to ATF2 targets, silencing transcription at these sites [84]; other studies have implicated SS18-SSX fusion genes in epigenetic regulation and modification of target genes [85, 86]. Treatment with a selective inhibitor of the histone methyltransferase EZH2, the enzymatic component of the PRC2, reverses gene expression of synovial sarcomas and leads to growth inhibition and cell death in SS18-SSX-positive cells [87].

Most recently, two studies have further elucidated mechanisms underlying the retargeting of SS18-SSX-containing BAF complexes. Using CRISPR/Cas9-mediated epitope tagging, Banito et al. were able to investigate SS18-SSX1 occupancy and its effects on gene expression genome-wide. They observed that SS18-SSX1 is recruited to unmethylated CpG-rich sequences on DNA through interaction with lysine demethylase 2B (KDM2B), a core component of the non-canonical PRC1.1, also known as the BCOR complex. Recruitment of SS18-SSX to these PRC1.1 targets results in abnormal induction of genes that constitute a gene signature of Synovial sarcoma, including transcription factors associated with neurogenesis and development [88]. Second, McBride et al. have shown that SS18-SSX targets BAF complexes in bivalent chromatin regions to genes marked by H3K4me3 and H3K27me3, repressing PRC2 and abnormally activating a gene program essential for Synovial sarcoma survival. Loss of SS18-SSX results in decreased binding of the BAF complex to genes that depend on the fusion for their continued expression decreased chromatin accessibility at these sites, and mesenchymal differentiation [89].

5. Targeting fusion oncoproteins

Fusion proteins of the sarcomas shown here appear to block the differentiation potential of these cells. This is achieved by hijacking transcriptional regulatory mechanisms to maintain the expression of stem cell transcriptional programs or by repressing differentiation programs. In Ewing sarcomas, the EWSR1-FLI1 protein upregulates EZH2 by binding to its promoter, thereby blocking its endothelial and neuronal differentiation capabilities [90]. Recent data show that in this process EZH2-containing PRC2 complexes interact with HDAC1, 2 and this HDAC activity mediates the immature, tumorigenic phenotype of Ewing sarcoma [91]. However, in the alveolar RMS HDAC1,2,3 also appears to serve an essential function of P3F-driven super-enhancers, as appropriate inhibitors disrupt the activity of these tumor-specific super-enhancers [92].

Transcription factors such as EWSR1-FLI1 can bind to DNA target sites on chromatin and initiate chromatin remodeling by recruiting other transcription factors and coactivator complexes. One way to achieve this chromatin remodeling is through association with BAF complexes. These multimembered complexes use ATP to move, displace, or exchange nucleosomes on chromatin. In Ewing sarcomas, BAF complexes can directly interact with the N-terminal EWSR1 protein of the fusion protein to promote and direct its tumor-specific activity at GGAA microsatellites. This binding activity is attributed to a specific prion-like domain in the N-terminal EWSR1 protein that is sufficient to drive chromatin remodeling and oncogenic gene transcription when fused to FLI1 [37]. In alveolar RMS, no direct interaction of P3F with the BAF complex has yet been shown. However, prion-like domains are suspected in a growing class of genes involved in oncogenic fusions, including FOXO1 and SS18 [93]. In synovial sarcomas, the SS18-SSX fusion also relocalizes and disrupts the BAF complex. The SS18-SSX fusion protein not only displaces wild-type SS18 binding and the tumor suppressor BAF47 from the complex [79]. Moreover, the SS18-SSX-containing BAF complexes interact with various repressive polycomb complexes in a context-dependent manner, thereby promoting the transcription of oncogenic genes [89], or alternatively, SS18-SSX and the BAF complex can localize and activate target genes via interaction with KDM2B and the PRC1.1 complex [88], as described above.

Despite these preclinical and clinical data, to date, there are few examples of targeted therapies that directly target these fusion transcription factors in solid tumors. However, all of these examples do not directly target structures of these chimeric transcription factors that are considered undruggable but attempt to identify processes or proteins that are essential for the activity or stability of these fusion proteins. An example is the observed interaction of EWSR1-FLI1 with RNA helicase A: YK-4-279 interferes with the interaction of EWSR1-FLI1 with RNA helicase A and thereby efficiently impairs both the activity of the fusion protein and cell proliferation of Ewing sarcoma cells [40]. Based on these data, the derivative TK-216 is now being tested in a clinical trial in patients with relapsed or refractory Ewing sarcoma. Another example is BAF complexes in which the SS18-SSX fusion protein is present in synovial sarcomas. Recent studies have shown that targeting the BRD9 protein, which is a component of SS18-SSX-containing complexes, provides potent antitumor effects in this context [94, 95]. BRD9 and SS18-SSX bind together to regions of the synovial sarcoma genome, and small molecule-triggered targeted degradation of BRD9 prevents oncogenic transcriptional programs in cell lines and blocks tumor progression in vivo [94]. These results will form the basis for future clinical trials in patients with synovial sarcomas. Furthermore, efforts are underway to identify downstream target genes that have critical roles in mediating the oncogenic effects of fusion transcription factors. Examples of these are described below.

6. Combining targeted drugs with protein degradation

To identify potential targeted therapeutic compounds that can promote fusion protein degradation, high-throughput chemical (HTS) screening can be used in a model system that reports on the stability of the target protein [96]. Thus, cell-based systems expressing a fluorescent dye-labeled protein of interest and a different color fluorescent control can be used for image-based screening that can identify compounds that measure the stability of the fluorescently labeled protein. The identified compounds can be further investigated and the mechanism affecting protein stability can be identified [96].

An example of the successful use of such a system was recently published for Ewing sarcomas: Using a high-throughput drug screen (HTS) enriched with FDA-approved drugs coupled with global protein stability (GPS) approach revealed that the dual HDAC and phosphatidylinositol 3-kinase (PI3K) inhibitor Fimepinostat (CUDC-907) is an excellent candidate to modulate EWSR1-FLI1 stability. Fimepinostat greatly reduced the amount of fusion protein, decreased the viability of several Ewing sarcoma cell lines and PDX primary cells, and delayed tumor growth in a xenograft mouse model, while not significantly affecting healthy cells. They demonstrated that EWSR1-FLI1 protein levels were mainly regulated by the HDAC activity of Fimepinostat [97].

A second approach to degradation of fusion oncoproteins is their targeted protein degradation mediated by degradation molecules or proteolysis targeting chimeras (PROTACs). While there are several strategies for targeted protein degradation [98–100], PROTACs are small molecule-based and thus a drug-like method to degrade a target protein of interest. The methodology combines small molecules that can bind directly to E3 ligases such as CRBN and VHL [101–103] with molecules that bind to the desired target protein-coupled through a chemical linker such as polyethylene glycol. Thus, these compounds bring the target protein and an E3 ligase complex into close proximity, resulting in polyubiquitination of the target protein, followed by proteasome-mediated degradation [100].

This strategy requires a small molecule that can bind to the desired fusion protein but does not necessarily need to enter the enzyme pocket or specifically inhibit the activity of the target protein, which has historically been an obstacle to the development of drugs targeting transcription factors. Small molecule inhibitors of proteins with bromodomains and extra terminal domains (BET) such as JQ1 and OTX015 have been successfully converted into degraders [104, 105].

On the other hand, there are ways to directly tag fusion proteins for proteasomal degradation. For example, it has been shown that EWSR1-FLI1 degradation involves polyubiquitination at lysine-380, which marks the fusion protein for proteasomal degradation [106]. Lysine-380 is located within the DNA-binding domain and is also present in wild-type FLI1 and conserved in several other members of the ETS family like ETS1. However, this may limit specificity [107]. Although, given the short half-life of EWSR-FLI1, a PROTAC targeting a lysine-380-containing motif could create a therapeutic window [106]. On the other hand, EWSR1-FLI1-specific PROTACs have not yet been developed. However, PROTACs targeting fusion protein interacting with BET or CK proteins have been successfully tested in Ewing sarcoma cells [108, 109].

In the search for small molecules that can bind to a protein of interest, the HTS method is now being used very successfully. A wide variety of target-specific HTS methods and assay formats can be used (see review in Coussens et al. [110]). With improvements in stability and delivery of PROTACS targeting fusion proteins, they may represent a viable approach to identify new drugs for targeted therapy of FP sarcomas.

7. Ways to block oncogenic transcription

The basic mechanism by which fusion-positive sarcomas promote and maintain tumorigenicity is through the activation of pathogenic transcriptional programs. They mediate this (as described above) through direct regulation of genes at promoters, the establishment of de novo enhancers, and aberrant recruitment of transcription cofactors [111]. Pathogenic transcriptional activity is also achieved through dysregulation of epigenetic programs, including the generation of super-enhancers characterized by extended stretches of acetylation at histone H3 lysine 27 (H3K27ac) [112]. These histone marks are recognized by members of the BET family (BRD2, BRD3, BRD4) [113]. They have an essential role in regulating transcription by interacting with various proteins such as RNA polymerase II [114]. This allows multiple approaches to intervene pharmacologically in this pathogenic transcriptional program. For example, the first published inhibitor of BET proteins, JQ1, has also shown much noted antitumor activity against various tumor cells [115]. We demonstrated that the BET inhibitor JQ1 reverses the EWSR1-FLI1 transcriptional signature of Ewing sarcoma cells and inhibits tumor growth of Ewing sarcoma xenografts [116]. These results have been confirmed or further investigated in other studies [109, 117–119] Thus, Jacques et al. confirmed the effect of JQ1 on Ewing sarcoma xenografts and additionally observed their decreased vascularization [117]. The effect on angiogenesis was confirmed by another study that examined rhabdomyosarcoma in addition to Ewing sarcomas and showed a reduction in the expression of tumor-associated angiogenic factors [118]. Finally, EWSR1-FLI1 or EWSR1-ERG were studied in a functional complex with BRD4, MED1, and RNAPII [109], and impairment of this complex was observed either by RNA interference of BRD4 expression or by BET inhibitors [109]. In alveolar rhabdomyosarcoma, PAX3-FOXO1 was shown to recruit BRD4 to establish de novo super-enhancers at myogenic transcription factors. These FP-RMS cells were highly sensitive to JQ1, as it selectively silenced PAX3-FOXO1-driven transcription [55].

Another way to interfere with the pathogenic transcriptional program of FP sarcomas is to pharmacologically inhibit transcription-dependent cyclin kinases (CDKs) CDK7, 8, 9, 12, and 13. These CDKs have an essential role in transcription by phosphorylating the C-terminal domain of RNA polymerase II, thereby regulating transcription initiation and elongation [120]. Indeed, profiling of cancer cell lines with the covalent CDK7/12/13 inhibitor, THZ1, showed exceptional sensitivity in cancer cell lines dependent on dysregulated transcriptional programs [121]. Using chemical genomics screening, Iniguez et al. 2018 found that Ewing sarcomas are particularly sensitive to THZ1. Further, they observed that the selective CDK12/13 inhibitor THZ531 elicited DNA damage repair in an EWSR1-FLI1-dependent manner. Combining these molecules with the PARP inhibitor Olaparib resulted in tumor volume reduction and prolonged survival in both cell lines and patient-derived xenografts without hematopoietic toxicity [122].

Synergistic effects were also observed with a sequential targeting approach using the histone demethylase inhibitor GSK-J4 and the CDK inhibitor THZ1 [123]. We observed that CDK9 binds to EWSR1-FLI1 via the BET protein BRD4. The combination of the CDK9 inhibitor CDKI-73 with the BET inhibitor JQ1 was more effective in reducing Ewing sarcoma cell proliferation and tumor volume in xenografts than either agent alone [124]. Another study also demonstrated synergy between the EWSR1-FLI inhibitor mithramycin and the CDK9 inhibitor PHA-767491. Importantly, the synergy was observed at clinically relevant concentrations of mithramycin [125]. Finally, in synovial sarcomas, Li et al. 2019 observed that inhibition of CDK9, with either siRNA or the CDK9 inhibitor LDC067, impaired synovial sarcoma cell growth and proliferation in a dose-dependent manner. This was also associated with a decrease in RNA polymerase II phosphorylation and an increase in the expression of anti-apoptotic proteins. In addition, inhibition of CDK9 decreased sarcoma cell spheroid formation and cell motility [126].

8. Inhibition of key players of the fusion-positive interactome

Fusion oncoproteins remodel the transcriptional machinery of cells, silencing genes and activating others by creating new enhancers, remodeling chromatin, and critically altering the epigenetic profile of sarcoma cells. By cooperating with histone deacetylases (HDACs) in transcriptional regulatory complexes, fusion oncoproteins affect histone acetylation and chromatin remodeling. For these chromatin remodeling complexes, they recruit BAF complexes as in the case of Ewing sarcoma [37] or alter their function as in the case of synovial sarcoma [79] to enforce pathogenic transcriptional programs. Binding of EWSR1-FLI1 to GGAA mSATs leads to the binding of histone acetyltransferase p300 at many of these sites and an increase in H3K27ac [35, 36]. On the other hand, the PAX3-FOXO1 fusion oncogene of alveolar rhabdomyosarcoma recruits master transcription factors MYOG, MYOD, and MYCN to activated gene loci and alters their histone acetylation which enables binding and manipulation of reader proteins such as BRD4 [55]. In synovial sarcomas, SS18-SSX fusion oncogenes, cause epigenetic restructuring involving HDACs [127]. Conversely, EWSR1-FLI1 translocation recruits histone deacetylases and histone demethylase LSD1 to specific gene loci through direct interaction with the NuRD complex, thereby suppressing their expression in Ewing sarcoma [39].

However, downstream processes also appear to be important for the epigenetic expression profile in FP sarcomas. For example, EWSR1-FLI1 binds to the promoter of the histone methyltransferase EZH2, upregulating its expression and thereby blocking its endothelial and neuronal differentiation abilities [90, 128]. But, chemical inhibitors of EZH2 activity cannot reproduce the results after RNA interference (unpublished). Yet, recent data show that EZH2-containing PRC2 complexes interact with HDAC1, 2 and this HDAC activity mediates the immature, tumorigenic phenotype of Ewing sarcoma [91].

The involvement of HDACs in key mechanisms of sarcoma cell transformation has paved the way for the investigation of HDACi for therapeutic intervention. Preclinical studies have not found significant therapeutic benefits in solid tumors, including sarcomas. Nevertheless, in combination therapies based on HDACi, sarcomas were represented in most cases as an unclassified group [129]. More recent studies are now specifically examining individual sarcomas and attempting to identify meaningful combination therapies based on known/identified mechanisms: In Ewing sarcomas, we observed that CRISPR/Cas9 knockout of individual HDACs such as HDAC1 and HDAC2 inhibited the invasiveness of Ewing sarcomas and blocked local tumor growth of xenografts. RNA analyses showed that treatment with single HDAC inhibitors (HDACi) blocked an EWSR1-FLI1-specific expression profile, and EwS cells in the presence of HDAC inhibitors (HDACi) such as entinostat and romidepsin had increased susceptibility to treatment with chemotherapeutic agents including doxorubicin. HDACi acted synergistically with the EED inhibitor A-395 and together inhibited tumor growth of Ewing sarcoma xenografts [91]. Similarly, the dual HDAC and phosphatidylinositol 3-kinase (PI3K) inhibitor Fimepinostat can thus also provide simultaneous and sustained inhibition of multiple oncogenic pathways in Ewing sarcoma and reduce EWSR1-FLI1 levels and transcriptional activity [97]. Inhibition of HDAC activity largely affects Ewing sarcoma cell proliferation and survival, alone or in combination with DNA-damaging agents, through a variety of pathways that include induction of apoptosis, cell cycle arrest, and prevention of tumor invasion and metastasis [130–133]. Fimepinostat is currently being tested in children and young adults with relapsed or refractory solid tumors (NCT03893487).

In alveolar RMS, class I HDACs such as HDAC1, 2, and 3 appear to play an essential function in PAX3-FOXO1 driven super-enhancers, as corresponding inhibitors disrupt the activity of these tumor-specific super-enhancers and block transcription and cell proliferation [92]. Recent data show that entinostat affects in vivo growth of FP-RMS and inhibits PAX3-FOXO1 via a multistep and indirect process through an HDAC3-SMARCA4-miR-27a axis [134]. Interestingly, the HDAC inhibitor Entinostat is now being clinically tested in pediatric rhabdomyosarcomas (NCT02780804).

Previous studies have shown that HDAC inhibitors disrupt the oncoprotein complex of synovial sarcoma, leading them to apoptosis. Transcriptome analysis showed that HDAC inhibition blocks the cell cycle, neuronal differentiation promotes polycomb repressor complexes and proapoptotic factors were reactivated. HDAC inhibition resulted in a lower tumor burden in the mouse model [135]. In another study, the response of synovial sarcoma to HDACi was consistently characterized by activation of ERKs, EGR1, and the β-endoglycosidase heparanase. Disruption of HDAC-induced ERK-EGR1-heparanase pathway by concomitant treatment of cells with an MEK inhibitor (trametinib) or a heparanase inhibitor (SST0001/Roneparstat) enhanced the antiproliferative and proapoptotic effects. HDAC and heparanase inhibitors had opposite effects on histone acetylation and heparanase core levels. The combination of SAHA with SST0001 prevented the upregulation of ERK-EGR1 heparanase, induced by HDACi, and promoted caspase-dependent cell death. In the mouse model, combined treatment with SAHA and SST0001 enhanced the antitumor effect compared with single-agent administration [127]. Thus, it seems very reasonable to advance mediators of epigenetic processes as treatment targets for FP sarcomas. Pracinostat (SB939) a potent pan-HDAC inhibitor is now being tested in pediatric patients with refractory solid tumors and leukemias (NCT01184274).

9. Conclusions

The FP sarcomas presented here are characterized by chromosomal rearrangements that generate pathognomonic fusion transcripts and oncoproteins. It is certainly desirable to primarily block or destroy the translocation products of the sarcomas themselves with targeted therapeutic approaches. However, this has not yet been possible for the fusion transcription factors EWSR1-ETS, PAX3/7-FOXO1, and the SS18-SSX fusion oncogene. But it seems promising to prevent important binding partners of these fusion oncogenes, which are essential for mediating the oncogenic processes, from successfully binding to these fusion oncogenes. An example of this is the observed blockade of the interaction of EWSR1-FLI1 with RNA helicase A by YK-4-279, and the results of initial therapeutic interventions are of great interest here.

Currently, the greatest progress seems to be promised by approaches that address mediators of the fusion-positive interactome. Essential here seems the pathological takeover of the transcriptional machinery by these fusion oncogenes and the manifestation of their epigenetic state by histone deacetylases. Approaches that block epigenetic reader proteins such as BRD4 or transcription-specific cyclin kinases such as CDK 9 and 12 indicate promising results. The remarkable efficacy of HDAC inhibitors is highly interesting. Also, the use of these inhibitors seems to significantly reduce the stability of fusion oncogenes. On the other hand, particularly high therapeutic effects were achieved experimentally where these inhibitors were used in combination. It can therefore be assumed that targeted therapeutic approaches will be particularly successful in the future where they specifically address pathological processes of the fusion oncogenes and block several identified processes simultaneously. In doing so, the existing plasticity of the tumor must be kept in mind or synergistic processes must be identified by combining the drugs, which will probably make it possible to reduce their concentration and thus toxicity of individual doses.

Acknowledgements

The author would like to thank Angelika Eggert, Nicole Hübener, Katharina Pardon, and Beat W. Schäfer for their support. This work was supported by grants from the Berliner Krebsgesellschaft (RIFF201913), and KINDerLEBEN e.V. Berlin. It is part of the EpiCycle Consortium(01KC2012E), Funding Program of the Federal Ministry of Education and Research (BMBF), Germany.

Conflict of interest

The author declares no conflict of interest.

Abbreviations

APC	Adenomatous Polyposis Coli regulator of WNT signaling pathway
AKT	AKT serine/threonine kinase
ARF	ADP-ribosylation factor
ATF2	Activating transcription factor 2
ATP	Adenosin-triphosphate
AYA	adolescents, and young adults
BAF	ATP-dependent BRG1/BRM associated factor
BAF47	is SMARCB1: SWI/SNF related, matrix associated, actin dependent regulator of chromatin, subfamily b, member 1
BET	Bromodomain and extraterminal domain
BRG	BRM/SWI2-related gene is SMARCA4 SWI/SNF related, matrix associated, actin dependent regulator of chromatin, subfamily a, member 4
BRD	Bromodomain containing
BRM	Brahma is a core, ATPase subunit of the chromatin-remodeling complex
Cas9	Type II CRISPR RNA-guided endonuclease
CDK	Cyclin dependent kinase
Co-IP	Co-immuno-precipitation
CRBN	Cereblon
CRISPR	Clustered regularly interspaced short palindromic repeats
CTNNB1	Catenin beta 1
DEAD	Contains the amino acid sequence D-E-A-D (asp-glu-ala-asp)
EED	Embryonic ectoderm development
ERG	Erythroblast transformation specific (ETS) related gene
ETV	ETS variant transcription factor
EWSR1	Ewing sarcoma breakpoint region 1/EWS RNA binding protein 1
EZH2	Enhancer of zeste 2 polycomb repressive complex 2 subunit
FET	Fused in sarcoma (FUS) RNA binding protein, EWSR1 and TATA-box binding protein associated factor 15 (TAF15) family of genes
FEV	Fifth Ewing variant transcription factor, ETS family member
FGFR4	Fibroblast growth factor receptor 4
FLI1	Friend leukemia virus integration 1 proto-oncogene, ETS transcription factor
FOXO1	Forkhead box O1
HDAC	Histone deacetylase
Hippo	Protein kinase hippo (hpo) is part of a signaling pathway that controls organ size through the regulation of cell proliferation and apoptosis
IGF2	Insulin like growth factor 2
INI1	Integrase interactor 1 (INI1) is SMARCAB1
LSD1	Lysine-specific demethylase 1A
KDM2B	Lysine (K)-specific demethylase 2B
KRAS	Kirsten rat sarcoma viral oncogene homolog (KRAS) proto-oncogene, GTPase
LOX	Lysyl oxidase
MET	Mesenchymal-epithelial transition factor (MET) proto-oncogene, receptor tyrosine kinase

miR-27a	microRNA-27a
MYCN	MYCN proto-oncogene, BHLH transcription factor
MYOD	Myogenic differentiation
MYOG	Myogenin
PAX	Paired box
p21	is CDKN1A: cyclin dependent kinase inhibitor 1A
PCR2	Polycomb repressor complex 2
PI3K	Phosphatidylinositol 3-kinase
PIK3CA	Phosphatidylinositol-4,5-bisphosphate 3-kinase catalytic subunit alpha
PTEN	Phosphatase and tensin homolog
RAS	Rat sarcoma proto-oncogene, GTPase
RNAi	RNA interference
RNAPII	RNA Polymerase II
SAHA	Suberoylanilide hydroxamic acid
SMARCA4	SWI/SNF related, matrix associated, actin dependent regulator of chromatin, subfamily A, member 4
SMARCB1	SWI/SNF related, matrix associated, actin dependent regulator of chromatin, subfamily b, member 1
SNF5	Sucrose nonfermenting 5 is SMARCB1
SS18	Synovial sarcoma translocation, chromosome 18, subunit of BAF chromatin remodeling complex
SSX	Synovial sarcoma, X breakpoint
STAG2	Stromal antigen 2
SWI/SNF	SWItch/Sucrose Non-Fermentable is a subfamily of ATP-dependent chromatin remodeling complexes
TGFBR2	Transforming growth factor-beta receptor 2
TP53	Tumor protein 53
TGF-β	Transforming growth factor beta
VHL	von Hippel-Lindau tumor suppressor

Author details

Günther H.S. Richter
Department of Pediatrics, Division of Oncology and Hematology,
Charité—Universitätsmedizin Berlin, Berlin, Germany

*Address all correspondence to: guenther.richter@charite.de

References

[1] Stiller CA, Trama A, Serraino D, Rossi S, Navarro C, Chirlaque MD, et al. Descriptive epidemiology of sarcomas in Europe: Report from the RARECARE project. European Journal of Cancer. 2013;**49**(3):684-695

[2] Baldauf MC, Gerke JS, Orth MF, Dallmayer M, Baumhoer D, de Alava E, et al. Are EWSR1-NFATc2-positive sarcomas really Ewing sarcomas? Modern Pathology. 2018;**31**(6):997-999

[3] Koelsche C, Hartmann W, Schrimpf D, Stichel D, Jabar S, Ranft A, et al. Array-based DNA-methylation profiling in sarcomas with small blue round cell histology provides valuable diagnostic information. Modern Pathology. 2018;**31**(8):1246-1256

[4] Watson S, Perrin V, Guillemot D, Reynaud S, Coindre JM, Karanian M, et al. Transcriptomic definition of molecular subgroups of small round cell sarcomas. The Journal of Pathology. 2018;**245**(1):29-40

[5] Grunewald TG, Alonso M, Avnet S, Banito A, Burdach S, Cidre-Aranaz F, et al. Sarcoma treatment in the era of molecular medicine. EMBO Molecular Medicine. 2020;**12**(11):e11131

[6] Sultan I, Qaddoumi I, Yaser S, Rodriguez-Galindo C, Ferrari A. Comparing adult and pediatric rhabdomyosarcoma in the surveillance, epidemiology and end results program, 1973 to 2005: An analysis of 2,600 patients. Journal of Clinical Oncology: Official Journal of the American Society of Clinical Oncology. 2009;**27**(20):3391-3397

[7] Downing JR, Wilson RK, Zhang J, Mardis ER, Pui CH, Ding L, et al. The pediatric cancer genome project. Nature Genetics. 2012;**44**(6):619-622

[8] Rahal Z, Abdulhai F, Kadara H, Saab R. Genomics of adult and pediatric solid tumors. American Journal of Cancer Research. 2018;**8**(8):1356-1386

[9] Seidal T, Mark J, Hagmar B, Angervall L. Alveolar rhabdomyosarcoma: A cytogenetic and correlated cytological and histological study. Acta Pathologica, Microbiologica, et Immunologica Scandinavica. Section A. 1982;**90**(5):345-354

[10] Delattre O, Zucman J, Plougastel B, Desmaze C, Melot T, Peter M, et al. Gene fusion with an ETS DNA-binding domain caused by chromosome translocation in human tumours. Nature. 1992;**359**(6391):162-165

[11] Rabbitts TH. Commonality but diversity in cancer gene fusions. Cell. 2009;**137**(3):391-395

[12] Mertens F, Antonescu CR, Mitelman F. Gene fusions in soft tissue tumors: Recurrent and overlapping pathogenetic themes. Genes, Chromosomes & Cancer. 2016;**55**(4):291-310

[13] Mertens F, Johansson B, Fioretos T, Mitelman F. The emerging complexity of gene fusions in cancer. Nature Reviews. Cancer. 2015;**15**(6):371-381

[14] Grobner SN, Worst BC, Weischenfeldt J, Buchhalter I, Kleinheinz K, Rudneva VA, et al. The landscape of genomic alterations across childhood cancers. Nature. 2018;**555**(7696):321-327

[15] Crompton BD, Stewart C, Taylor-Weiner A, Alexe G, Kurek KC, Calicchio ML, et al. The genomic landscape of pediatric

Ewing sarcoma. Cancer Discovery. 2014;**4**(11):1326-1341

[16] Lawrence MS, Stojanov P, Polak P, Kryukov GV, Cibulskis K, Sivachenko A, et al. Mutational heterogeneity in cancer and the search for new cancer-associated genes. Nature. 2013;**499**(7457):214-218

[17] Shern JF, Chen L, Chmielecki J, Wei JS, Patidar R, Rosenberg M, et al. Comprehensive genomic analysis of rhabdomyosarcoma reveals a landscape of alterations affecting a common genetic axis in fusion-positive and fusion-negative tumors. Cancer Discovery. 2014;**4**(2):216-231

[18] Tirode F, Surdez D, Ma X, Parker M, Le Deley MC, Bahrami A, et al. Genomic landscape of Ewing sarcoma defines an aggressive subtype with co-association of STAG2 and TP53 mutations. Cancer Discovery. 2014;**4**(11):1342-1353

[19] Vlenterie M, Hillebrandt-Roeffen MH, Flucke UE, Groenen PJ, Tops BB, Kamping EJ, et al. Next generation sequencing in synovial sarcoma reveals novel gene mutations. Oncotarget. 2015;**6**(33):34680-34690

[20] Koelsche C, Schrimpf D, Stichel D, Sill M, Sahm F, Reuss DE, et al. Sarcoma classification by DNA methylation profiling. Nature Communications. 2021;**12**(1):498

[21] Vogelstein B, Papadopoulos N, Velculescu VE, Zhou S, Diaz LA Jr, Kinzler KW. Cancer genome landscapes. Science. 2013;**339**(6127):1546-1558

[22] Gaspar N, Hawkins DS, Dirksen U, Lewis IJ, Ferrari S, Le Deley MC, et al. Ewing Sarcoma: Current management and future approaches through collaboration. Journal of Clinical Oncology: Official Journal of the American Society of Clinical Oncology. 2015;**33**(27):3036-3046

[23] Pappo AS, Dirksen U. Rhabdomyosarcoma, Ewing Sarcoma, and Other Round Cell Sarcomas. Journal of Clinical Oncology: Official Journal of the American Society of Clinical Oncology. 2018;**36**(2):168-179

[24] Grunewald TGP, Cidre-Aranaz F, Surdez D, Tomazou EM, de Alava E, Kovar H, et al. Ewing sarcoma. Nature Reviews. 2018;**4**(1):5

[25] Anderson ND, de Borja R, Young MD, Fuligni F, Rosic A, Roberts ND, et al. Rearrangement bursts generate canonical gene fusions in bone and soft tissue tumors. Science. 2018;**361**:6405

[26] Agelopoulos K, Richter GH, Schmidt E, Dirksen U, von Heyking K, Moser B, et al. Deep sequencing in conjunction with expression and functional analyses reveals activation of FGFR1 in Ewing Sarcoma. Clinical Cancer Research: An Official Journal of the American Association for Cancer Research. 2015;**21**(21):4935-4946

[27] Henssen AG, Koche R, Zhuang J, Jiang E, Reed C, Eisenberg A, et al. PGBD5 promotes site-specific oncogenic mutations in human tumors. Nature Genetics. 2017;**49**(7):1005-1014

[28] Henssen AG, Reed C, Jiang E, Garcia HD, von Stebut J, MacArthur IC, et al. Therapeutic targeting of PGBD5-induced DNA repair dependency in pediatric solid tumors. Science Translational Medicine. 2017;**9**:44

[29] Sheffield NC, Pierron G, Klughammer J, Datlinger P, Schonegger A, Schuster M, et al. DNA methylation heterogeneity defines a disease spectrum in Ewing sarcoma. Nature Medicine. 2017;**23**(3):386-395

[30] Tirode F, Laud-Duval K, Prieur A, Delorme B, Charbord P, Delattre O. Mesenchymal stem cell features of Ewing tumors. Cancer Cell. 2007;**11**(5):421-429

[31] von Levetzow C, Jiang X, Gwye Y, von Levetzow G, Hung L, Cooper A, et al. Modeling initiation of Ewing sarcoma in human neural crest cells. PLoS One. 2011;**6**(4):e19305

[32] Kovar H, Hyde D. The two faces of the FUS/EWS/TAF15 protein family. Sarcoma. 2011;**2011**:837474

[33] Sharrocks AD. The ETS-domain transcription factor family. Nature Reviews. Molecular Cell Biology. 2001;**2**(11):827-837

[34] Franzetti GA, Laud-Duval K, van der Ent W, Brisac A, Irondelle M, Aubert S, et al. Cell-to-cell heterogeneity of EWSR1-FLI1 activity determines proliferation/migration choices in Ewing sarcoma cells. Oncogene. 2017;**36**(25):3505-3514

[35] Riggi N, Knoechel B, Gillespie SM, Rheinbay E, Boulay G, Suva ML, et al. EWS-FLI1 utilizes divergent chromatin remodeling mechanisms to directly activate or repress enhancer elements in Ewing sarcoma. Cancer Cell. 2014;**26**(5):668-681

[36] Tomazou EM, Sheffield NC, Schmidl C, Schuster M, Schonegger A, Datlinger P, et al. Epigenome mapping reveals distinct modes of gene regulation and widespread enhancer reprogramming by the oncogenic fusion protein EWS-FLI1. Cell Reports. 2015;**10**(7):1082-1095

[37] Boulay G, Sandoval GJ, Riggi N, Iyer S, Buisson R, Naigles B, et al. Cancer-Specific Retargeting of BAF Complexes by a Prion-like Domain. Cell. 2017;**171**(1):163-178

[38] Musa J, Grunewald TGP. Interaction between somatic mutations and germline variants contributes to clinical heterogeneity in cancer. Molecular & Cellular Oncology. 2020;**7**(1):1682924

[39] Sankar S, Bell R, Stephens B, Zhuo R, Sharma S, Bearss DJ, et al. Mechanism and relevance of EWS/FLI-mediated transcriptional repression in Ewing sarcoma. Oncogene. 2013;**32**(42):5089-5100

[40] Erkizan HV, Kong Y, Merchant M, Schlottmann S, Barber-Rotenberg JS, Yuan L, et al. A small molecule blocking oncogenic protein EWS-FLI1 interaction with RNA helicase A inhibits growth of Ewing's sarcoma. Nature Medicine. 2009;**15**(7):750-756

[41] Cai W, Xiong Chen Z, Rane G, Satendra Singh S, Choo Z, Wang C, et al. Wanted DEAD/H or alive: Helicases winding up in cancers. Journal of National Cancer Institute. 2017;**109**(6):1-15

[42] Parham DM. Pathologic classification of rhabdomyosarcomas and correlations with molecular studies. Modern Pathology. 2001;**14**(5):506-514

[43] Hettmer S, Li Z, Billin AN, Barr FG, Cornelison DD, Ehrlich AR, et al. Rhabdomyosarcoma: Current challenges and their implications for developing therapies. Cold Spring Harbor Perspectives in Medicine. 2014;**4**(11):a025650

[44] Raney RB, Maurer HM, Anderson JR, Andrassy RJ, Donaldson SS, Qualman SJ, et al. The Intergroup Rhabdomyosarcoma Study Group (IRSG): Major Lessons From the IRS-I Through IRS-IV Studies as Background for the Current IRS-V Treatment Protocols. Sarcoma. 2001;**5**(1):9-15

[45] Galili N, Davis RJ, Fredericks WJ, Mukhopadhyay S, Rauscher FJ 3rd,

Emanuel BS, et al. Fusion of a fork head domain gene to PAX3 in the solid tumour alveolar rhabdomyosarcoma. Nature Genetics. 1993;**5**(3):230-235

[46] Shapiro DN, Sublett JE, Li B, Downing JR, Naeve CW. Fusion of PAX3 to a member of the forkhead family of transcription factors in human alveolar rhabdomyosarcoma. Cancer Research. 1993;**53**(21):5108-5112

[47] Coomans de Brachene A, Demoulin JB. FOXO transcription factors in cancer development and therapy. Cellular and Molecular Life Sciences. 2016;**73**(6):1159-1172

[48] Fletcher CD. The evolving classification of soft tissue tumours—An update based on the new 2013 WHO classification. Histopathology. 2014;**64**(1):2-11

[49] Loupe JM, Miller PJ, Bonner BP, Maggi EC, Vijayaraghavan J, Crabtree JS, et al. Comparative transcriptomic analysis reveals the oncogenic fusion protein PAX3-FOXO1 globally alters mRNA and miRNA to enhance myoblast invasion. Oncogene. 2016;5(7):e246

[50] Pandey PR, Chatterjee B, Olanich ME, Khan J, Miettinen MM, Hewitt SM, et al. PAX3-FOXO1 is essential for tumour initiation and maintenance but not recurrence in a human myoblast model of rhabdomyosarcoma. The Journal of Pathology. 2017;**241**(5):626-637

[51] Bennicelli JL, Advani S, Schafer BW, Barr FG. PAX3 and PAX7 exhibit conserved cis-acting transcription repression domains and utilize a common gain of function mechanism in alveolar rhabdomyosarcoma. Oncogene. 1999;**18**(30):4348-4356

[52] Davis RJ, Barr FG. Fusion genes resulting from alternative chromosomal translocations are overexpressed by gene-specific mechanisms in alveolar rhabdomyosarcoma. Proceedings of the National Academy of Sciences of the United States of America. 1997;**94**(15):8047-8051

[53] Bennicelli JL, Fredericks WJ, Wilson RB, Rauscher FJ 3rd, Barr FG. Wild type PAX3 protein and the PAX3-FKHR fusion protein of alveolar rhabdomyosarcoma contain potent, structurally distinct transcriptional activation domains. Oncogene. 1995;**11**(1):119-130

[54] Fredericks WJ, Galili N, Mukhopadhyay S, Rovera G, Bennicelli J, Barr FG, et al. The PAX3-FKHR fusion protein created by the t(2;13) translocation in alveolar rhabdomyosarcomas is a more potent transcriptional activator than PAX3. Molecular and Cellular Biology. 1995;**15**(3):1522-1535

[55] Gryder BE, Yohe ME, Chou HC, Zhang X, Marques J, Wachtel M, et al. PAX3-FOXO1 establishes myogenic super enhancers and confers BET bromodomain vulnerability. Cancer Discovery. 2017;**7**(8):884-899

[56] Missiaglia E, Williamson D, Chisholm J, Wirapati P, Pierron G, Petel F, et al. PAX3/FOXO1 fusion gene status is the key prognostic molecular marker in rhabdomyosarcoma and significantly improves current risk stratification. Journal of Clinical Oncology: Official Journal of the American Society of Clinical Oncology. 2012;**30**(14):1670-1677

[57] Williamson D, Missiaglia E, de Reynies A, Pierron G, Thuille B, Palenzuela G, et al. Fusion gene-negative alveolar rhabdomyosarcoma is clinically and molecularly indistinguishable from embryonal rhabdomyosarcoma. Journal of Clinical Oncology: Official Journal of the American Society of Clinical Oncology. 2010;**28**(13):2151-2158

[58] Barr FG. Gene fusions involving PAX and FOX family members in alveolar rhabdomyosarcoma. Oncogene. 2001;**20**(40):5736-5746

[59] Kikuchi K, Tsuchiya K, Otabe O, Gotoh T, Tamura S, Katsumi Y, et al. Effects of PAX3-FKHR on malignant phenotypes in alveolar rhabdomyosarcoma. Biochemical and Biophysical Research Communications. 2008;**365**(3):568-574

[60] Graf Finckenstein F, Shahbazian V, Davicioni E, Ren YX, Anderson MJ. PAX-FKHR function as pangenes by simultaneously inducing and inhibiting myogenesis. Oncogene. 2008;**27**(14):2004-2014

[61] Keller C, Hansen MS, Coffin CM, Capecchi MR. Pax3:Fkhr interferes with embryonic Pax3 and Pax7 function: Implications for alveolar rhabdomyosarcoma cell of origin. Genes & Development. 2004;**18**(21):2608-2613

[62] Naini S, Etheridge KT, Adam SJ, Qualman SJ, Bentley RC, Counter CM, et al. Defining the cooperative genetic changes that temporally drive alveolar rhabdomyosarcoma. Cancer Research. 2008;**68**(23):9583-9588

[63] Chen L, Shern JF, Wei JS, Yohe ME, Song YK, Hurd L, et al. Clonality and evolutionary history of rhabdomyosarcoma. PLoS Genetics. 2015;**11**(3):e1005075

[64] Cao L, Yu Y, Bilke S, Walker RL, Mayeenuddin LH, Azorsa DO, et al. Genome-wide identification of PAX3-FKHR binding sites in rhabdomyosarcoma reveals candidate target genes important for development and cancer. Cancer Research. 2010;**70**(16):6497-6508

[65] Crose LE, Galindo KA, Kephart JG, Chen C, Fitamant J, Bardeesy N, et al. Alveolar rhabdomyosarcoma-associated PAX3-FOXO1 promotes tumorigenesis via Hippo pathway suppression. The Journal of clinical investigation. 2014;**124**(1):285-296

[66] Ginsberg JP, Davis RJ, Bennicelli JL, Nauta LE, Barr FG. Up-regulation of MET but not neural cell adhesion molecule expression by the PAX3-FKHR fusion protein in alveolar rhabdomyosarcoma. Cancer Research. 1998;**58**(16):3542-3546

[67] Walters ZS, Villarejo-Balcells B, Olmos D, Buist TW, Missiaglia E, Allen R, et al. JARID2 is a direct target of the PAX3-FOXO1 fusion protein and inhibits myogenic differentiation of rhabdomyosarcoma cells. Oncogene. 2014;**33**(9):1148-1157

[68] Schmitt-Ney M, Camussi G. The PAX3-FOXO1 fusion protein present in rhabdomyosarcoma interferes with normal FOXO activity and the TGF-beta pathway. PLoS One. 2015;**10**(3):e0121474

[69] Wang S, Song R, Sun T, Hou B, Hong G, Mallampati S, et al. Survival changes in patients with Synovial Sarcoma, 1983-2012. Journal of Cancer. 2017;**8**(10):1759-1768

[70] Sultan I, Rodriguez-Galindo C, Saab R, Yasir S, Casanova M, Ferrari A. Comparing children and adults with synovial sarcoma in the Surveillance, Epidemiology, and End Results program, 1983 to 2005: An analysis of 1268 patients. Cancer. 2009;**115**(15):3537-3547

[71] Clark J, Rocques PJ, Crew AJ, Gill S, Shipley J, Chan AM, et al. Identification of novel genes, SYT and SSX, involved in the t(X;18)(p11.2;q11.2) translocation found in human synovial sarcoma. Nature Genetics. 1994;**7**(4):502-508

[72] de Leeuw B, Balemans M, Olde Weghuis D. Geurts van Kessel A.

Identification of two alternative fusion genes, SYT-SSX1 and SYT-SSX2, in t(X;18)(p11.2;q11.2)-positive synovial sarcomas. Human Molecular Genetics. 1995;**4**(6):1097-1099

[73] Skytting B, Nilsson G, Brodin B, Xie Y, Lundeberg J, Uhlen M, et al. A novel fusion gene, SYT-SSX4, in synovial sarcoma. Journal of the National Cancer Institute. 1999;**91**(11):974-975

[74] Merchant MS, Mackall CL. Current approach to pediatric soft tissue sarcomas. The Oncologist. 2009;**14**(11):1139-1153

[75] Joseph CG, Hwang H, Jiao Y, Wood LD, Kinde I, Wu J, et al. Exomic analysis of myxoid liposarcomas, synovial sarcomas, and osteosarcomas. Genes, Chromosomes & Cancer. 2014;**53**(1):15-24

[76] Haldar M, Hancock JD, Coffin CM, Lessnick SL, Capecchi MR. A conditional mouse model of synovial sarcoma: Insights into a myogenic origin. Cancer Cell. 2007;**11**(4):375-388

[77] Nagai M, Tanaka S, Tsuda M, Endo S, Kato H, Sonobe H, et al. Analysis of transforming activity of human synovial sarcoma-associated chimeric protein SYT-SSX1 bound to chromatin remodeling factor hBRM/hSNF2 alpha. Proceedings of the National Academy of Sciences of the United States of America. 2001;**98**(7):3843-3848

[78] Carmody Soni EE, Schlottman S, Erkizan HV, Uren A, Toretsky JA. Loss of SS18-SSX1 inhibits viability and induces apoptosis in synovial sarcoma. Clinical Orthopaedics and Related Research. 2014;**472**(3):874-882

[79] Kadoch C, Crabtree GR. Reversible disruption of mSWI/SNF (BAF) complexes by the SS18-SSX oncogenic fusion in synovial sarcoma. Cell. 2013;**153**(1):71-85

[80] Tamaki S, Fukuta M, Sekiguchi K, Jin Y, Nagata S, Hayakawa K, et al. SS18-SSX, the Oncogenic Fusion Protein in Synovial Sarcoma, Is a Cellular Context-Dependent Epigenetic Modifier. PLoS One. 2015;**10**(11):e0142991

[81] Middeljans E, Wan X, Jansen PW, Sharma V, Stunnenberg HG, Logie C. SS18 together with animal-specific factors defines human BAF-type SWI/SNF complexes. PLoS One. 2012;**7**(3):e33834

[82] Thaete C, Brett D, Monaghan P, Whitehouse S, Rennie G, Rayner E, et al. Functional domains of the SYT and SYT-SSX synovial sarcoma translocation proteins and co-localization with the SNF protein BRM in the nucleus. Human Molecular Genetics. 1999;**8**(4):585-591

[83] Soulez M, Saurin AJ, Freemont PS, Knight JC. SSX and the synovial-sarcoma-specific chimaeric protein SYT-SSX co-localize with the human Polycomb group complex. Oncogene. 1999;**18**(17):2739-2746

[84] Su L, Sampaio AV, Jones KB, Pacheco M, Goytain A, Lin S, et al. Deconstruction of the SS18-SSX fusion oncoprotein complex: Insights into disease etiology and therapeutics. Cancer Cell. 2012;**21**(3):333-347

[85] de Bruijn DR, Allander SV, van Dijk AH, Willemse MP, Thijssen J, van Groningen JJ, et al. The synovial-sarcoma-associated SS18-SSX2 fusion protein induces epigenetic gene (de)regulation. Cancer Research. 2006;**66**(19):9474-9482

[86] Garcia CB, Shaffer CM, Eid JE. Genome-wide recruitment to Polycomb-modified chromatin and activity

regulation of the synovial sarcoma oncogene SYT-SSX2. BMC Genomics. 2012;**13**:189

[87] Kawano S, Grassian AR, Tsuda M, Knutson SK, Warholic NM, Kuznetsov G, et al. Preclinical evidence of anti-tumor activity induced by EZH2 inhibition in human models of Synovial Sarcoma. PLoS One. 2016;**11**(7):e0158888

[88] Banito A, Li X, Laporte AN, Roe JS, Sanchez-Vega F, Huang CH, et al. The SS18-SSX Oncoprotein Hijacks KDM2B-PRC1.1 to Drive Synovial Sarcoma. Cancer Cell. 2018;**34**(2):346-348

[89] McBride MJ, Pulice JL, Beird HC, Ingram DR, D'Avino AR, Shern JF, et al. The SS18-SSX Fusion Oncoprotein Hijacks BAF complex targeting and function to drive Synovial Sarcoma. Cancer Cell. 2018;**33**(6):1128-1141

[90] Richter GH, Plehm S, Fasan A, Rossler S, Unland R, Bennani-Baiti IM, et al. EZH2 is a mediator of EWS/FLI1 driven tumor growth and metastasis blocking endothelial and neuro-ectodermal differentiation. Proceedings of the National Academy of Sciences of the United States of America. 2009;**106**(13):5324-5329

[91] Schmidt O, Nehls N, Prexler C, von Heyking K, Groll T, Pardon K, et al. Class I histone deacetylases (HDAC) critically contribute to Ewing sarcoma pathogenesis. Journal of Experimental & Clinical Cancer Research. 2021;**40**(1):322

[92] Gryder BE, Wu L, Woldemichael GM, Pomella S, Quinn TR, Park PMC, et al. Chemical genomics reveals histone deacetylases are required for core regulatory transcription. Nature Communications. 2019;**10**(1):3004

[93] March ZM, King OD, Shorter J. Prion-like domains as epigenetic regulators, scaffolds for subcellular organization, and drivers of neurodegenerative disease. Brain Research. 1647;**2016**:9-18

[94] Brien GL, Remillard D, Shi J, Hemming ML, Chabon J, Wynne K, et al. Targeted degradation of BRD9 reverses oncogenic gene expression in synovial sarcoma. eLife. 2018;**7**:1-26

[95] Michel BC, D'Avino AR, Cassel SH, Mashtalir N, McKenzie ZM, McBride MJ, et al. A non-canonical SWI/SNF complex is a synthetic lethal target in cancers driven by BAF complex perturbation. Nature Cell Biology. 2018;**20**(12):1410-1420

[96] Blay V, Tolani B, Ho SP, Arkin MR. High-throughput screening: Today's biochemical and cell-based approaches. Drug Discovery Today. 2020;**25**(10):1807-1821

[97] Pedot G, Marques JG, Ambuhl PP, Wachtel M, Kasper S, Ngo QA, et al. Inhibition of HDACs reduces Ewing sarcoma tumor growth through EWS-FLI1 protein destabilization. Neoplasia. 2022;**27**:100784

[98] Bondeson DP, Crews CM. Targeted protein degradation by small molecules. Annual Review of Pharmacology and Toxicology. 2017;**57**:107-123

[99] Toure M, Crews CM. Small-molecule PROTACS: New approaches to protein degradation. Angewandte Chemie (International Ed. in English). 2016;**55**(6):1966-1973

[100] Nalawansha DA, Crews CM. PROTACs: An emerging therapeutic modality in precision medicine. Cell Chemical Biology. 2020;**27**(8):998-1014

[101] Buckley DL, Van Molle I, Gareiss PC, Tae HS, Michel J, Noblin DJ,

et al. Targeting the von Hippel-Lindau E3 ubiquitin ligase using small molecules to disrupt the VHL/HIF-1alpha interaction. Journal of the American Chemical Society. 2012;**134**(10):4465-4468

[102] Kronke J, Udeshi ND, Narla A, Grauman P, Hurst SN, McConkey M, et al. Lenalidomide causes selective degradation of IKZF1 and IKZF3 in multiple myeloma cells. Science. 2014;**343**(6168):301-305

[103] Lu G, Middleton RE, Sun H, Naniong M, Ott CJ, Mitsiades CS, et al. The myeloma drug lenalidomide promotes the cereblon-dependent destruction of Ikaros proteins. Science. 2014;**343**(6168):305-309

[104] Lu J, Qian Y, Altieri M, Dong H, Wang J, Raina K, et al. Hijacking the E3 ubiquitin ligase cereblon to efficiently target BRD4. Chemistry & Biology. 2015;**22**(6):755-763

[105] Winter GE, Buckley DL, Paulk J, Roberts JM, Souza A, Dhe-Paganon S, et al. DRUG DEVELOPMENT. Phthalimide conjugation as a strategy for in vivo target protein degradation. Science. 2015;**348**(6241):1376-1381

[106] Gierisch ME, Pfistner F, Lopez-Garcia LA, Harder L, Schafer BW, Niggli FK. Proteasomal degradation of the EWS-FLI1 fusion protein is regulated by a single lysine residue. The Journal of Biological Chemistry. 2016;**291**(52):26922-26933

[107] Ducker C, Shaw PE. Ubiquitin-mediated control of ETS transcription factors: Roles in cancer and development. International Journal of Molecular Science. 2021;**22**(10):1-17

[108] Su S, Chen J, Jiang Y, Wang Y, Vital T, Zhang J, et al. SPOP and OTUD7A Control EWS-FLI1 Protein Stability to Govern Ewing Sarcoma Growth. Advanced Science (Weinh). 2021;**8**(14):e2004846

[109] Gollavilli PN, Pawar A, Wilder-Romans K, Natesan R, Engelke CG, Dommeti VL, et al. EWS/ETS-Driven Ewing Sarcoma Requires BET Bromodomain Proteins. Cancer Research. 2018;**78**(16):4760-4773

[110] Coussens NP, Braisted JC, Peryea T, Sittampalam GS, Simeonov A, Hall MD. Small-molecule screens: A gateway to cancer therapeutic agents with case studies of food and drug administration-approved drugs. Pharmacological Reviews. 2017;**69**(4):479-496

[111] Bradner JE, Hnisz D, Young RA. Transcriptional addiction in cancer. Cell. 2017;**168**(4):629-643

[112] Whyte WA, Orlando DA, Hnisz D, Abraham BJ, Lin CY, Kagey MH, et al. Master transcription factors and mediator establish super-enhancers at key cell identity genes. Cell. 2013;**153**(2):307-319

[113] Zeng L, Zhou MM. Bromodomain: An acetyl-lysine binding domain. FEBS Letters. 2002;**513**(1):124-128

[114] Bechter O, Schoffski P. Make your best BET: The emerging role of BET inhibitor treatment in malignant tumors. Pharmacology & Therapeutics. 2020;**208**:107479

[115] Loven J, Hoke HA, Lin CY, Lau A, Orlando DA, Vakoc CR, et al. Selective inhibition of tumor oncogenes by disruption of super-enhancers. Cell. 2013;**153**(2):320-334

[116] Hensel T, Giorgi C, Schmidt O, Calzada-Wack J, Neff F, Buch T, et al. Targeting the EWS-ETS transcriptional program by BET bromodomain

inhibition in Ewing sarcoma. Oncotarget. 2016;**7**(2):1451-1463

[117] Jacques C, Lamoureux F, Baud'huin M, Rodriguez Calleja L, Quillard T, Amiaud J, et al. Targeting the epigenetic readers in Ewing sarcoma inhibits the oncogenic transcription factor EWS/Fli1. Oncotarget. 2016;**7**(17):24125-24140

[118] Bid HK, Phelps DA, Xaio L, Guttridge DC, Lin J, London C, et al. The bromodomain BET inhibitor JQ1 suppresses tumor angiogenesis in models of childhood sarcoma. Molecular Cancer Therapeutics. 2016;**15**(5):1018-1028

[119] Loganathan SN, Tang N, Fleming JT, Ma Y, Guo Y, Borinstein SC, et al. BET bromodomain inhibitors suppress EWS-FLI1-dependent transcription and the IGF1 autocrine mechanism in Ewing sarcoma. Oncotarget. 2016;**7**(28):43504-43517

[120] Larochelle S, Amat R, Glover-Cutter K, Sanso M, Zhang C, Allen JJ, et al. Cyclin-dependent kinase control of the initiation-to-elongation switch of RNA polymerase II. Nature Structural & Molecular Biology. 2012;**19**(11):1108-1115

[121] Kwiatkowski N, Zhang T, Rahl PB, Abraham BJ, Reddy J, Ficarro SB, et al. Targeting transcription regulation in cancer with a covalent CDK7 inhibitor. Nature. 2014;**511**(7511):616-620

[122] Iniguez AB, Stolte B, Wang EJ, Conway AS, Alexe G, Dharia NV, et al. EWS/FLI confers tumor cell synthetic lethality to CDK12 inhibition in Ewing Sarcoma. Cancer Cell. 2018;**33**(2):202-216

[123] Heisey DAR, Jacob S, Lochmann TL, Kurupi R, Ghotra MS, Calbert ML, et al. Pharmaceutical interference of the EWS-FLI1-driven transcriptome by cotargeting H3K27ac and RNA polymerase activity in Ewing Sarcoma. Molecular Cancer Therapeutics. 2021;**20**(10):1868-1879

[124] Richter GHS, Hensel T, Schmidt O, Saratov V, von Heyking K, Becker-Dettling F, et al. Combined inhibition of epigenetic readers and transcription initiation targets the EWS-ETS transcriptional program in Ewing Sarcoma. Cancers. Basel; 2020;**12**(2):1-17

[125] Flores G, Everett JH, Boguslawski EA, Oswald BM, Madaj ZB, Beddows I, et al. CDK9 blockade exploits context-dependent transcriptional changes to improve activity and limit toxicity of Mithramycin for Ewing Sarcoma. Molecular Cancer Therapeutics. 2020;**19**(5):1183-1196

[126] Li X, Seebacher NA, Xiao T, Hornicek FJ, Duan Z. Targeting regulation of cyclin dependent kinase 9 as a novel therapeutic strategy in synovial sarcoma. Journal of Orthopaedic Research. 2019;**37**(2):510-521

[127] Lanzi C, Favini E, Dal Bo L, Tortoreto M, Arrighetti N, Zaffaroni N, et al. Upregulation of ERK-EGR1-heparanase axis by HDAC inhibitors provides targets for rational therapeutic intervention in synovial sarcoma. Journal of Experimental & Clinical Cancer Research. 2021;**40**(1):381

[128] Burdach S, Plehm S, Unland R, Dirksen U, Borkhardt A, Staege MS, et al. Epigenetic maintenance of stemness and malignancy in peripheral neuroectodermal tumors by EZH2. Cell Cycle. 2009;**8**(13):1991-1996

[129] Lanzi C, Cassinelli G. Combinatorial strategies to potentiate the efficacy of HDAC inhibitors in fusion-positive sarcomas. Biochemical Pharmacology. 2022;**198**:114944

[130] Tang F, Choy E, Tu C, Hornicek F, Duan Z. Therapeutic applications of histone deacetylase inhibitors in sarcoma. Cancer Treatment Reviews. 2017;**59**:33-45

[131] Souza BK, da Costa Lopez PL, Menegotto PR, Vieira IA, Kersting N, Abujamra AL, et al. Targeting histone deacetylase activity to arrest cell growth and promote neural differentiation in Ewing Sarcoma. Molecular Neurobiology. 2018;**55**(9):7242-7258

[132] El-Naggar AM, Somasekharan SP, Wang Y, Cheng H, Negri GL, Pan M, et al. Class I HDAC inhibitors enhance YB-1 acetylation and oxidative stress to block sarcoma metastasis. EMBO Reports. 2019;**20**(12):e48375

[133] Sampson VB, Vetter NS, Kamara DF, Collier AB, Gresh RC, Kolb EA. Vorinostat enhances cytotoxicity of SN-38 and temozolomide in Ewing Sarcoma cells and activates STAT3/AKT/MAPK pathways. PLoS One. 2015;**10**(11):e0142704

[134] Bharathy N, Berlow NE, Wang E, Abraham J, Settelmeyer TP, Hooper JE, et al. The HDAC3-SMARCA4-miR-27a axis promotes expression of the PAX3:FOXO1 fusion oncogene in rhabdomyosarcoma. Science Signaling. 2018;**11**(557):1-13

[135] Laporte AN, Poulin NM, Barrott JJ, Wang XQ, Lorzadeh A, Vander Werff R, et al. Death by HDAC inhibition in synovial sarcoma cells. Molecular Cancer Therapeutics. 2017;**16**(12):2656-2667

Chapter 8

Statins: Are Lipid-lowering Drugs Useful in Sarcomas?

José M. García-Castellano, Nerea Martínez-Aragón, David García-Padrón, Borja Guerra, Margarita Ramírez-Sánchez, Vicente Vera-Gutiérrez, Gerardo Garcés-Martín and Leandro Fernández-Pérez

Abstract

Sarcomas are rare tumors that are difficult to treat. Many of them are chemoresistant and with a high tendency to recur. Hence, finding new treatments is imperative in these tumors. Metabolic changes in tumor biology have become an essential characteristic in carcinogenesis processes, highlighting among them the role of lipids in these events, mainly cholesterol biosynthesis. Statins, inhibitors of 3-hydroxy-3-methylglutaryl coenzyme A (HMGCoAR), a key enzyme in the mevalonate pathway responsible for cholesterol synthesis, have an effect beyond the reduction in plasma cholesterol levels. These are the so-called pleiotropic effects of statins, responsible for some of the antitumor action of statins. Although there are considerable epidemiological and preclinical evidences that support the use of these medicaments in the treatment of sarcomas as adjuvant reprofiled drugs, clinical trials are disparate and heterogeneous, and do not provide enough information to help determine the convenience of their use, being necessary more studies to evaluate the efficacy and safety of statins in sarcomas. The purpose of this review is to update the role played by the reprofiled statins in the treatment of sarcomas.

Keywords: sarcoma, cholesterol metabolism, mevalonate, HMGCoAR, statin, reprofiling

1. Introduction

Sarcomas are malignant uncommon heterogeneous tumors [1] derived from mesenchymal tissues [2, 3]. There are mainly bone and soft tissue sarcomas (4:1), accounting for 1% of all cancers [2]. They are responsible for 19%–21% of cancer deaths [2]. Low frequency, high diversity, and limited knowledge about the underlying biological mechanisms make it difficult to treat sarcomas [1, 2]. Chemoresistance, local recurrences (10–20%) [4], and metastatic disease (33%) are still unresolved clinical problems with no new critical improvement in sarcomas treatment [2]. In these tumors about one-third of sarcoma patients die, so it is imperative to find new therapeutic strategies for sarcomas. Since lipids, especially those derived from the cholesterol pathway, play an important role in tumorigenesis, the purpose of this review is to update the function played by cholesterol in the treatment of sarcomas and to assess whether statins can have a place in the therapeutic treatment of sarcomas.

2. Role of lipid metabolism in tumorigenesis

Changes in cancer cell metabolism are essential in tumor behavior, but it is not known how they interrelate (**Figure 1**). The high proliferative capacity of tumor cells generates high metabolic demands [5]. Lipids are necessary for cell survival, proliferation, differentiation, motility, cell structure, and cell signaling [6, 7]. Cholesterol stands out in cancer progression because tumor cells require more cholesterol than normal cells to achieve various functions [4, 8–10]. To reach this, some tumors overexpress genes from the cholesterol biosynthetic pathway to accomplish this goal [11].

2.1 Physiology of cholesterol synthesis

Cholesterol, synthesized in the mevalonate pathway from HMGCoAR (**Figure 2**) [3], is regulated in response to different stimuli [3]. This pathway also generates [1, 2] farnesyl pyrophosphate (FPP), precursor of sterols, such as cholesterol; ubiquinone, necessary for the mitochondrial electron transport chain; dolichols, for the protein N-glycosylation; carotenoids, free radical scavengers; isoprenoids, to anchor proteins to cell membranes [2]; and geranylgeranyl pyrophosphate (GGPP), involved in a wide

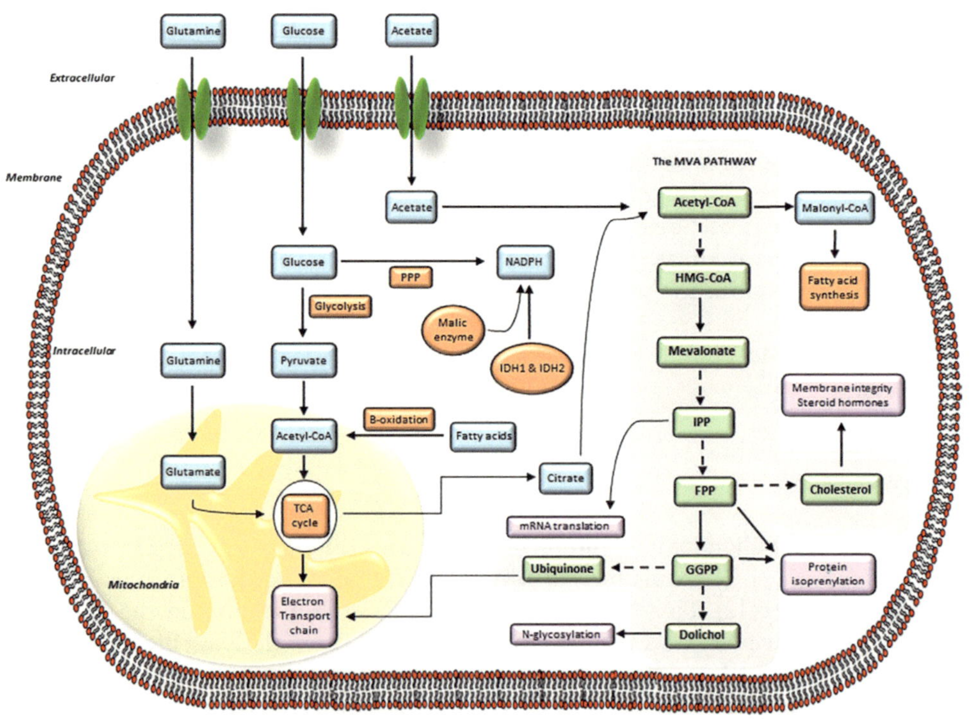

Figure 1.
The mevalonate (MVA) pathway and its connection to intracellular energy metabolism signaling. The fatty acid synthesis and β-oxidation pathway; glycolysis and the TCA cycle are noteworthy among other.

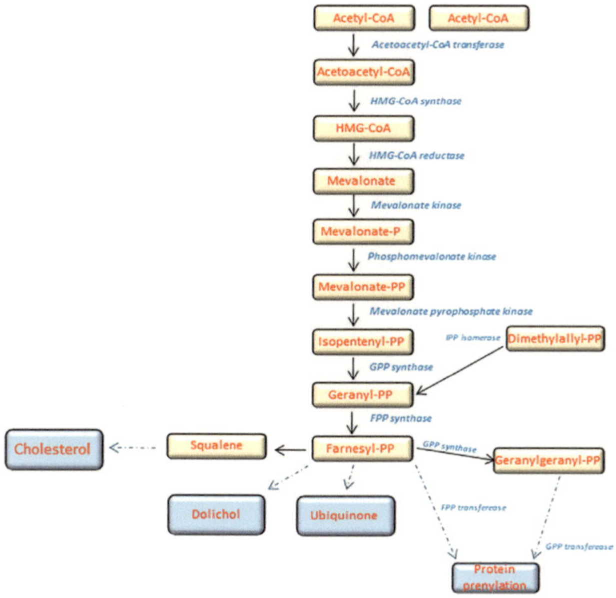

Figure 2.
Diagram of the MVA pathway. Acetyl-CoA is converted to hydroxymethylglutaryl-CoA (HMG-CoA) used by HMGC reductase (HMGCR) to synthesize MVA. MVA generates farnesyl pyrophosphate (FPP), precursor of some sterols, such as membrane cholesterol; as well as ubiquinone (Coenzyme Q) from the mitochondrial electron transport chain; dolichols, for protein N-glycosylation; carotenoids, free radicals' scavenger; and isoprenoids, for membranal protein anchoring. FPP is converted into geranylgeranyl pyrophosphate (GGPP), both essential in prenylation processes.

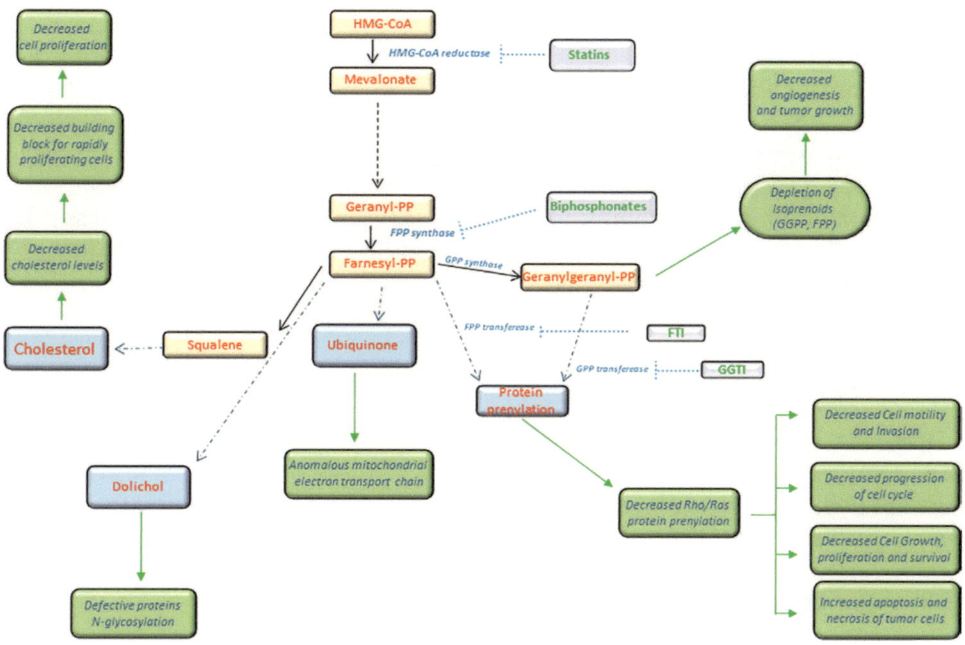

Figure 3.
Antitumoral effects of MVA pathway inhibition. MVA pathway inhibition inhibits tumor growth and progression through reduction in MVA synthesis, which decreases isoprenoid levels, preventing protein prenylation, translocation of Rho and Ras to the cell membrane, and inhibition of cholesterol synthesis.

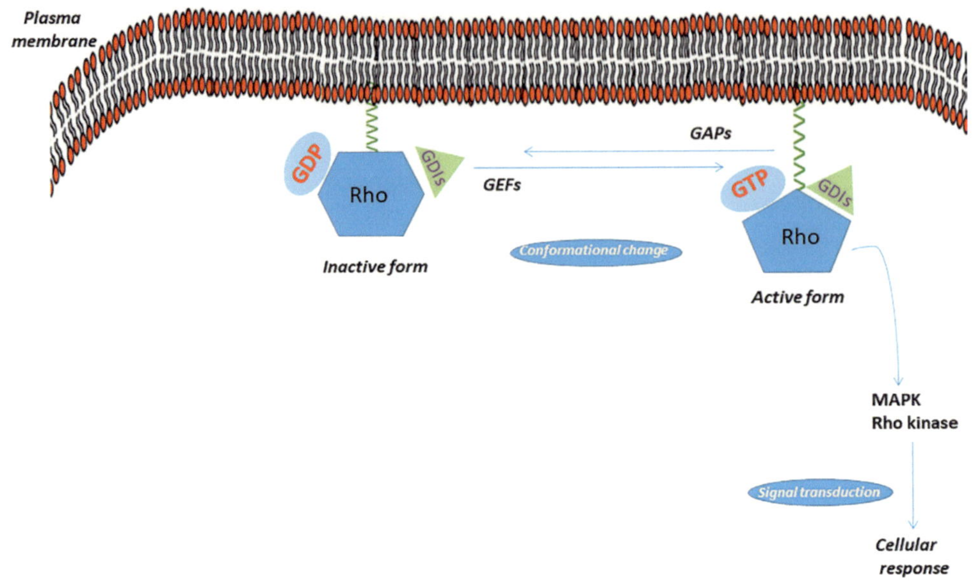

Figure 4.
*Signal transduction through Rho-GTP proteins. Rho proteins are present in an active state, bound to GTP, and an inactive state, bound to GDP. When GTP binds to Rho proteins, a change in protein structure is produced that allows information to be processed and the signal to be propagated within the cell. The Rho proteins change cyclically between their active and inactive forms, these reactions being catalyzed by the "guanine-nucleotide-exchange factors" proteins (GEFs); by the "GTPase-activating proteins" (GAPs), and by the "guanine-nucleotide" "proteins-dissociation inhibitors" (GDIs). Among the effectors downstream of Rho (**Figure 4**), the Rho-dependent kinase (ROCK) family of MAP kinase proteins stands out.*

range of cellular processes (**Figure 3**) [3]. Prenyltransferases farnesyl transferase (FTase) and geranylgeranilatransferase (GGTase I and II) activate the functions of some FPP or GGPP-dependent proteins in the cell membrane [3, 5, 12]. Thus, Ras protein regulates cell differentiation and proliferation; Rho controls the cytoskeleton and cell growth progression (**Figure 4**) [3, 13]; Rab, acts in the transport of intracellular vesicles; Rap, is essential in cell replication, platelet activation and generation of oxygen radicals; and G proteins, necessary in the signal transduction process [6]. Therefore, blocking the mevalonate pathway would lead to dysfunctional proteins due to disruption of the prenylation process (**Figure 3**) [3, 7].

2.2 HMGCoAR inhibition by statins

Statins inhibit the enzyme HMGCoAR, binding to the enzyme active site instead of HMGCoA [14]. There are differential effects of statins according to the specific tissue analyzed (liver *vs* non-hepatic) or polarity (hydrophilic *vs* lipophilic) [15]. The more lipophilic, the higher levels in non-hepatic tissues [16], while the hydrophilic are more hepato-selective [17].

2.3 Increased cholesterol needed in tumor cells

Increased cholesterol synthesis requires a rise in HMGCoAR activity; enhanced absorption of low-density lipoprotein (LDL); and/or both mechanisms [18].

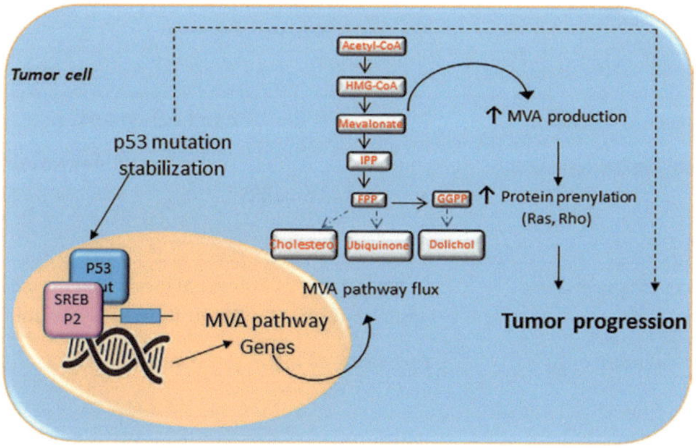

Figure 5.
The mevalonate (MVA) pathway in cancer progression. The MVA pathway is dysregulated in several cancer cells due to mutations or abnormal signaling of different proteins/pathways. Upregulation of MVA pathway drives increased protein prenylation thus promoting a malignant phenotype of cancer cells with uncontrolled cell invasive growth and survival. In cancer cells expressing a mutation of tumor protein p53, there is a positive-feedback loop where p53 interacts with sterol regulatory element-binding protein (SREBP), leading to increased activation of the MVA pathway activity and therefore higher levels of MVA. This MVA leads to the stabilization of p53 mutation as well as promotes protein prenylation, thus accelerating cancer progression.

2.3.1 Expression of HMGCoAR in tumors

Overexpression or activation of HMGCoAR [10] produces the isoprenoids necessary to maintain pro-tumor benefits (**Figure 5**) [19]. High levels of HMGCoAR, present in various types of tumors [20–22], are associated with favorable prognostic criteria [20], such as prolonged relapse-free survival [23, 24] or predicted response to treatment [24].

2.3.2 LDL receptor expression

Physiologically, plasma cholesterol transported in LDL is internalized into the cell upon contact with its receptor. If the cell needs cholesterol, it increases its synthesis and LDL receptor activity; otherwise, both activities decrease [24]. In tumor cells, higher cholesterol requirements cause an increase in LDL receptor concentration, associated with an increased plasma LDL activity and absorption [25–27].

3. Pleiotropic effects of statins beyond lowering cholesterol levels

Statins, regulators of small GTPases prenylation [26], are essential in multiple cellular processes [4, 27]. These pleiotropic effects of statins [1] are modulated either by HMGCoAR-dependent (canonical) or HMGCoAR-independent (non-canonical) ways [28]. We will focus on HMGCoAR-dependent processes, which prevent the isoprenylation of small GTPases Rho, Ras, Rac, and Cdc24 [1, 29].

3.1 Non-tumor pleiotropic effects of statins

Statins can affect several tissue functions [30]. The different pleiotropic effects are summarized in **Table 1**.

Pleiotropic effect	Main mechanism of action	Ref.
Brain		
Reduction of incidence of dementia	Reduction of embolic and ischemic stroke	[31]
Improvement psychological well-being	Cumulative reduction of levels of depression, anxiety and hostility	[32]
Vascular		
Endothelial function enhancement	Education seric cholesterol levels. Decreased vascular relaxation Restoration of NO production	[33]
Reduction of blood pressure	Reduction of blood pressure and peripheral vascular resistance	[34]
Reduction of thrombogenicity	Reduction of platelet aggregation - Reduction (TxA2) -Increase in prostacyclin synthesis	[35]
Endocrine		
Reduction of incidence of type II diabetes	Inhibition of cellular pathway insulin-dependent	[35]
Immunology		
Reduced transplanted organ rejection	Inhibition of the expression of the MTF and reduction of hypercoagulability. Decrease of TNF α, IL-6 and NBP	[36, 37]
Cardiology		
Reduction of vascular events	Ischemia reduction: -Coronary arteries, Cerebrovascular; Kidney arteries	[36, 38]
Improved VE fraction function in HF	VE fraction improvement	[32]
Bone		
Reduction of osteoporosis and the fracture risk	Stimulates ECM genes expression	[39]
	Prevention of bone resorption	[35]
	Stimulation of bone formation	[39]
	Promotes differentiation and proliferation	[39]
	Enhances bone mineral density	[39]

Table 1.
Non-tumor pleiotropic effects of statin.

3.2 Tumor pleiotropic effects of statins

3.2.1 Pleiotropic effects of statins in non-mesenchymal tumors

Inhibition of mevalonate pathway by statins (**Table 2**) (**Figure 5**) [10] prevents Rho protein isoprenylation and consequently produces apoptosis [47], decreases cell proliferation [49] and tumor cells invasiveness [42], but not in non-tumoral cells [43].

3.2.2 Pleiotropic effects of statins in mesenchymal tumors

Cholesterol is involved in the sarcomagenesis process, with an inverse relationship between increased cholesterol synthesis activity and decreased survival of patients with sarcoma [11, 55].

Pleiotropic effect	Main mechanism of action	Ref.
Cell proliferation and cell cycle arrest	Suppression of cell proliferation. Promotion of cells differentiation	[25]
	Activation (phosphorylation) of IF2α, JNK and c-Jun	[40]
	Arrest in the G0/G1 and the S phase with changes in p53, $p21^{Cip1}$, CDK1	[40]
Loss of cell viability and apoptosis	Osteosarcoma, chondrosarcoma, rhabdomyosarcoma, Ewing's sarcoma.	[22, 41–43]
	Cell detachment (anoikis) and induction of apoptosis	[27, 30]
	Increase in the bax/bcl-2 ratio (decreased expression of bcl-2)	[21, 28, 29, 41–44]
Enhancement of chemotherapeutic effect	Doxorubicin and cisplatin enhancement in osteosarcoma and rhabdomyosarcoma	[29, 45]
	Potentiating the inhibitory effect of cell migration	[45]
	Less released troponin T by cardiomyocytes in doxorubicin-treated mice	[46]
Effect on cell differentiation and ECM	Promotion of cell differentiation in Ewing's sarcoma	[44]
	Modulation of PTHrP/Ras/MAPK pathway in osteoblasts	[47]
	Increases in collagen, alkaline phosphatase, osteocalcin or BMP-2	[24]
Effect on migration and invasiveness	Reduction of cell migratory ability in sarcoma cells	[30, 48]
	Anti-angiogenic role decreasing the expression of VEGF, bFGF, HGF and TGF-β	[45, 48]
	In osteosarcoma inhibition of migration, invasiveness and metastasis	[49]
	Down-regulation in osteosarcoma of MMP-2, 9 and 14 and TIMP2 expression or activity	[50]
	MMP-3, −13, −2, −9 and TIMP-2 down-regulation in chondrosarcoma and in fibrosarcoma	[48]
	In osteosarcomas alteration of RhoA-JNK-c-Jun-MMP2 pathway	[48, 51]
	Decreased Jak2/Stat5 phosphorylation and increased expression of SOCS3 in osteosarcomas	[30]
	Growth inhibition of fibrosarcoma in animal models	[52]
	Control of tumor growth and pulmonary metastasis of rat fibrosarcoma	[22]
	In vivo potentiation of doxorubicin or cisplatin	[53]
	In a xenograft model of osteosarcoma synergy of MTX with simvastatin	[54]

Table 2.
Pleiotropic effects of statin on mesenchymal tumors.

3.2.2.1 Effects of statins on cell proliferation and cell cycle

Statins, essentially lipophilic ones [56], suppress cell proliferation [57], promote cell differentiation *in vitro* [56], mainly in tumor cells [56], and prevent the prenylation of Ras and Rho. These effects are due to the increased phosphorylation of IF2α,

JNK and c-Jun, and alteration of the p53, $p21^{Cip1}$ and CDK1 gene expression [58, 59], which arrest cells in the G0/G1 and the S phases.

3.2.2.2 Effect of statins on cell viability and apoptosis

Statin induces loss of cell viability [56, 60] and anoikis [61, 62], followed by p53 translocation, cytochrome c release [63], decreased expression of bcl-2 [64], caspase 9 and 3 activation [65], apoptosis and cell differentiation [66].

3.2.2.3 Enhancement of chemotherapeutic effect

Statins enhance the antitumor effects of chemotherapy [67]. Thus, lovastatin enhances the effect of doxorubicin on NIH-3 T3 sarcoma cells [65], and in osteosarcomas, stimulates apoptosis and invasive behavior [68]. Sublethal doses of simvastatin potentiate the cytotoxicity of doxorubicin in rhabdomyosarcomas [65], reducing *in vivo* cardiac toxicity in mice [69, 70]. It is believed that these effects are produced by the action of the p53 protein (**Figure 5**); the JNK phosphorylation [67]; the decreased MMP-2 activity [68], the decrease in drug resistance regulated by the p-glycoprotein/ABCB1 gene [71], whose expression is associated with a poor prognosis in children diagnosed with soft tissue sarcoma [62].

3.2.2.4 Effect of statins on cell differentiation and ECM composition

Simvastatin modulates cell differentiation through the IL-6-dependent PTHrP/Ras/MAPK pathway in human osteoblasts and MG-63 osteosarcoma cells, increasing the level of bone differentiation markers like alkaline phosphatase activity and/or osteocalcin [72]. BMP-2-dependent osteoblast differentiation is stimulated by lipophilic statins, while the hydrophilic statin pravastatin does not [72], also modifying osteoblast differentiation markers collagen, alkaline phosphatase, and osteocalcin [73]. Statins also promote cell differentiation of Ewing's sarcoma [66].

3.2.2.5 Effect of statins on invasive behavior

Statins, increasing the non-isoprenylated cytosolic form of Ras [64], and helped by its antiangiogenic effect and inhibition of the ECM degradation, reduce sarcoma cell invasive ability [74]. Therefore, in osteosarcoma, statin decreases the expression of the angiogenic factors secreted by the tumor VEGF, bFGF, HGF, and TGF-β [75] and inhibits the neo-vascularization. Moreover, statins inhibit invasiveness [68, 76] by MMP-3, −13, −2, −9, −14 and TIMP-2 genes down-regulation, involved in the ECM degradation, in the chondrosarcoma cell line SW1353 and in HT1080 fibrosarcoma cells [76, 77]. Among some signaling pathways [32], the RhoA-JNK-c-Jun-MMP2 pathway [76] or the Jak2/Stat5/SOCS3 pathway [74] controlled by GGPP-prenylated RhoA [78]. In animal models, statins inhibit the growth of primary tumor fibrosarcoma [50] and prevent tumor growth and pulmonary metastatic development of rat fibrosarcoma [60]. Besides, statins enhance the effect of doxorubicin or cisplatin [67]. In a xenograft model of osteosarcoma, simvastatin synergistically potentiates the action of methotrexate, enhancing tumor volume reduction, decreasing side effects, and drastically reducing lung metastases [33].

4. Mechanisms of action of statins

4.1 Effects derived from lipophilicity of statins

Lipophilicity of statins is an important factor in the effectiveness of these drugs. Lipophilic statins diffuse passively through the plasma membranes, but hydrophilic statins need transporters to cross them. Hydrophilic statins act mostly in the liver, and lipophilic statins are mainly in extra-hepatic cells [15, 79]. Lipophilicity affects antitumor actions of statins [41] inducing a cell cycle arrest in osteosarcoma [40]. Viability and apoptosis are dependent on lipophilicity, in osteosarcoma [24], chondrosarcoma [41], or rhabdomyosarcoma [43], but no clinical data related to the differential effect of lipophilic *vs* hydrophilic statin in sarcomas were found. Data from other types of tumors show this action [80], being lipophilic statins more effective.

4.2 Role of isoprenoid lipids, GTPases, and Rho in sarcomas

Members of the Rho family of small GTPases are involved in important functions involved in malignant transformation and progression, like actin reorganization, cell motility, or cell-cell and cell-ECM [55]. Rho proteins are promising targets as a novel anticancer drug in several cancers [56] including sarcoma [28]. Rho GTPases localized at membranes become activated upon stimulation of cell surface receptors. So, Rho GEFs are often oncogenic, and the expression level of Rho GTPases frequently increases with malignancy. A possible drawback of isoprenylation inhibitors is their poor selectivity for individual Rho GTPases. High levels of RhoA and/or RhoC have been observed to indicate a poor prognosis [81]. In addition, RhoA is involved in tumor progression invasion [57] and RhoC in tumor invasion. Cell growth arrest and proliferation inhibition in osteosarcoma depend on GGPP prenylation, rather than FPP and farnesylation [19]. Similarly, treatment of NIH3T3 sarcoma cells with GGTI-298 or lovastatin stops the cell cycle [82]; but FTI-277 has no such effect. So, geranylgeranylated proteins play a critical role in the cell cycle [83]. Statin-induced apoptosis is also associated with changes in RhoA protein geranylgeranylation in human chondrosarcoma [41] and osteosarcoma cell lines. Besides, in osteosarcoma cells, simvastatin induced mevalonate-dependent apoptosis [30], mediated by the MAPK-RhoA-p42/p44-bcl-2 mechanism [28]; or by activation of AMPK and p38 MAPK [84]; or is associated with the RhoA/Stat1/bcl-2 signaling pathway [24, 30]. Inhibition of geranylation by statins is also responsible for apoptosis in sarcomas [85]. Thus, in osteosarcoma and chondrosarcoma cell lines [41], geranylgeranylation inhibition induces apoptosis, which can be restored by adding GGPP, but not FPP. Similar results have been observed after treating sarcomas with GGTI-298, but not with FTI-277. This different effect of isoprenoid lipids on sarcoma cells may be due to the fact that GGPP is derived from the condensation of FPP and isopentenyl pyrophosphate (IPP). Since IPP could not be synthesized in cells treated with simvastatin, FPP could not be converted into GGPP.

4.3 Autophagic cell death

Autophagic cell death or programmed cell death (PCD) type II is a constitutively active self-degradative process of cellular constituents [86]. It is responsible for maintaining cellular homeostasis [87] under stressful conditions, such as nutrient starvation, hypoxia, growth factor insufficiency, acidosis, or drug exposure [87]. Autophagy begins with an isolation membrane that engulfs intracellular cargo [88], degraded by lysosomal acid proteases. These lysosomal permeases and transporters export amino acids and other by-products of degradation back out to the cytoplasm, where they can be reused for building macromolecules and for metabolism [88]. Autophagy is regulated by the target of rapamycin (TOR) kinase, which is regulated by some effectors [89]. Upstream of TOR, activation of AMP-activated protein kinase AMPK in response to low ATP levels. Downstream, reduced Akt activity represses TOR kinase [89] and induces autophagy, stimulating catabolism and reducing its growth. Cholesterol depletion induced by statins produces inactivation of mTOR, which then induces autophagy [18] and also can promote cancer cell death after stimulation of ERK1/2 and Akt pathways [58]. In sarcomas, autophagy plays an important role in the pro-survival response to therapies and stress, and in the therapeutic resistance of sarcoma [87]. The cell cycle arrest and apoptosis process start with the GGPP depletion, which leads to a disrupted RhoA function, which activates AMPK and consequently inactivates mTOR [84]. Finally, statin accumulated p53 at the nucleus and induces autophagy through phosphorylation of HMGCoAR [59].

5. Evidence of the antitumor effect of statins

5.1 Epidemiological evidence of the antitumor activity of statins

Epidemiological studies have shown that statins reduce cancer mortality [74]. There is also a positive correlation between statin use and a reduction in cancer incidence [60, 74, 78]. However, other authors have not found this connection between taking statins and cancer risk [74]. Nevertheless, these epidemiological studies have been criticized for having intrinsic limitations and a retrospective approach [74]. In addition, another criticism is that the studies have been designed to evaluate the reduction of cholesterol levels and not the role it plays in oncogenesis [60], including sarcomas. Besides, clinical studies of statins and their antitumor action are few, limited, and inconclusive [61]. In addition, there is a discrepancy between data from preclinical and epidemiology regarding the lack of response to combination therapy in clinical trials. Moreover, unfortunately, clinical trials with statins and sarcomas were not found.

5.2 Combined treatment of statins with chemotherapy

Statins can be administered at high doses to cancer patients (i.e. 15 mg/kg/day for simvastatin; 25 mg/kg/day for lovastatin), but the expected effects have not been observed [62]. However, statins sensitize the tumor cells to the action of chemotherapy, improving antitumor efficacy, due to the synergism of these drugs, enhancing cytotoxicity [60], increasing the therapeutic window of statins, and reducing toxicity [63]. In sarcomas, statins increase the anti-tumor efficacy of doxorubicin or cisplatin on human osteo- and fibrosarcoma in an additive manner [53]. Besides, atorvastatin potentiates the effect on viability, migration, and cell invasion in human osteosarcoma cells [45]. In a xenograft model of human sarcoma, lovastatin enhances doxorubicin efficacy, reducing acute doxorubicin-induced heart damage [22, 46]. In the same model with osteosarcoma cells, simvastatin increased methotrexate cytotoxic effect, being necessary for lower doses of this drug and decreasing the toxicity in the mice. Besides, increased the reduction in tumor volume caused by methotrexate and markedly decreased the rate of lung metastases [54]. In this sense, there are also some positive reports showing the efficacy of the combination of these drugs [64]. Therefore, in a patient with rhabdomyosarcoma refractory to chemotherapy, statins contributed to the improvement of the patient after receiving radiotherapy and being treated with bevacizumab [90]. However, it has also been described in other drugs that patient survival did not improve with this strategy [65].

5.3 Disadvantages and inappropriate effects of using statins

Several advantages have been associated with statin therapy, but some drawbacks have also been described. For instance, the low bioavailability of statins (5%–20%) limits their effectiveness [63, 66]. For this reason, nanocarriers have been developed [67] to overcome the lower oral bioavailability of statins [66]. Another drawback of statins may be myopathies [91], due to direct effect of statins on muscle or autoimmune responses from autoantibodies against HMGCoAR [68]. Also, statins could increase the risk of developing diabetes mellitus (in 10%–20% of patients receiving statins) [69], increase of the rate of hemorrhagic stroke when blood cholesterol levels are reduced [70], or increased liver enzymes, although hepatotoxicity is rarely observed [92].

6. Discussion

Is there enough evidence to say that statins are useful in the treatment of sarcomas? From the epidemiological studies' point of view, the results are not clear enough to advise their use since the conclusions are not homogeneous and are objectionable. Most studies are observational and retrospective [71], mainly phase I and/or phase II clinical trials, with small sample size and poor statistical support [93]. The few prospective articles published cannot assess the true extent of statins in cancer treatment. It is also difficult to draw valid conclusions from heterogeneous articles, therapeutic regimens with different types and doses of statins; not systematized frequency of administration; dispensing or not concomitantly with chemotherapy; lipophilic *vs* hydrophilic statins, etc. In addition, it is also necessary to investigate what dose and how long statin treatment is needed to prevent cancer; or what mechanism of death (apoptosis *vs* autophagy) is responsible for the observed effects [94]. In addition, it is not well known whether statins reduce the degree of tumor aggressiveness [71] or allow them to be diagnosed earlier [95]. Second, the response to statins may depend on interindividual variability that may explain the variation in pharmacological response to them [93]. HMGCoAR expression is known as a tumor biomarker. Thus, in ovarian cancer, is associated with greater survival without recurrence [96]. In colorectal cancer, the chemopreventive capacity of statins depends on polymorphisms in the HMGCoAR gene [72]. Even so, population studies have shown chemopreventive and survival benefits of statins in several types of cancer [93]. Thus, in a case-control study, cancer was diagnosed less frequently among patients who took statins (28%) [78]. Also, the use of statins in cancer patients is associated with a reduction in cancer-related mortality [74]. But in a clinical trial, designed to evaluate the effect of pravastatin combined with sorafenib on hepatocellular carcinoma, no improvement in survival was observed in these patients [73]. On the other hand, is the use of statins effective and safe in the treatment of these neoplasms? While epidemiological studies are contradictory, preclinical studies confirm the anticancer efficacy of statins in controlling metastatic disease [20, 93] due to growth inhibition and cell death, both *in vitro* and *in vivo* [20]. These contradictory epidemiological data generate uncertainty regarding the role of cholesterol in the development of cancer [97]. Based on data from long-term studies of cardiovascular disease, neither taking statins nor lowering serum cholesterol levels increases cancer risk [76]. These discrepant data may be due to inadequate methodological designs (retrospective *vs* prospective), insufficient follow-up, and/or the different types of statins used [98]. In this sense, some mechanisms can alter cholesterol homeostasis and lead to cancer development [97]. Are statins safe or do they have any degree of toxicity? Toxicity caused by statins it is more selective in tumor than in healthy cells [99]. This fact has been observed in osteosarcoma cell lines with simvastatin [24]; or in Ewing's sarcoma cells, with lovastatin [75]. These data are critical, because these drugs are safe and well tolerated, and the achievable plasma concentration (0.1–4 μM) at a dose of 24 mg/kg/day corresponds to the dose range that can trigger apoptosis in vitro [100]. Moreover, treatment with atorvastatin, evaluated for 3 years in growing patients diagnosed with heterozygous familial hypercholesterolemia, was effective, safe, and well tolerated [9], with no impact on child growth or maturation, with only a few adverse events responsible for a 2.2% treatment withdrawal. With respect to the toxic effects of fluvastatin in terminal pediatric Ewing's sarcoma patients, fluvastatin showed that can be used safely at a dose of 8 mg/kg/day in this population [77].

In conclusion, for the above-mentioned reasons, even though many aspects remain to be resolved, we consider statins to be good potential candidates for being reprofiled in sarcomas. However, further studies in sarcoma patients, with large phase III prospective randomized controlled trials are warranted to establish the effect of statins in cancer prevention and treatment [93], and to answer the question of whether statins can be used to prevent and/or treat various types of cancer [71], including sarcomas.

Abbreviations

HMGCoAR	3-hydroxy-3-methylglutaryl coenzyme A reductase
FPP	farnesyl pyrophosphate
GGPP	geranylgeranyl pyrophosphate
FTase	farnesyl transferase
GGTase	geranylgeranyl transferase
LDL	low-density lipoprotein
Gen de ABCB1	gen del casete de unión de B1 a ATP

Author details

José M. García-Castellano[1,2,3,4*], Nerea Martínez-Aragón[2†], David García-Padrón[2†], Borja Guerra[3], Margarita Ramírez-Sánchez[5], Vicente Vera-Gutiérrez[6], Gerardo Garcés-Martín[4] and Leandro Fernández-Pérez[3*]

1 Orthopedic Surgery and Traumatology, Maternal and Child University Hospital Complex of Gran Canaria (C.H.U.I.M.I.), Las Palmas de Gran Canaria, Spain

2 Molecular Oncology Laboratory, Research Unit (C.H.U.I.M.I.), Spanish Sarcoma Research Group (GEIS), Las Palmas de Gran Canaria, Spain

3 Molecular and Translational Pharmacology Group, University Institute of Biomedical and Health Research (IUIBS), University of Las Palmas de Gran Canaria, Spain

4 Department of Medical and Surgical Sciences, University of Las Palmas de Gran Canaria, Spain

5 Physical Medicine and Rehabilitation Service, University Hospital of Gran Canaria Doctor Negrín, Las Palmas de Gran Canaria, Spain

6 Orthopedic Surgery and Traumatology, University Hospital of Gran Canaria Doctor Negrín, Las Palmas de Gran Canaria, Spain

*Address all correspondence to: jmgc_61@yahoo.com and leandrofco.fernandez@ulpgc.es

† Both authors contributed equally to this work.

References

[1] Yeganeh B et al. Targeting the mevalonate cascade as a new therapeutic approach in heart disease, cancer and pulmonary disease. Pharmacology & Therapeutics. 2014;**143**(1):87-110

[2] Goldstein JL, Brown MS. Regulation of the mevalonate pathway. Nature. 1990;**343**(6257):425-430

[3] Likus W et al. Could drugs inhibiting the mevalonate pathway also target cancer stem cells? Drug Resistance Updates. 2016;**25**:13-25

[4] Clendening JW et al. Dysregulation of the mevalonate pathway promotes transformation. Proceedings of the National Academy of Sciences of the United States of America. 2010;**107**(34):15051-15056

[5] Maurer-Stroh S, Washietl S, Eisenhaber F. Protein prenyltransferases. Genome Biology. 2003;**4**(4):212

[6] Faggiotto A, Paoletti R. State-of-the-Art lecture. Statins and blockers of the renin-angiotensin system: Vascular protection beyond their primary mode of action. Hypertension. 1999;**34**(4 Pt 2):987-996

[7] Yang W, Urano J, Tamanoi F. Protein farnesylation is critical for maintaining normal cell morphology and canavanine resistance in Schizosaccharomyces pombe. The Journal of Biological Chemistry. 2000;**275**(1):429-438

[8] Luu W et al. The role of signalling in cellular cholesterol homeostasis. IUBMB Life. 2013;**65**(8):675-684

[9] Gorin A, Gabitova L, Astsaturov I. Regulation of cholesterol biosynthesis and cancer signaling. Current Opinion in Pharmacology. 2012;**12**(6):710-716

[10] Huang C, Freter C. Lipid metabolism, apoptosis and cancer therapy. International Journal of Molecular Sciences. 2015;**16**(1):924-949

[11] Ribas V, García-Ruiz C, Fernández-Checa JC. Mitochondria, cholesterol and cancer cell metabolism. Clinical and Translational Medicine. 2016;**5**(1):22

[12] Zhang FL, Casey PJ. Protein prenylation: Molecular mechanisms and functional consequences. Annual Review of Biochemistry. 1996;**65**:241-269

[13] Sebti SM. Protein farnesylation: Implications for normal physiology, malignant transformation, and cancer therapy. Cancer Cell. 2005;**7**(4):297-300

[14] Laufs U, Liao JK. Direct vascular effects of HMG-CoA reductase inhibitors. Trends in Cardiovascular Medicine. 2000;**10**(4):143-148

[15] Hamelin BA, Turgeon J. Hydrophilicity/lipophilicity: Relevance for the pharmacology and clinical effects of HMG-CoA reductase inhibitors. Trends in Pharmacological Sciences. 1998;**19**(1):26-37

[16] Liao JK. Isoprenoids as mediators of the biological effects of statins. The Journal of Clinical Investigation. 2002;**110**(3):285-288

[17] Vitols S et al. Expression of the low-density lipoprotein receptor, HMG-CoA reductase, and multidrug resistance (Mdr1) genes in colorectal carcinomas. Biochemical Pharmacology. 1996;**52**(1):127-131

[18] Cheng J et al. Cholesterol depletion induces autophagy. Biochemical and Biophysical Research Communications. 2006;**351**(1):246-252

[19] Vitols S et al. Multilevel regulation of low-density lipoprotein receptor and 3-hydroxy-3-methylglutaryl coenzyme A reductase gene expression in normal and leukemic cells. Blood. 1994;**84**(8):2689-2698

[20] Chan KK, Oza AM, Siu LL. The statins as anticancer agents. Clinical Cancer Research. 2003;**9**(1):10-19

[21] Lee SK, Kim YS. Phosphorylation of eIF2α attenuates statin-induced apoptosis by inhibiting the stabilization and translocation of p53 to the mitochondria. Life Science Alliance. 2013;**42**(3):810-816

[22] Jakobisiak M, Golab J. Potential antitumor effects of statins (Review). International Journal of Oncology. 2003;**23**(4):1055-1069

[23] Park C, Lee I, Kang WK. Lovastatin-induced E2F-1 modulation and its effect on prostate cancer cell death. Carcinogenesis. 2001;**22**(10):1727-1731

[24] Benítez Cabrera NE. Papel de los inhibidores de la 3-hidroxi-3metilglutaril coenzima a reductasa (estatinas) en líneas celulares de osteosarcoma. Estudio in vitro [Doctoral Thesis]. Universidad de Las Palmas de Gran Canaria; 2008

[25] Warita K et al. Statin-induced mevalonate pathway inhibition attenuates the growth of mesenchymal-like cancer cells that lack functional E-cadherin mediated cell cohesion. Scientific Reports. 2014;**4**:7593

[26] Sandoval-Usme MC et al. Efectos antitumorales de la simvastatina sobre la linea cellular de osteosarcoma UMR-106. Revista de la Academia Colombiana de Ciencias Exactas, Fisicas y Naturales. 2011;**35**(136):287-295

[27] Chan HS et al. Immunohistochemical detection of P-glycoprotein: Prognostic correlation in soft tissue sarcoma of childhood. Journal of Clinical Oncology. 1990;**8**(4):689-704

[28] Fromigué O et al. RhoA GTPase inactivation by statins induces osteosarcoma cell apoptosis by inhibiting p42/p44-MAPKs-Bcl-2 signaling independently of BMP-2 and cell differentiation. Cell Death and Differentiation. 2006;**13**(11):1845-1856

[29] Werner M, Sacher J, Hohenegger M. Mutual amplification of apoptosis by statin-induced mitochondrial stress and doxorubicin toxicity in human rhabdomyosarcoma cells. British Journal of Pharmacology. 2004;**143**(6):715-724

[30] Sandoval-Usme MC et al. Simvastatin impairs growth hormone-activated signal transducer and activator of transcription (STAT) signaling pathway in UMR-106 osteosarcoma cells. PLoS One. 2014;**9**(1):e87769

[31] Waldman A, Kritharides L. The pleiotropic effects of HMG-CoA reductase inhibitors: Their role in osteoporosis and dementia. Drugs. 2003;**63**(2):139-152

[32] Young-Xu Y et al. Long-term statin use and psychological well-being. Journal of the American College of Cardiology. 2003;**42**(4):690-697

[33] Liao JK. Beyond lipid lowering: The role of statins in vascular protection. International Journal of Cardiology. 2002;**86**(1):5-18

[34] Susic D et al. Beneficial pleiotropic vascular effects of rosuvastatin in two hypertensive models. Journal of the American College of Cardiology. 2003;**42**(6):1091-1097

[35] McFarlane SI et al. Clinical review 145: Pleiotropic effects of statins: Lipid

reduction and beyond. The Journal of Clinical Endocrinology and Metabolism. 2002;**87**(4):1451-1458

[36] Kobashigawa JA et al. Effect of pravastatin on outcomes after cardiac transplantation. The New England Journal of Medicine. 1995;**333**(10):621-627

[37] Mehra MR et al. Comparative beneficial effects of simvastatin and pravastatin on cardiac allograft rejection and survival. Journal of the American College of Cardiology. 2002;**40**(9):1609-1614

[38] Schwartz GG et al. Effects of atorvastatin on early recurrent ischemic events in acute coronary syndromes: The MIRACL study: A randomized controlled trial. JAMA. 2001;**285**(13):1711-1718

[39] Garrett IR, Mundy GR. The role of statins as potential targets for bone formation. Arthritis Research & Therapy. 2002;**4**(4):1-4

[40] Kany S et al. Simvastatin exerts anticancer effects in osteosarcoma cell lines via geranylgeranylation and c-Jun activation. International Journal of Oncology. 2018;**52**(4):1285-1294

[41] López UT. Efecto de la inhibición de la isoprenilación de la proteína RhoA por las estatinas lipofílicas sobre la supervivencia celular de líneas celulares de condrosarcoma [Doctoral Thesis]. 2015

[42] Moriceau G et al. Zoledronic acid potentiates mTOR inhibition and abolishes the resistance of osteosarcoma cells to RAD001 (Everolimus): Pivotal role of the prenylation process. Cancer Research. 2010;**70**(24):10329-10339

[43] Maiguma T et al. Cell-specific toxicity of fibrates in human embryonal rhabdomyosarcoma cells. Naunyn-Schmiedeberg's Archives of Pharmacology. 2003;**367**(3):289-296

[44] Kim JS et al. Lovastatin induces apoptosis in a primitive neuroectodermal tumor cell line in association with RB down-regulation and loss of the G1 checkpoint. Oncogene. 2000;**19**(52):6082-6090

[45] Fromigué O, Hamidouche Z, Marie PJ. Statin-induced inhibition of 3-hydroxy-3-methyl glutaryl coenzyme a reductase sensitizes human osteosarcoma cells to anticancer drugs. The Journal of Pharmacology and Experimental Therapeutics. 2008;**325**(2):595-600

[46] Feleszko W et al. Lovastatin potentiates antitumor activity and attenuates cardiotoxicity of doxorubicin in three tumor models in mice. Clinical Cancer Research. 2000;**6**(5):2044-2052

[47] Sugiyama M et al. Compactin and simvastatin, but not pravastatin, induce bone morphogenetic protein-2 in human osteosarcoma cells. Biochemical and Biophysical Research Communications. 2000;**271**(3):688-692

[48] Fromigué O, Hamidouche Z, Marie PJ. Blockade of the RhoA-JNK-c-Jun-MMP2 cascade by atorvastatin reduces osteosarcoma cell invasion. The Journal of Biological Chemistry. 2008;**283**(45):30549-30556

[49] Garcia-Castellano JM. et al. Role of the IL-6/Jak/Stat Pathway in Tumor Angiogenesis: Influence of Estrogen Status. DOI: 10.5772/intechopen.104102

[50] Kushlinsky N et al. Matrix metalloproteinases 2, 7, 9 and tissue inhibitor of matrix metalloproteinase-1 in the sera of patients with bone tumors. Bulletin of Experimental Biology and Medicine. 2010;**149**(2):233-235

[51] Kido A et al. Overexpression of matrix metalloproteinase (MMP)-9 correlates

with metastatic potency of spontaneous and 4-hydroxyaminoquinoline 1-oxide (4-HAQO)-induced transplantable osteosarcomas in rats. Cancer Letters. 1999;**137**(2):209-216

[52] Matar P et al. Lovastatin inhibits tumor growth and metastasis development of a rat fibrosarcoma. Cancer Biotherapy & Radiopharmaceuticals. 1998;**13**(5):387-393

[53] Nilsson S, Huelsenbeck J, Fritz G. Mevalonate pathway inhibitors affect anticancer drug-induced cell death and DNA damage response of human sarcoma cells. Cancer Letters. 2011;**304**(1):60-69

[54] García-Castellano JMH-P, García-Padrón O, David Guerra-Hernández C, Fernández-Pérez LB. Potenciación del efecto del MTX por la simvastatina en el tratamiento del osteosarcoma experimental. Estudio in vitro e in vivo. Review Soc Can Traumatology Ortopeadics. 2021;**2**(1):65-72

[55] Karlsson R et al. Rho GTPase function in tumorigenesis. Biochimica et Biophysica Acta. 2009;**1796**(2):91-98

[56] Jung H, Yoon SR. Dysregulation of Rho GTPases in Human. Cancers. 2020;**12**(5):1179. DOI: 10.3390/cancers12051179

[57] Malliri A, Collard JG. Role of Rho-family proteins in cell adhesion and cancer. Current Opinion in Cell Biology. 2003;**15**(5):583-589

[58] Shi Y et al. Differential effects of lovastatin on cisplatin responses in normal human mesothelial cells versus cancer cells: Implication for therapy. PLoS One. 2012;**7**(9):e45354

[59] Ghavami S et al. Mevalonate cascade regulation of airway mesenchymal cell autophagy and apoptosis: A dual role for p53. PLoS One. 2011;**6**(1):e16523

[60] Barkas F et al. Beyond cholesterol reduction, the pleiotropic effects of statins: Is their use in cancer prevention hype or hope? Clinical Lipidology. 2013;**8**(3):273-277

[61] Jeong GH et al. Statin and cancer mortality and survival: An umbrella systematic review and meta-analysis. Journal of Clinical Medicine. 2020;**9**(2):326

[62] Sondergaard TE et al. A phase II clinical trial does not show that high dose simvastatin has beneficial effect on markers of bone turnover in multiple myeloma. Hematological Oncology. 2009;**27**(1):17-22

[63] Guerra B et al. The mevalonate pathway, a metabolic target in cancer therapy. Frontiers in Oncology. 2021;**11**:626971

[64] Fiala O et al. Statins augment efficacy of EGFR-TKIs in patients with advanced-stage non-small cell lung cancer harbouring KRAS mutation. Tumour Biology. 2015;**36**(8):5801-5805

[65] Konings IR et al. The addition of pravastatin to chemotherapy in advanced gastric carcinoma: A randomised phase II trial. European Journal of Cancer. 2010;**46**(18):3200-3204

[66] Meola TR et al. Enhancing the oral bioavailability of simvastatin with silica-lipid hybrid particles: The effect of supersaturation and silica geometry. European Journal of Pharmaceutical Sciences. 2020;**150**:105357

[67] Korani S et al. Application of nanotechnology to improve the therapeutic benefits of statins. Drug Discovery Today. 2019;**24**(2):567-574

[68] Gorabi AM et al. Implications on the therapeutic potential of statins via

modulation of autophagy. Oxidative Medicine and Cellular Longevity. 2021;**2021**

[69] Sattar N et al. Statins and risk of incident diabetes: A collaborative meta-analysis of randomised statin trials. The Lancet. 2010;**375**(9716):735-742

[70] Sanz-Cuesta BE, Saver JL. Lipid-lowering therapy and hemorrhagic stroke risk: Comparative meta-analysis of statins and PCSK9 inhibitors. Stroke. 2021;**52**(10):3142-3150

[71] Bradford WD et al. Effects of direct-to-consumer advertising of hydroxymethylglutaryl coenzyme a reductase inhibitors on attainment of LDL-C goals. Clinical Therapeutics. 2006;**28**(12):2105-2118 discussion 2104

[72] Medina MW. The relationship between HMGCR genetic variation, alternative splicing, and statin efficacy. Discovery Medicine. 2010;**9**(49):495-499

[73] Jouve JL et al. Pravastatin combination with sorafenib does not improve survival in advanced hepatocellular carcinoma. Journal of Hepatology. 2019;**71**(3):516-522

[74] Nielsen SF, Nordestgaard BG, Bojesen SE. Statin use and reduced cancer-related mortality. New England Journal of Medicine. 2012;**367**(19):1792-1802

[75] Dulak J, Józkowicz A. Anti-angiogenic and anti-inflammatory effects of statins: Relevance to anti-cancer therapy. Current Cancer Drug Targets. 2005;**5**(8):579-594

[76] Bjerre LM, LeLorier J. Do statins cause cancer? A meta-analysis of large randomized clinical trials. The American Journal of Medicine. 2001;**110**(9):716-723

[77] López-Aguilar E et al. Security and maximal tolerated doses of fluvastatin in pediatric cancer patients. Archives of Medical Research. 1999;**30**(2):128-131

[78] Blais L, Desgagné A, LeLorier J. 3-Hydroxy-3-methylglutaryl coenzyme A reductase inhibitors and the risk of cancer: A nested case-control study. Archives of Internal Medicine. 2000;**160**(15):2363-2368

[79] Karp I et al. Statins and cancer risk. The American Journal of Medicine. 2008;**121**(4):302-309

[80] Cheung KS, Yeung YWM, Wong WS, Li B, Seto WK, Leung WK. Statins associate with lower risk of biliary tract cancers: A systematic review and meta-analysis. Cancer Medicine. 2022:1-12. DOI: 10.1002/cam4.494

[81] Demierre MF et al. Statins and cancer prevention. Nature Reviews. Cancer. 2005;**5**(12):930-942

[82] Vogt A et al. The geranylgeranyl transferase-I inhibitor GGTI-298 arrests human tumor cells in G0/G1 and induces p21(WAF1/CIP1/SDI1) in a p53-independent manner. The Journal of Biological Chemistry. 1997;**272**(43):27224-27229

[83] Vogt A et al. Protein geranylgeranylation, not farnesylation, is required for the G1 to S phase transition in mouse fibroblasts. Oncogene. 1996;**13**(9):1991-1999

[84] Kamel WA et al. Simvastatin-induced apoptosis in osteosarcoma cells: A key role of RhoA-AMPK/p38 MAPK signaling in antitumor activity. Molecular Cancer Therapeutics. 2017;**16**(1):182-192

[85] Göbel A et al. Cholesterol and beyond-the role of the mevalonate pathway in cancer biology. Biochimica et Biophysica Acta (BBA)-Reviews on Cancer. 2020;**1873**(2):188351

[86] Shapira KE et al. Autophagy is induced and modulated by cholesterol depletion through transcription of autophagy-related genes and attenuation of flux. Cell Death Discovery. 2021;7(1):1-11

[87] Min L et al. Autophagy as a potential target for sarcoma treatment. Biochimica et Biophysica Acta (BBA)-Reviews on Cancer. 2017;**1868**(1):40-50

[88] Mizushima N. Autophagy: Process and function. Genes & Development. 2007;**21**(22):2861-2873

[89] Sabatini DM. mTOR and cancer: Insights into a complex relationship. Nature Reviews. Cancer. 2006;**6**(9):729-734

[90] Lindén O et al. Chemorefractory rhabdomyosarcoma treated with radiotherapy, bevacizumab, statins and surgery and maintenance with bevacizumab and chemotherapy. Onkologie. 2008;**31**(7):391-393

[91] Ward NC, Watts GF, Eckel RH. Statin toxicity: Mechanistic insights and clinical implications. Circulation Research. 2019;**124**(2):328-350

[92] Bjornsson E, Kalaitzakis E, Niklasson A. Hepatotoxicity associated with statins: Reports of idiosyncratic liver injury post-marketing. Gastroenterology. 2011;**5**(140):S-975

[93] Altwairgi AK. Statins are potential anticancerous agents (review). Oncology Reports. 2015;**33**(3):1019-1039

[94] Zhang J et al. Statins, autophagy and cancer metastasis. The International Journal of Biochemistry & Cell Biology. 2013;**45**(3):745-752

[95] Poynter JN et al. Statins and the risk of colorectal cancer. The New England Journal of Medicine. 2005;**352**(21):2184-2192

[96] Brennan DJ et al. Tumour-specific HMG-CoAR is an independent predictor of recurrence free survival in epithelial ovarian cancer. BMC Cancer. 2010;**10**(1):1-9

[97] Kuzu OF, Noory MA, Robertson GP. The role of cholesterol in cancer. Cancer Research. 2016;**76**(8):2063-2070

[98] Moorman PG, Hamilton RJ. Statins and cancer risk: What do we know and where do we go from here? Epidemiology. 2007;**18**(2):194-196

[99] Karlic H et al. Statin and bisphosphonate induce starvation in fast-growing cancer cell lines. International Journal of Molecular Sciences. 2017;**18**(9)

[100] Wong WW et al. HMG-CoA reductase inhibitors and the malignant cell: The statin family of drugs as triggers of tumor-specific apoptosis. Leukemia. 2002;**16**(4):508-519

Chapter 9

Perspective Chapter: Ameloblastoma – Present and Future Concepts of Managing

Dragana Gabrić, Roko Bjelica, Mato Sušić and Marko Vuletić

Abstract

Ameloblastoma is a benign odontogenic tumor of epithelial origin with locally aggressive behavior. It affects a broad age range of patients and it is most commonly found in the mandible, especially posterior area. The majority of ameloblastomas are conventional (multicystic), which are more difficult to eradicate than the unicystic or peripheral types. Although most of ameloblastoma cases can be treated predictably with radical surgical treatment, the management of recurrent and metastasizing ameloblastomas remains a major challenge. Surgical treatment is standard, but the extent of resection is controversial. Radical resection with segmental and marginal mandibulectomy or curettage and enucleation with better quality of life, but with higher recurrence rate. Besides the conventional surgical treatment, novel therapy options like neoadjuvant molecular targeted therapy and decompression in young patients could make a significant improvement in the management of the disease. The aim of this chapter was to determine the present and future concepts of treatment and discuss significant factors responsible for recurrence.

Keywords: ameloblastoma, odontogenic tumors, surgical procedures, molecular targeted therapy, recurrence

1. Introduction

Odontogenic tumors are considered as relatively rare and destructive neoplasms of the jaw bones. They are derived from the remnants of odontogenic tissue and each odontogenic tumor represents the abnormality in odontogenesis [1].

Ameloblastomas belong to benign odontogenic tumors with locally aggressive behavior. Although the incidence of odontogenic tumors varies from 1% to 32% of all jawbone tumors, ameloblastoma, alongside odontoma, is the most common benign odontogenic tumor [2]. It is predominantly found in the mandible (up to 80%) and most patients diagnosed with ameloblastoma are aged between 30 and 60 years [3].

The current, 5th World Health Organization (WHO) classification from 2022 distinguishes five different types of benign ameloblastoma as described hereafter [4]. They most commonly manifest as slow-growing and asymptomatic swelling with the ability to expand and perforate cortical bone. Slow-growing character and lack of symptoms are considered responsible for delayed diagnosis of the ameloblastoma which is an ongoing problem, especially in developing countries [3].

Throughout history, primary treatment was, and still is, surgical with controversial extent of resection [5]. Taking into consideration severe clinical implications with high recurrence rate it is of utmost importance to provide sufficient guidelines and standardize surgical approach. In addition, recent literature has provided us with breakthrough in the understanding of genetic mutations and signaling pathways crucial in ameloblastoma pathogenesis [6]. Thus, novel therapy options like neoadjuvant molecular targeted therapy could significantly contribute to the management of the disease.

This chapter will address evidence-based treatment options and contemporary concepts of managing ameloblastoma.

2. Etiopathogenesis

The exact etiological factors associated with ameloblastoma are not yet completely understood. Up to 2014, little was known about exact molecular pathogenesis and a variety of etiological factors existed, including trauma, inflammation, dental caries and nutritional deficiencies [3, 7]. Considering ectodermal origin of ameloblastoma and its development from cells of the dental lamina, it is anticipated that enamel organ, cell rests of Malessez, cell rests of Serres and remnants of odontogenic epithelium are linked to etiopathogenesis of ameloblastoma [8].

As the genetic understanding increased, valuable findings have been brought to light regarding molecular pathogenesis of ameloblastoma. In 2014, it was confirmed that recurrent somatic and activating mutations in the mitogen-activated protein kinase (MAPK) plays a prominent role in the pathogenesis of the disease [6, 9, 10]. Additionally, there is evidence that mutations in non-MAPK signaling pathways, especially sonic hedgehog (SHH) pathway are also associated with ameloblastoma [11].

Mutations related to MAPK pathway include BRAF, fibroblast growth factor receptor 2 (FGFR2) and RAS genes [6, 9, 10]. BRAF is a serine/threonine protein kinase which activates the MAPK/ERK signaling pathway with consequential increase in cell proliferation and neoplastic transformation [6]. BRAF V600E mutations were firstly found in ameloblastoma clinical samples by Kurppa et al. [6] using real-time PCR enhanced by Sanger sequencing. These authors observed a high frequency of BRAF V600E mutations (63%). Subsequently, more recent studies described occurrence of the mutations ranging from 43% to 82% [7, 12, 13]. RAS is a protein that normally activates BRAF, therefore acts upstream of BRAF. In addition, the activation of RAS is normally triggered by the activation of FGFR2 which is a membrane-bound activator of MAPK signaling [14]. FGFR2 and RAS mutations were identified in up to 20% ameloblastoma cases [7]. Together, all the mentioned mutations are present in vast majority of ameloblastomas, suggesting that activation of the MAPK signaling pathway represents a critical event in the pathogenesis of ameloblastoma [2].

Several non-MAPK mutations have also been associated with ameloblastoma. The most important is nonclassical G protein-coupled receptor, the smoothened (SMO) gene. It is a signaling receptor that mediates SHH signaling pathway. Frequency rates of SMO mutations are lower than those in MAPK pathways, but these mutations have a greater tendency to appear in the maxillary ameloblastomas. Furthermore, SHH mutations including SMO appear to be associated with higher recurrence of the disease [7, 10].

3. Classification

WHO has recently provided the 5th edition of Classification of Head and Neck Tumours. Ameloblastoma classification is almost identical to that of 2017, with one new entity that will be mentioned in further text [4].

Ameloblastoma is primarily divided into five types:

- Conventional
- Unicystic
- Extraosseous/Peripheral
- Metastasizing
- Adenoid

Conventional ameloblastoma, earlier known as multicystic or solid ameloblastoma, is the most common type and comprises about 90% of cases. Clinically, it is a slow growing, benign neoplasm with locally aggressive behavior [3]. It is of vital importance to distinguish radiographic features of ameloblastoma to the earlier mentioned term of multicystic ameloblastoma. Multilocular radiographic presentation of ameloblastoma in no way should be considered as the reason why conventional type was named multicystic in the past classifications. On the contrary, it was reported that ameloblastomas appear equally as multilocular or unilocular radiolucencies [15, 16]. However, opinions about radiographic features contradict and radiographic evaluation alone is in no case sufficient for adequate diagnostics (**Figure 1**). Histologically, a decent number of ameloblastoma variants have been found, such as follicular, plexiform, acanthomatous, desmoplastic, basaloid and granular cell. Plexiform and follicular are the two most prevalent histological patterns. It is worth mentioning that ameloblastoma can simultaneously display both histological patterns [3]. Additionally,

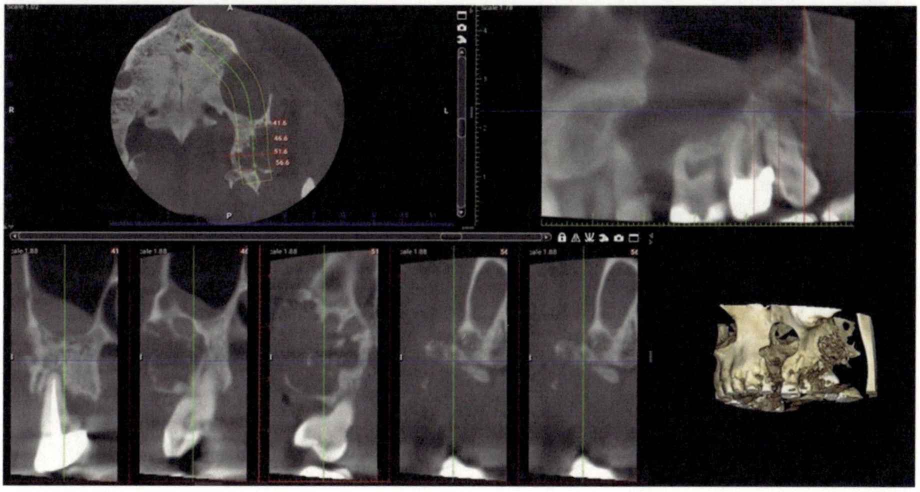

Figure 1.
Conventional ameloblastoma of distal part of maxillae.

desmoplastic ameloblastoma is from 2017 no longer recognized as separate type, but is classified as histological variant because of its distinctive histological appearance. It possesses a pathognomonic histological feature of extensive stromal dysplasia, epithelial islands within a highly collagenous connective tissue, and metaplastic bone formations in some cases [2, 3].

Unicystic type is the second most common ameloblastoma making from 5% to 15% of all cases. This type is most frequently found in younger patients, with different clinical, radiological and histopathological features from conventional type [16]. Unicystic ameloblastomas can be predominantly found in the posterior mandible and are often associatied with an unerupted tooth, resembling dentigerous cyst (**Figure 2**). It is thought to be less aggressive and has a lower recurrence rate, which mainly depends on the histological variant. Luminal and intraluminal variants have a good response to conservative treatment with approximately 10% of recurrence, but conservatively treated mural variant has a high recurrence comparable to that of conventional type [2].

Peripheral or extraosseous ameloblastoma is rare variant that has about 1% ratio among all ameloblastomas [17]. This variant has gone through a terminological

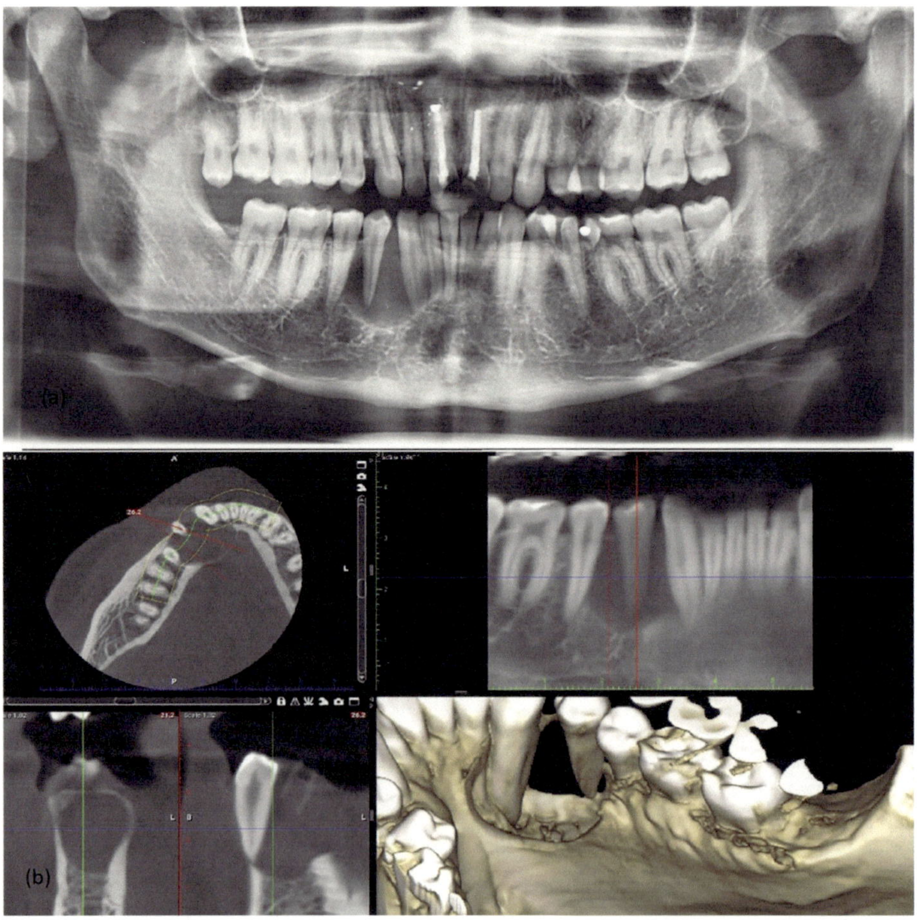

Figure 2.
Radiological features of unicystic ameloblastoma in the mandible: (a) orthopantomographic image; and (b) CBCT image.

evolution from its first appearance in late nineteenth century until 1959, when the term "peripheral ameloblastoma" was used for the first time [18]. Stanley and Krogh [19] introduced this term in their study and from that point on, "epithelial epulis" and "alveolar border ameloblastoma" fell out of favor. This type mostly affects middle-aged patients with higher prevalence in the mandible. It is considered to be amenable to conservative surgical therapy, recurring in a small number of cases [2]. From histological point of view, it has a similar pattern to conventional ameloblastoma consisting of ameloblastic epithelium islands [3].

Metastasizing ameloblastoma was defined as a histologically benign type of ameloblastoma which metastasizes to distant sites by WHO classification from 2017 [14]. It is particularly rare type of ameloblastoma and despite its affiliation with benign tumors, it metastasizes to distant sites and makes treatment unpredictable with a high recurrence rate [20]. It is most commonly found in lungs, but other sites, such as brain and kidneys have also been reported [21].

According to the 5th edition of Classification of Head and Neck Tumors by WHO, adenoid ameloblastoma is introduced as a new entity. It is described as epithelial odontogenic tumor with cribriform architecture, ameloblastoma-like component and presence of duct-like structures. It is also characterized by possible presence of dentinoid, ghost and clear cells [22]. The hybrid histological pattern including both ameloblastoma and adenomatoid odontogenic tumor characteristics was reported in approximately 40 cases in the literature [23]. Moreover, adenoid ameloblastoma is considered as more biologically aggressive type with higher recurrence rate than conventional ameloblastoma. In contrast to other ameloblastoma types, BRAF V600E mutations are not present in the adenoid type [23].

4. Contemporary treatment options

Current management concept of ameloblastoma is still controversial. To date, standard treatment is radical resection with a wide bone margin. However, various treatment methods have been recommended with respect to many factors, such as type and clinical presentation of tumor [5]. Regardless of the type, the management of ameloblastoma is either surgical or non-surgical. Surgical approach can be furtherly divided into radical and conservative surgery. These approaches often intertwine, and conservative methods such as decompression are valuable in preoperative reduction of tumor volume [24]. Non-surgical methods include radiotherapy and/or chemotherapy. Recent advances in signaling pathways and genetic understanding related to pathogenesis of ameloblastoma resulted with the development of molecular targeted therapies as a valuable treatment option in management of the disease [3, 25]. Details on the contemporary surgical approach and aforementioned treatment methods will be provided in the following subchapters.

4.1 Diagnostic protocol

Standard diagnostic protocol of ameloblastoma is by no means different from other odontogenic tumors [26]. Thorough clinical examination combined with adequate radiological imaging and histopathological analysis are mandatory to successful diagnosis and further management. A variety of radiological procedures are available to provide surgeon with precise structural expanse of ameloblastoma. Different methods are often combined, starting with orthopantomogram as a usual starting

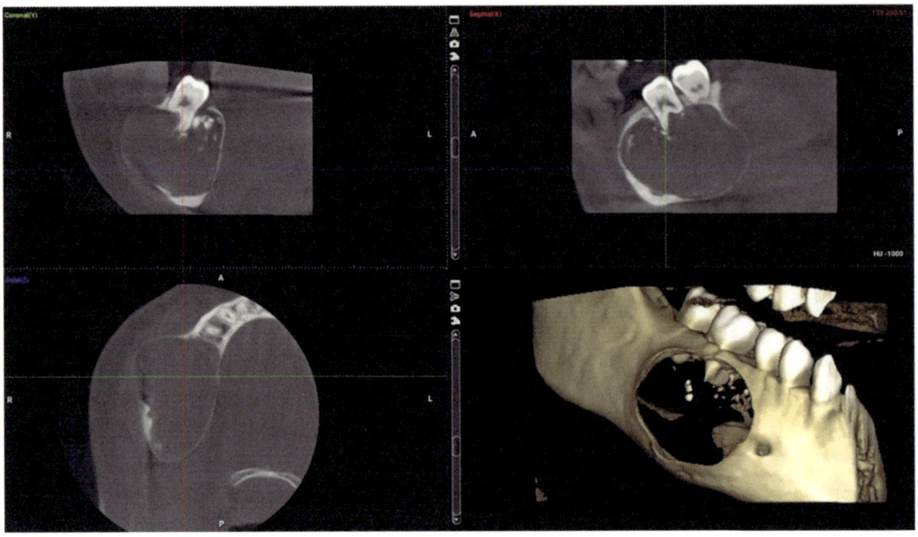

Figure 3.
Preoperative CBCT image of ameloblastoma found on the right side of the mandible.

point. Three-dimensional analysis is further performed by conventional computed tomography (CT), cone-beam computed tomography (CBCT) or magnetic resonance imaging (MRI). Taking into consideration potential malignancy of ameloblastoma, positron emission tomography combined with CT (PET/CT) can be used for diagnosing distant metastasis [3]. CBCT is considered as a standard three-dimensional imaging modality prior to further therapeutic procedures (**Figure 3**). Nevertheless, it is worth pointing out that MRI provides superior soft-tissue contrast, which makes it a useful imaging modality for diagnosing tumors with soft-tissue components [27]. This is especially applicable for depicting the extension of ameloblastoma to adjacent anatomical structures. Finally, definitive diagnosis cannot be made by clinical and/or radiological findings alone, thus it is imperative to obtain a biopsy for histopathological analysis.

4.2 Surgical treatment.

4.2.1 Radical surgical approach

Still a gold standard in ameloblastoma treatment, radical surgery is favored for all aggressive types of primary and recurrent ameloblastomas [3]. Radical resection implies *en bloc* tumor removal with a wide bone margin followed by immediate or delayed bony reconstruction of the defect with tissue grafts and/or prosthetic appliance [28]. In the mandible, resection can be performed through segmental osteotomy which involves the loss of continuity and requires reconstruction or can be marginal preserving the lower border with consequential maintenance of bone continuity [29]. Even though radical treatment is favored according to the contemporary literature [5, 30–32], several factors such as age, clinical presentation and ameloblastoma type should be considered when determining the course of therapy. Surgery can impair facial growth and development of pediatric patients, thus a conservative approach may be preferred [5]. Patient wishes regarding surgically induced facial deformations and psychological effects affecting the quality of life are also important factors that should not be overlooked.

Relatively high recurrence rate of ameloblastoma presents a major challenge. The recurrence rate of aggressively treated ameloblastomas is approximately 12%, which is significantly lower than that for conservative treatment, with post-treatment recurrence of 30% [33]. In a retrospective review by Ooi et al. [31] patients with conventional and unicystic ameloblastoma treated with segmental mandibulectomy and free fibula flap reconstruction were observed. The treatment showed no recurrence in a 5-year follow-up period with overall patient satisfactory regarding esthetic and functional results. 40% of the patients did not receive any form of prosthodontic rehabilitation and only 3 patients underwent dental implant insertion, showing that low uptake of dental rehabilitation did not adversely affect outcome and patient satisfaction. Another retrospective study by Bianchi et al. [34] confirmed positive outcomes of radical therapy. The study comprised 34 patients with histologically confirmed mandibular ameloblastomas, treated with segmental mandibular resection, fibula or iliac crest free flap reconstruction, and immediate or delayed dental implant placement. The duration of follow-up was from 18 to 120 months and no patient showed radiological or clinical signs of recurrence. Furthermore, recurrence rates up to 80% were reported after enucleation of conventional ameloblastoma, indicating the necessity for segmental resection with at least 1 cm of margin to the bone, including an adjacent soft tissue margin [35]. Moreover, the importance of adequate treatment choice is evident in the study by Hertog et al. [36]. The experience with the treatment of recurrent ameloblastoma previously treated by enucleation over a 40-year period was reported. Of all patients who underwent radical surgery, not a single recurrence was found during 10.5 years follow-up period. The remaining patients treated with conservative approach all developed one or more new recurrences. Observing a localization of tumor alone, it is believed that the best treatment option for maxillary ameloblastoma is radical resection [37]. Maxillary tumors are believed to be more aggressive than those found in the mandible due to the bone histomorphology, which is spongier providing a weak wall of defense against local spread (**Figure 4**). Moreover, the proximity of important anatomical structures such as the orbit, infratemporal fossa, pterygopalatine fossa, nasal fossa and base of the skull makes the treatment more difficult

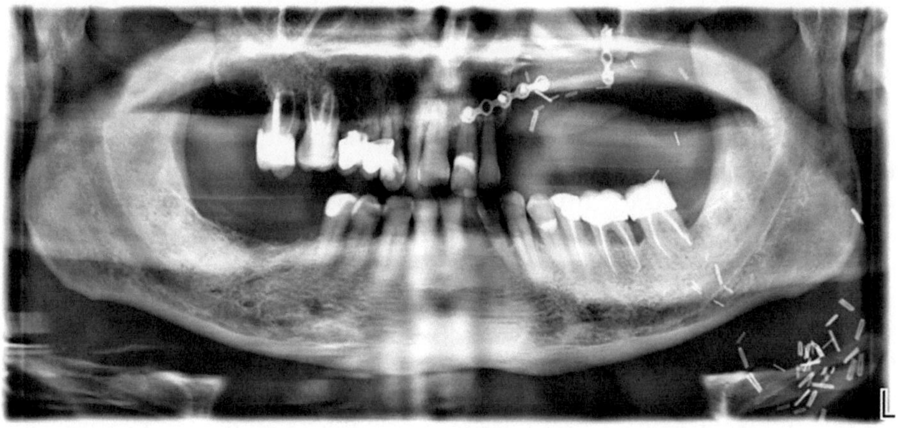

Figure 4.
Postoperative orthopantomographic image after segmental resection of left maxillae.

and mutilating [38]. These tumors can be resected via various midface approaches, resulting with defect that unifies oral cavity, nasal cavity and paranasal sinuses causing alterations in phonation, mastication and deglutition [32]. The remaining defects can be fitted with an obturator, allowing surgeons an easy access for clinical examination [2].

With the development of bone grafting and osteomyocutaneous free flaps, loss of function and esthetics can finally be considered relics of the past. Patients undergoing extensive tumor removals are now enabled to receive improved postoperative course with preserved essential functions such as mastication, deglutition and phonation together with a satisfactory esthetic outcome [39]. Nowadays, the emphasis is increasingly placed on the use of *computer-aided design/computer-aided manufacturing* (CAD/CAM) technology in reconstructive surgery. Virtual surgical planning and 3D printing techniques are used to preoperatively shape free flap dimensions or individually fabricate titanium meshes and fixation plates [40]. In a recent study by Lv et al. [41], guiding plate system for precise mandibular reconstruction was introduced with thorough postoperative evaluation. Mandibular and fibular osteotomy guides for tumor resection and simultaneous donor site bone segment shaping were designed and fabricated using CAD/CAM technology. All patients underwent successful surgery with 100% overall survival rate of flaps. Postoperative esthetic assessment was rated as excellent and quantitative evaluation was performed by measuring different parameters such as discrepancy in osteotomy lines, mandibular resemblance and symmetry. The cohort included patients undergoing traditional resection and reconstruction. There was significant difference between cohort and test group in all the mentioned parameters.

Last but not least important step in surgical management of ameloblastoma is postoperative follow-up. Various examples of recurrences emphasize the inevitable need for prolonged follow-up visits after surgery [42]. Adebayo et al. [42] presented a case of soft tissue recurrence 21 years after radical surgery in the mandible which leads to conclusion that radiological follow-up should be carried out throughout life in ameloblastoma patients.

4.2.2 Conservative surgical approach

Conservative treatment has found its purpose in treating less aggressive types of ameloblastoma [2]. It involves one or more of the following procedures: enucleation, curettage, physicochemical treatment (cryotherapy or Carnoy's solution), marsupialization and decompression (**Figure** 5) [43]. The main advantages of the conservative approach are: preservation of adjacent healthy tissues, avoidance of facial disfiguration and, consequentially, better postoperative quality of life. Pediatric patients are, for instance, very approach sensitive and radical surgery may affect the growth dynamics of the dentition, soft tissues and entire craniofacial skeleton [44]. Therefore, a conservative approach is often the treatment of choice in children. However, ameloblastoma type and histological pattern must be taken into account during the planning and selection of the adequate treatment. These are mandatory factors influencing the surgeon's decision with a primary goal of minimizing the possibility of recurrence and avoiding under- or overtreatment [16].

Considering the high recurrence rate of conservatively treated conventional type of ameloblastoma it is crucial to emphasize the right indication [33]. Firstly, histopathological analysis is necessary to confirm the type of ameloblastoma curable with conservative approach. Only less aggressive types such as unicystic or peripheral are

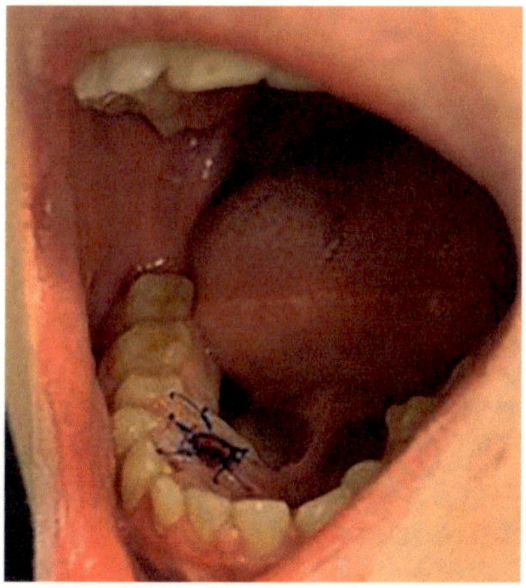

Figure 5.
Preoperative decompression of the unicystic ameloblastoma in the mandible of young patient.

suitable to be treated by this type of approach [35]. In a study by Seintou et al. [43], a thorough review of clinical, radiological, and histopathological characteristics of unicystic ameloblastoma in children was presented with findings that treatment is still controversial. However, it was concluded that conservative treatment was preferable due to better postoperative quality of life, despite a slightly higher recurrence rate. Huang et al. [45] also claim that radical treatment should be reserved for recurrent and more aggressive types of ameloblastoma, with important statement that recurrence is probably not a major consideration for pediatric patients and should not be considered as equivalent to failure. On the other hand, some authors [46, 47] believe that radical resection should still be a treatment of choice whenever follow-up examinations are limited. This applies usually to developing countries, but any other limiting factors are not excluded. Even though the radical treatment results with less recurrence, a majority of ameloblastoma cases in pediatric patients

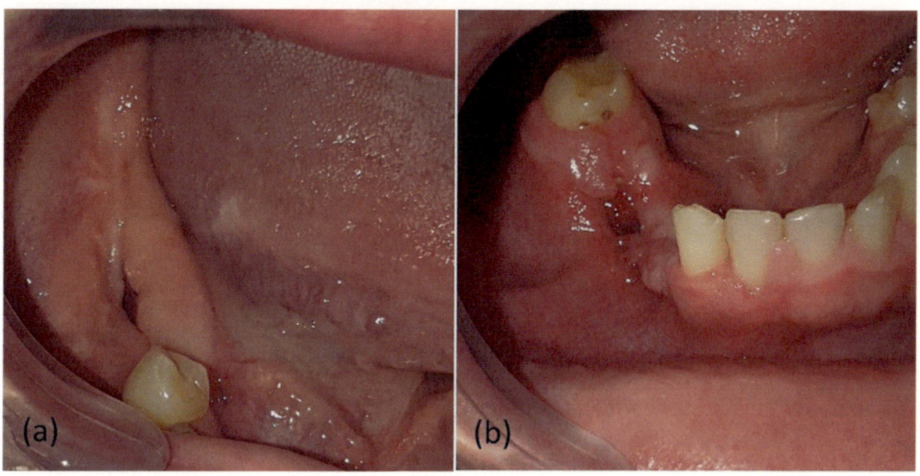

Figure 6.
Postoperative healing after conservative surgical treatment of ameloblastoma in adolescent patient (a), and patient in the middle of 20's (b).

are unicystic [43, 44]. Less aggressive behavior and lower recurrence rate are factors that furtherly support the conservative treatment of ameloblastoma in these patients (**Figure 6**). In addition, peripheral ameloblastoma is another entity successfully treatable with conservative therapy. It is most frequently present in the gingival tissues and the conservative approach with narrow margins of unaffected tissue is treatment of choice [48].

Altogether, opinions on the treatment of conventional ameloblastoma are still divergent with valid arguments regarding both radical and conservative approaches. It is of vital importance to know the differences between various types of conservative procedures. A simple enucleation is considered as inadequate with unacceptably high recurrence rate of up to 60% in unicystic ameloblastoma and up to 80% in conventional ameloblastoma [35]. Enucleation followed by curettage and/or physicochemical treatment has been suggested as standard conservative approach (**Figures** 7 and **8**) [43].

It is necessary to eradicate intraosseous ameloblastoma cells that can be found up to 8 mm from the clinical and radiographic margin of the lesion (**Figure 9**).

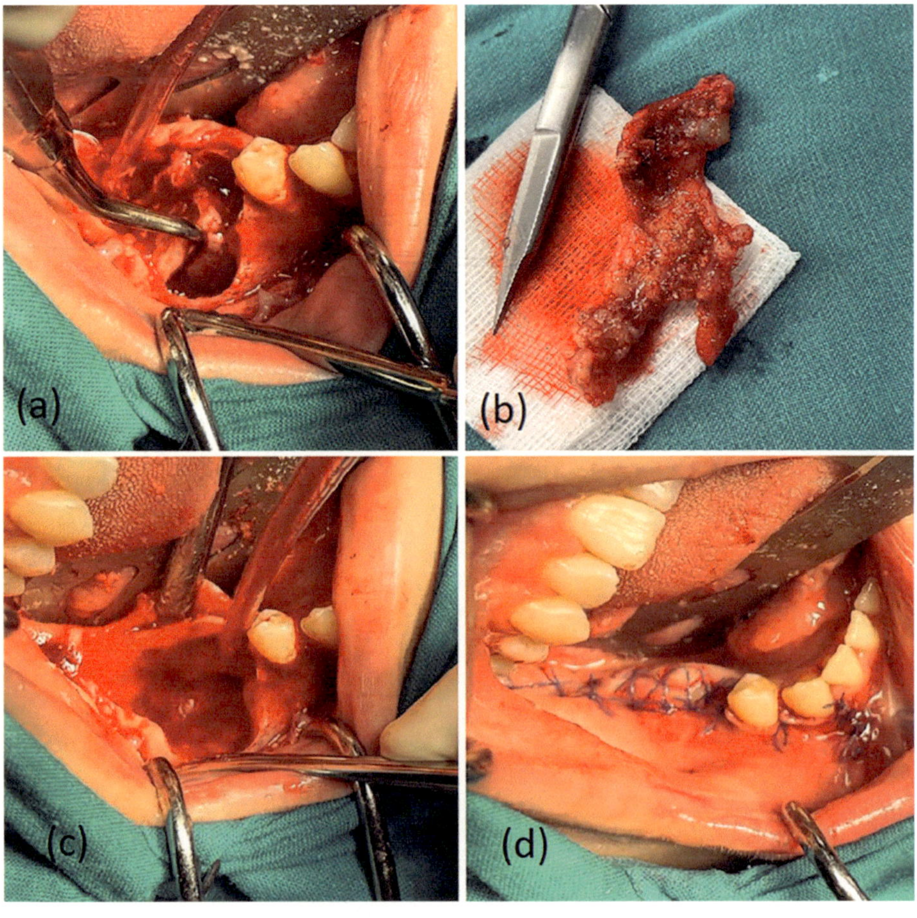

Figure 7.
Conservative surgical treatment of ameloblastoma in an adolescent patient with CBCT image presented in **Figure 3***: (a) enucleation of tumor mass; (b) enucleated ameloblastoma; (c) status post-enucleation and curettage; and (d) primary wound closure.*

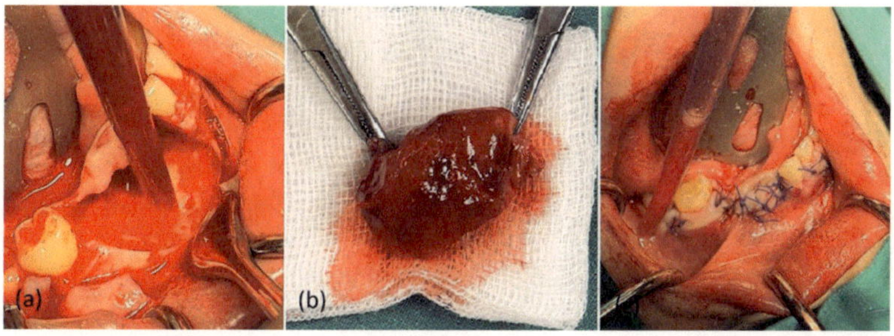

Figure 8.
Conservative surgical treatment of ameloblastoma in patient in the middle 20's with radiological status presented in **Figure 2***: (a) status post enucleation and curettage; (b) enucleated tumor mass; and (c) primary wound closure.*

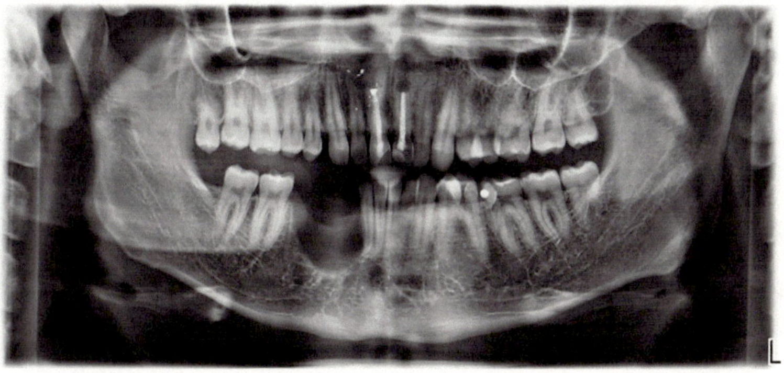

Figure 9.
Orthopantomographic image showing postoperative margins after conservative surgical treatment with decompression and subsequent enucleation and curettage. Preoperative radiological status is presented in **Figure 2**.

Physicochemical treatment of these cells can be performed with liquid nitrogen cryospray or with Carnoy's solution [30]. Carnoy's solution is a fixative initially proposed by Stoelinga and Bronkhorst [49]. It has ability to penetrate cancellous bone to a depth of 15 mm, so it is ideal for application after enucleation [35].

Decompression is a valuable method most commonly used to preoperatively reduce the size of cysts [50]. The size of the lesion is expected to be reduced by inserting a rubber tube or a stent through a previously created hole in the overlying bone and mucosa [51]. Huang et al. [45] have reported a significant reduction in ameloblastoma size using 6–12 months preoperative decompression. Furthermore, Park et al. [51] reported a 36.7% reduction in size of unicystic ameloblastoma after 13 months of decompression in 5 patients with mean age of 18.6 years (**Figures 10** and **11**). They also highlighted that the patient's age is inversely proportional to the relative velocity of shrinkage. Additionally, contemporary methods including active decompression and distraction osteogenesis have been developed for the treatment of odontogenic cystic entities [52]. Active decompression and distraction osteogenesis involve the use of active negative pressure inside a cyst to increase the velocity of cystic lesion shrinkage and to stimulate the regeneration of bone [52]. There is still no evidence of its clinical use in literature, thus the further research is required to verify the effect of active decompression on pathophysiology of ameloblastoma.

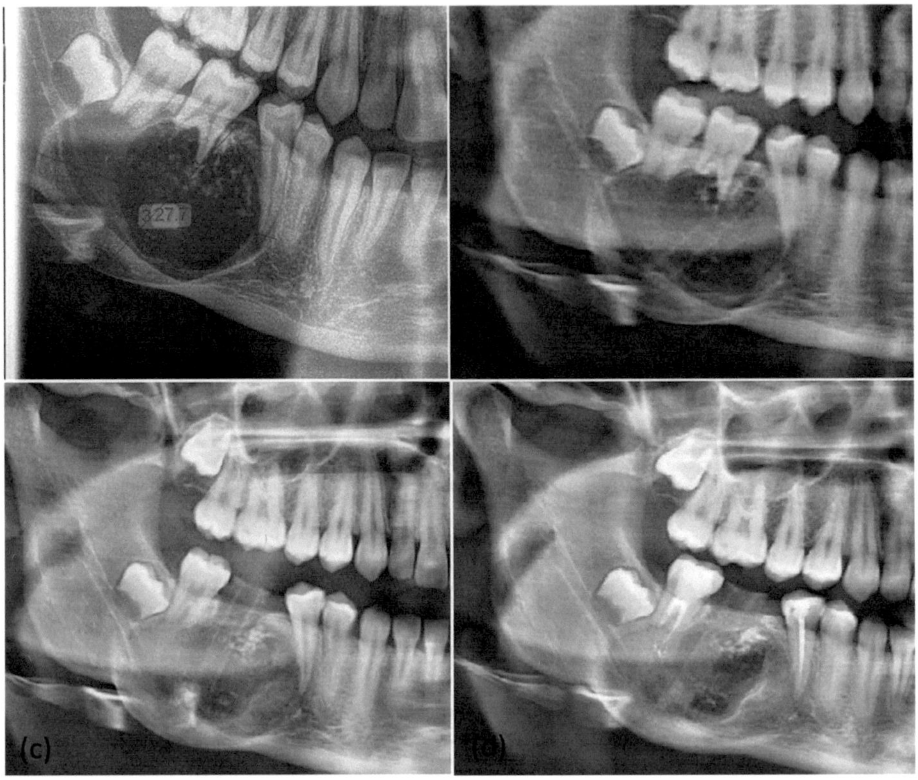

Figure 10.
Decompression in a pediatric patient with unicystic ameloblastoma of the mandible. Preoperative radiographic follow-up (surgical procedure is presented in **Figure 7***: (a) initial situation of a large ameloblastoma; (b) 2 months after rubber tube insertion; (c) 4 months after tube insertion; and (d) 9 months after tube insertion.*

4.3 Non-surgical treatment

4.3.1 Chemotherapy and radiotherapy

Radiation therapy and chemotherapy have played no significant part in the management of ameloblastoma [35]. Ameloblastoma was, together with ameloblastic carcinoma, believed to be radioresistant tumor, as older methods failed to improve outcome of the disease [53]. Nevertheless, more recent literature suggest radiotherapy may be utilized for preventing recurrence in patients with microscopic positive margins or those with inoperable disease [54]. As malignant ameloblastomas or ameloblastic carcinomas are rare, data reporting radiotherapy effects remain scarce. Kennedy et al. [53] achieved local control in 4 of 6 patients treated with radiotherapy alone or postoperatively after radical surgery. Koukourakis et al. [55] concluded that image-guided radiation therapy, intensity-modulated radiation therapy or proton beam irradiation may be beneficial in adjuvant setting after surgical treatment for local control. Results of chemotherapy are also unpredictable with a lack of research [56]. Amzerin et al. [56] used combination of doxorubicin and cisplatin in patient with recurrent ameloblastoma with lung metastases. Pain disappearance, local stabilization and lung lesions shrinkage of 30% were reported. Gall et al. [57] evaluated effectiveness of three chemotherapeutic agents (methotrexate, cyclophosphamide,

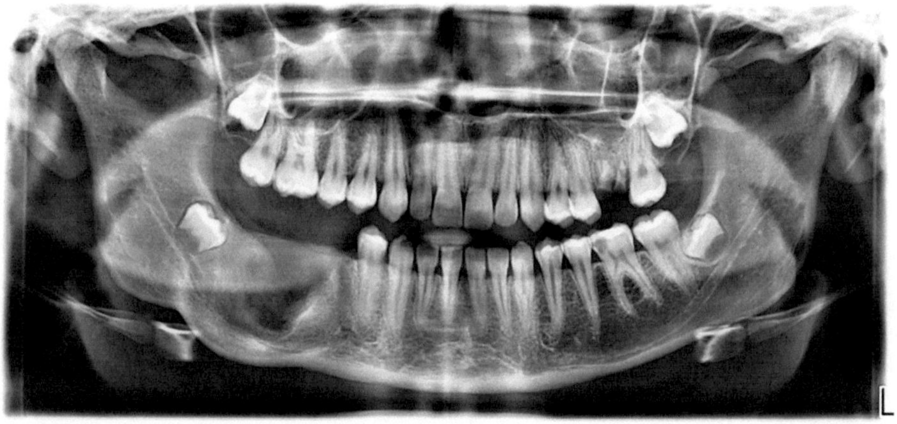

Figure 11.
Postoperative image of the patient presented in **Figure** 7. *Conservative surgery with enucleation and curettage was performed after 12 months of decompression.*

and doxorubicin) with no regression of tumor nodules in the lungs, but with major symptomatic improvements. These data suggest that chemotherapy may improve clinical symptoms in metastatic patients.

4.3.2 Molecular targeted therapy

Over the past decade, novel molecular targeted therapies are evolving alongside with dramatically improved understandings of biological behavior of ameloblastoma [58]. The main identified mutations are found in MAPK and SHH signaling pathways. These include BRAF, RAS and FGFR2 genes from MAPK pathway and SMO gene from SHH signaling pathway [2, 10]. Discovery and clarification of mentioned activated molecular pathways brought out the novel potentional targeted therapies in the management of ameloblastoma.

Drugs approved by US Food and Drug Administration which are predominantly used for treatment of metastasizing, unresectable or recurrent ameloblastoma are vemurafenib, dabrafenib and trametinib [59, 60]. Initially, vemurafenib was approved for use in treatment of metastatic or surgically non-treatable melanoma, while dabrafenib and trametinib for the treatment of metastatic non-small cell lung cancer with BRAF V600E mutations. Vemurafenib and dabrafenib are BRAF inhibitors, while trametinib is MEK inhibitor [59, 60]. Although the available literature is limited with a lack of clinical research, clinical effectiveness of using molecular targeted drugs for patients with ameloblastoma was reported in several case reports [61–66]. Fernandes et al. [61] presented a case of patient with recurrent ameloblastoma with confirmed BRAF V600E mutation. Vemurafenib therapy was prescribed and complete resolution of symptoms together with continuous shrinkage of lesion evidenced on MRI scans after 11 months of therapy were reported. Furthermore, Faden et al. [62] used dabrafenib reduced to a 50% of therapy dose to treat a patient with significant medical comorbidities. MRI analysis showed a 75% reduction in tumor mass after 8 months of therapy. Both authors [61, 62] recommended single agent therapy over dual therapy in ameloblastoma patients. However, adverse reaction to vemurafenib including arthralgia, nausea and rash has been reported after 12 months of therapy [63]. Adverse effects can be controlled by decreasing the dosage without adversely affecting outcomes of therapy. It has been found that neoadjuvant treatment with dabrafenib significantly reduces size of the primary tumor which could reduce the extent of the subsequent surgery [64]. On the other hand, Kaye et al. [65] reported a case of unresectable locally recurrent ameloblastoma of the mandible with lung metastases treated with dual targeted therapy. They used dabrafenib in combination with trametinib which resulted with significant reduction of tumor and metastases volume and utter resolution of symptoms after 20 weeks. Combination of dabrafenib and trametinib has also proven to have a significant influence resulting with complete remission in a study by Brunet et al. [66].

SMO inhibiting drugs, such as itraconazole and vismodegib, are considered less successful due to the mechanisms of resistance which disable their binding [10]. Cyclopamine is SHH signaling pathway antagonist and is more effective than SMO inhibitors [2]. However, it has ability to inhibit osteoblast proliferation and differentiation with negative effects on bone healing [67].

It is worth mentioning that matrix metalloproteinases (MMPs) have a role in local invasiveness of ameloblastoma [58]. MMPs are zinc-dependent proteinases that are important in extracellular matrix degradation and are associated with tumor growth and invasiveness [68]. MMP-2 and MMP-9 are expressed in various benign and malign tumors, including ameloblastoma. They are mainly involved in angiogenesis and tumor growth [69]. Consequently, invasion of adjacent tissues could be effectively controlled by regulation of MMPs. Still, they have a vital role in tissue remodeling and inhibition of their activity causes major side effects. Thus, further research is needed to reveal potential disease control by MMP inhibitors [58].

5. Conclusions

Despite the great strides that have recently been made in investigation of molecular factors and biological mechanisms responsible for ameloblastoma, the management continues to be the subject of debate among clinicians. Surgeons often empirically decide for radical treatment to reduce the risk of recurrence, affecting postoperative quality of life. Novel conservative surgical methods such as active decompression and distraction osteogenesis have the potential to vastly reduce the extent of surgery. The development of molecular targeted therapies implicates MAPK and SHH pathway inhibition as an effective treatment modality for ameloblastoma. Further clinical research is mandatory for standardization of treatment methods.

Conflict of interest

"The authors declare no conflict of interest."

Author details

Dragana Gabrić[1,2], Roko Bjelica[1], Mato Sušić[1,2] and Marko Vuletić[1,2*]

1 Department of Oral Surgery, School of Dental Medicine University of Zagreb, Zagreb, Croatia

2 Department of Dental Medicine, University Hospital Centre Zagreb, Zagreb, Croatia

*Address all correspondence to: mvuletic@sfzg.hr

References

[1] Silveira FM, Macedo CCS, Borges CMV, Mauramo M, Vasconcelos ACU, Soares AB, et al. Odontogenic tumors: An 11-year international multicenter study. Oral Diseases. 2021;**27**(2):320-324

[2] Shi HA, Ng CWB, Kwa CT, Sim QXC. Ameloblastoma: A succinct review of the classification, genetic understanding and novel molecular targeted therapies. The Surgeon. 2021;**19**:238-243

[3] Effiom OA, Ogundana OM, Akinshipo AO, Akintoye SO. Ameloblastoma: Current etiopathological concepts and management. Oral Diseases. 2018;**24**:307-316

[4] Soluk-Tekkesin M, Wright JM. The World Health Organization classification of odontogenic lesions: A summary of the changes of the 2022 (5th) edition. Turk Patoloji Dergisi. 2022;**38**:168-184

[5] Hendra FN, Natsir Kalla DS, van Cann EM, de Vet HCW, Helder MN, Forouzanfar T. Radical vs conservative treatment of intraosseous ameloblastoma: Systematic review and meta-analysis. Oral Diseases. 2019;**25**:1683-1696

[6] Kurppa KJ, Catón J, Morgan PR, Ristimäki A, Ruhin B, Kellokoski J, et al. High frequency of BRAF V600E mutations in ameloblastoma. The Journal of Pathology. 2014;**232**(5):492-498

[7] Brown NA, Betz BL. Ameloblastoma: A review of recent molecular Pathogenetic discoveries. Biomark Cancer. 2015;**7**(2):19-24

[8] Palanisamy JC, Jenzer AC. Ameloblastoma. In: StatPearls [Internet]. Treasure Island (FL): StatPearls Publishing; 2022

[9] Brown NA, Rolland D, McHugh JB, Weigelin HC, Zhao L, Lim MS, et al. Activating FGFR2-RAS-BRAF mutations in ameloblastoma. Clinical Cancer Research. 2014;**20**(21):5517-5526

[10] Sweeney RT, McClary AC, Myers BR, Biscocho J, Neahring L, Kwei KA, et al. Identification of recurrent SMO and BRAF mutations in ameloblastomas. Nature Genetics. 2014;**46**(7):722-725

[11] Mishra P, Panda A, Bandyopadhyay A, Kumar H, Mohiddin G. Sonic hedgehog signalling pathway and ameloblastoma—A review. Journal of Clinical and Diagnostic Research. 2015;**9**(11):10-13

[12] You Z, Liu SP, Du J, Wu YH, Zhang SZ. Advancements in MAPK signaling pathways and MAPK-targeted therapies for ameloblastoma: A review. Journal of Oral Pathology & Medicine. 2019;**48**(3):201-205

[13] González-González R, López-Verdín S, Lavalle-Carrasco J, Molina-Frechero N, Isiordia-Espinoza M, Carreón-Burciaga RG, et al. Current concepts in ameloblastoma-targeted therapies in B-raf proto-oncogene serine/threonine kinase V600E mutation: Systematic review. World Journal of Clinical Oncology. 2020;**11**(1):31-42

[14] Wright JM, Vered M. Update from the 4th edition of the World Health Organization classification of head and neck Tumours: Odontogenic and maxillofacial bone tumors. Head and Neck Pathology. 2017;**11**(1):68-77

[15] Dhanuthai K, Chantarangsu S, Rojanawatsirivej S, Phattarataratip E, Darling M, Jackson-Boeters L, et al. Ameloblastoma: A multicentric

study. Oral Surgery, Oral Medicine, Oral Pathology, Oral Radiology. 2012;**113**(6):782-788

[16] Bansal S, Desai RS, Shirsat P, Prasad P, Karjodkar F, Andrade N. The occurrence and pattern of ameloblastoma in children and adolescents: An Indian institutional study of 41 years and review of the literature. International Journal of Oral and Maxillofacial Surgery. 2015;**44**(6):725-731

[17] Siar CH, Lau SH, Han K. Ameloblastoma of the jaws: A retrospective analysis of 340 cases in a malaysian population. Journal of Oral and Maxillofacial Surgery. 2012;**70**(3):608-615

[18] Ide F, Ito Y, Miyazaki Y, Nishimura M, Kusama K, Kikuchi K. A new look at the history of peripheral Ameloblastoma. Head and Neck Pathology. 2020;**14**(4):1052-1057

[19] Stanley HR, Krogh HW. Peripheral ameloblastoma. Oral Surgery, Oral Medicine, and Oral Pathology. 1959;**12**(6):760-765

[20] Rizzitelli A, Smoll NR, Chae MP, Rozen WM, Hunter-Smith DJ. Incidence and overall survival of malignant ameloblastoma. PLoS One. 2015;**10**(2):1-9

[21] Yang X, Zhou K, Tao Y, Ge S, Shang W, Song K. Treatment efficacy and prognosis of pulmonary metastasizing ameloblastoma: A systematic review. International Journal of Oral and Maxillofacial Surgery. 2022;**51**(5):579-590

[22] Jo VY, Demicco EG. Update from the 5th edition of the World Health Organization classification of head and neck tumors: Soft tissue tumors. Head and Neck Pathology. 2022;**16**(1):87-100

[23] Jayasooriya PR, Abeyasinghe WAMUL, Liyanage RLPR, Uthpali GN, Tilakaratne WM. Diagnostic enigma of adenoid Ameloblastoma: Literature review based evidence to consider it as a new sub type of Ameloblastoma. Head and Neck Pathology. 2022;**16**(2):344-352

[24] Xavier SP, de Mello-Filho FV, Rodrigues WC, Sonoda CK, de Melo WM. Conservative approach: Using decompression procedure for management of a large unicystic ameloblastoma of the mandible. The Journal of Craniofacial Surgery. 2014;**25**(3):1012-1014

[25] Kreppel M, Zöller J. Ameloblastoma—Clinical, radiological, and therapeutic findings. Oral Diseases. 2018;**24**(1-2):63-66

[26] Liu Z, Liu J, Zhou Z, Zhang Q, Wu H, Zhai G, et al. Differential diagnosis of ameloblastoma and odontogenic keratocyst by machine learning of panoramic radiographs. International Journal of Computer Assisted Radiology and Surgery. 2021;**16**(3):415-422

[27] Fujita M, Matsuzaki H, Yanagi Y, Hara M, Katase N, Hisatomi M, et al. Diagnostic value of MRI for odontogenic tumours. Dento Maxillo Facial Radiology. 2013;**42**(5):1-9

[28] Shen YF, Rodriguez ED, Wei FC, Tsai CY, Chang YM. Aesthetic and functional mandibular reconstruction with immediate dental implants in a free fibular flap and a low-profile reconstruction plate: Five-year follow-up. Annals of Plastic Surgery. 2015;**74**(4):442-446

[29] Rastogi V, Pandilwar PK, Maitra S. Ameloblastoma: An evidence based study. Journal of Oral and Maxillofacial Surgery. 2010;**9**(2):173-177

[30] Neagu D, Escuder-de la Torre O, Vázquez-Mahía I, Carral-Roura N, Rubín-Roger G, Ángel P-V, et al. Surgical management of ameloblastoma. Review of literature. Journal of Clinical and Experimental Dentistry. 2019;**11**(1):70-75

[31] Ooi A, Feng J, Tan HK, Ong YS. Primary treatment of mandibular ameloblastoma with segmental resection and free fibula reconstruction: Achieving satisfactory outcomes with low implant-prosthetic rehabilitation uptake. Journal of Plastic, Reconstructive & Aesthetic Surgery. 2014;**67**(4):498-505

[32] Armocida D, Berra LV, Pucci R, Battisti A, della Monaca M, Valentini V, et al. Ameloblastoma and intracranial involvement: The current challenge of the radical surgical treatment. Comprehensive Review of the Literature and Institution experience. Journal of Oral and Maxillofacial Surgery. 2022;**21**:34-43

[33] Qiao X, Shi J, Liu J, Liu J, Guo Y, Zhong M. Recurrence rates of intraosseous Ameloblastoma cases with conservative or aggressive treatment: A systematic review and meta-analysis. Frontiers in Oncology. 2021;**11**:647-657

[34] Bianchi B, Ferri A, Ferrari S, Leporati M, Copelli C, Ferri T, et al. Mandibular resection and reconstruction in the management of extensive ameloblastoma. Journal of Oral and Maxillofacial Surgery. 2013;**71**(3):528-537

[35] Pogrel MA, Montes DM. Is there a role for enucleation in the management of ameloblastoma? International Journal of Oral and Maxillofacial Surgery. 2009;**38**(8):807-812

[36] Hertog D, Schulten EAJM, Leemans CR, Winters HAH, van der Waal I. Management of recurrent ameloblastoma of the jaws: A 40-year single institution experience. Oral Oncology. 2011;**47**(2):145-146

[37] Evangelou Z, Zarachi A, Dumollard JM, Peoc'h M, Komnos I, Kastanioudakis I, et al. Maxillary Ameloblastoma: A review with clinical, histological and prognostic data of a rare tumor. In Vivo. 2020;**34**(5):2249-2258

[38] Almeida RDAC, Andrade ESDS, Barbalho JC, Vajgel A, Vasconcelos BCDE. Recurrence rate following treatment for primary multicystic ameloblastoma: Systematic review and meta-analysis. International Journal of Oral and Maxillofacial Surgery. 2016;**45**(3):359-367

[39] Brown JS, Lowe D, Kanatas A, Schache A. Mandibular reconstruction with vascularised bone flaps: A systematic review over 25 years. The British Journal of Oral & Maxillofacial Surgery. 2017;**55**(2):113-126

[40] Hou JS, Chen M, Pan C b, Wang M, Wang JG, Zhang B, et al. Application of CAD/CAM-assisted technique with surgical treatment in reconstruction of the mandible. Journal of Cranio-Maxillo-Facial Surgery. 2012;**40**(8):432-437

[41] Lv M, Yang X, Gupta A, Shen Y, Li J, Sun J. Sequential application of novel guiding plate system for accurate transoral mandibular reconstruction. Oral Oncology. 2020;**111**:846-854

[42] Adebayo ET, Fomete B, Adekeye EO. Delayed soft tissue recurrence after treatment of ameloblastoma in a black African: Case report and review of the literature. Journal of Cranio-Maxillo-Facial Surgery. 2011;**39**:615-618

[43] Seintou A, Martinelli-Kläy CP, Lombardi T. Unicystic ameloblastoma in children: Systematic review of clinicopathological features and

treatment outcomes. International Journal of Oral and Maxillofacial Surgery. 2014;**43**:405-412

[44] Zhang J, Gu Z, Jiang L, Zhao J, Tian M, Zhou J, et al. Ameloblastoma in children and adolescents. The British Journal of Oral & Maxillofacial Surgery. 2010;**48**(7):549-554

[45] Huang IY, Lai ST, Chen CH, Chen CM, Wu CW, Shen YH. Surgical management of ameloblastoma in children. Oral Surgery, Oral Medicine, Oral Pathology, Oral Radiology, and Endodontology. 2007;**104**(4):478-485

[46] Arotiba GT, Ladeinde AL, Arotiba JT, Ajike SO, Ugboko VI, Ajayi OF. Ameloblastoma in Nigerian children and adolescents: A review of 79 cases. Journal of Oral and Maxillofacial Surgery. 2005;**63**(6):747-751

[47] Hammarfjord O, Roslund J, Abrahamsson P, Nilsson P, Thor A, Magnusson M, et al. Surgical treatment of recurring ameloblastoma, are there options? The British Journal of Oral & Maxillofacial Surgery. 2013;**51**(8):762-766

[48] Anpalagan A, Tzortzis A, Twigg J, Wotherspoon R, Chengot P, Kanatas A. Current practice in the management of peripheral ameloblastoma: A structured review. The British Journal of Oral & Maxillofacial Surgery. 2021;**59**(1):1-8

[49] Stoelinga PJW, Bronkhorst FB. The incidence, multiple presentation and recurrence of aggressive cysts of the jaws. Journal of Cranio-Maxillo-Facial Surgery. 1988;**16**(4):184-195

[50] Berretta LM, Melo G, Mello FW, Lizio G, Rivero ERC. Effectiveness of marsupialisation and decompression on the reduction of cystic jaw lesions: A systematic review. The British Journal of Oral & Maxillofacial Surgery. 2021;**23**:266-310

[51] Park HS, Song IS, Seo BM, Lee JH, Kim MJ. The effectiveness of decompression for patients with dentigerous cysts, keratocystic odontogenic tumors, and unicystic ameloblastoma. Journal of the Korean Association of Oral and Maxillofacial Surgeons. 2014;**40**(6):260-265

[52] Moreno-Rodríguez P, Guerrero LM, Gómez-Delgado A, Castro-Núñez J. Active decompression and distraction sugosteogenesis for the treatment of calcifying odontogenic cyst. Oral and Maxillofacial Surgery. 2021;**25**(1):89-97

[53] Kennedy WR, Werning JW, Kaye FJ, Mendenhall WM. Treatment of ameloblastoma and ameloblastic carcinoma with radiotherapy. European Archives of Oto-Rhino-Laryngology. 2016;**273**(10):3293-3297

[54] Petrovic ID, Migliacci J, Ganly I, Patel S, Xu B, Ghossein R, et al. Ameloblastomas of the mandible and maxilla. Ear, Nose, & Throat Journal. 2018;**97**(7):26-32

[55] Koukourakis GV, Miliadou A, Sotiropoulou-Lontou A. Ameloblastoma, a rare benign odontogenic tumour: An interesting tumour review targeting the role of radiation therapy. Clinical & Translational Oncology. 2011;**13**(11):793-797

[56] Amzerin M, Fadoukhair Z, Belbaraka R, Iraqui M, Boutayeb S, M'Rabti H, et al. Metastatic ameloblastoma responding to combination chemotherapy: Case report and review of the literature. Journal of Medical Case Reports. 2011;**5**:491-496

[57] Gall JA, Sartiano GP, Shreiner' DP. Ameloblastoma of the mandible with

pulmonary metastasis. Oncologia. 1975;**32**:118-126

[58] Fuchigami T, Ono Y, Kishida S, Nakamura N. Molecular biological findings of ameloblastoma. Japanese Dental Science Review. 2021;**57**:27-32

[59] Odogwu L, Mathieu L, Blumenthal G, Larkins E, Goldberg KB, Griffin N, et al. FDA approval summary: Dabrafenib and Trametinib for the treatment of metastatic non-small cell lung cancers harboring BRAF V600E mutations. The Oncologist. 2018;**23**(6):740-745

[60] Kim G, McKee AE, Ning YM, Hazarika M, Theoret M, Johnson JR, et al. FDA approval summary: Vemurafenib for treatment of unresectable or metastatic melanoma with the BRAFV600E mutation mutation. Clinical Cancer Research. 2014;**20**(19):4994-5000

[61] Fernandes GS, Girardi DM, Bernardes JPG, Fonseca FP, Fregnani ER. Clinical benefit and radiological response with BRAF inhibitor in a patient with recurrent ameloblastoma harboring V600E mutation. BMC Cancer. 2018;**18**(1):887-892

[62] Faden DL, Algazi A. Durable treatment of ameloblastomawith single agent BRAFi Re: Clinical and radiographic responsewith combined BRAF-targeted therapy in stage 4 ameloblastoma. Journal of the National Cancer Institute. 2016;**109**(1):190-192

[63] Broudic-Guibert M, Blay JY, Vazquez L, Evrard A, Karanian M, Taïeb S, et al. Persistent response to vemurafenib in metastatic ameloblastoma with BRAF mutation: A case report. Journal of Medical Case Reports. 2019;**13**(1):245-249

[64] Tan S, Pollack JR, Kaplan MJ, Colevas AD, West RB. BRAF inhibitor treatment of primary BRAF-mutant ameloblastoma with pathologic assessment of response. Oral Surgery, Oral Medicine, Oral Pathology, Oral Radiology. 2016;**122**(1):5-7

[65] Kaye FJ, Ivey AM, Drane WE, Mendenhall WM, Allan RW. Clinical and radiographic response with combined BRAF-targeted therapy in stage 4 ameloblastoma. Journal of the National Cancer Institute. 2014;**107**(1):378-381

[66] Brunet M, Khalifa E, Italiano A. Enabling precision medicine for rare head and neck tumors: The example of BRAF/MEK targeting in patients with metastatic Ameloblastoma. Frontiers in Oncology. 2019;**9**:1204-1207

[67] Stanton BZ, Peng LF. Small-molecule modulators of the sonic hedgehog signaling pathway. Molecular BioSystems. 2010;**6**:44-54

[68] Farias LC, Gomes CC, Rodrigues MC, de Castro WH, Lacerda JCT, Ferreira E, et al. Epigenetic regulation of matrix metalloproteinase expression in ameloblastoma. BMC Clinical Pathology. 2012;**12**:11-17

[69] de Vicente JC, Fresno MF, Villalain L, Vega JA, Hernández VG. Expression and clinical significance of matrix metalloproteinase-2 and matrix metalloproteinase-9 in oral squamous cell carcinoma. Oral Oncology. 2005;**41**(3):283-293